MW00611531

What they're saying – The unsolicited notes below were sent to Megaheart.com. Names and addresses of senders are on record. These and other notes also appear at megaheart.com/testimonialsbook.html

---

Your *No-Salt, Lowest-Sodium International Cookbook* is my daily bible. I love many of the breads and sauces!! The Ethiopian Spice bread is awesome. I have avoided blood pressure medication and NEVER want to go back to my old ways of not knowing what is in my daily diet. YOU ROCK!! – Pam Upchurch, USA

I teach the clinicals in our area in several clinical settings. The nursing home setting would be a great place to share your book. I have already ordered two of your books online, but I am sure that they would love to have one at work as well – Robyn, R.N., USA

I can't believe I found your Megaheart.com site. I started reading, devouring every bit of information, then I came to your part, your history, the astonishing low-sodium diet you follow and then the recipes!! Thank you. I sat there alone reading, I was overwhelmed, finally someone understood what I attempt to do for my husband. I am so frustrated and always bordering on panic of what to feed him. Maybe now it will be a little easier to find ways to prepare his meals. Thank you...Thank you – a loving and frightened wife, McBride, USA

Thank you for your great informative Web site and the support you have provided over the years. I have all your books and I am really looking forward to your new International Cookbook. Your recipes are very helpful. When I was first diagnosed my prognosis was poor and my doctor thought I would need a heart transplant. My heart function has gone from 20 - 24% to 45%. The Heart Failure Clinic in Toronto says I am their prize patient.– Patricia Miller, Canada

My grandpa has lost 38 pounds already just because I have been using your recipes, so THANK YOU THANK YOU THANK YOU! I really do appreciate your website and all that you do. You really are saving lives, and I am very grateful for you helping me save my grandfathers! – Kelly O'Brien, USA

"I started your regime in February. My bloods have been fantastic, and the centre said if my progress continues I may come off the transplant list at next check-up in Nov." – Gbeaco (U.K.)

Hi Don, I have CHF but your book gave me new life. I was on a heart transplant list.. After reading and using your book (life) is wonderful. My name has been removed from the list and I have not been back in the hospital in a year. I thank you. God bless. – Elbert Adams, USA

Just wanted to let you know how thrilled I am with the tortilla recipe from your International Low Sodium Cookbook. I prepared the recipe over the weekend and found it had excellent flavor. I have sorely missed being able to prepare flour tortilla recipes. Thanks so much. – Margaret A. Cox, USA

I'm a 35 year young woman with CHF, living in the Netherlands. Today I made your salad dressing with the dried cranberries…it's the best dressing I've ever tasted!!! And for dinner I made some chicken with your recipe for red onion marmalade. Without the salt, I taste so much more of the natural flavours in food, but you sure made my life even better! I think my family and friends can only agree on this, and I think they will be inviting themselves to dinner even more often than before. Thank you! – Marjon Savelsberg, The Netherlands

Thank you for the help with my Meniere's disease - eating low sodium works. I feel so much better and I'm enjoying eating food again. Please continue! - Diane Richmond, USA

Thank you again so very much for your good book and all your wonderful advice. Thank you, thank you, thank you!!! – Joan E. Krapf, Australia

I had to write. Two years now on your book's program. The guide in the back. Two years. Never a dull day, never a bad meal and now, get this. IMPROVEMENT. I am better. No transplant, no nothing but return to work. All thanks to you. Please accept this as my gratitude for what you have done for me and others. – D. Tremble, USA

Where have you been? Where? I've got a shelf full of books and now I find yours. For two weeks I've been baking and cooking and everyone LOVES your low sodium recipes. Both books are incredible! Thank you so much. My husband is the one who needs it and he's getting better already. But, get this. We're all eating his meals now...that's how good your books are. Thank you, thank you. – Janet M., USA

Wow, stopped using salt and my Meniere's dizziness is gone. So wonderful. Thank you. – Flip Manne, Director L.A. Jazz Assoc., wife of drummer Shelly Manne.

I wanted to write my appreciation. My husband and I will forever be grateful for the marvelous information and motivation you have provided. You have made a difference and hopefully I will be able to make one here in my little corner of the world as I become more knowledgeable.– Louise Cartagenise, Canada

I have made several recipes in your book for my Mom who suffers from acute hypertension and they are great! This cookbook is a real god-send! – Debbie Shanklin, USA

Thank you so much for all of your hard work and sharing information so that others have hope. – Martha Edwards, USA

Hi Chef Don.....this is Kathy Keegan again......I was very surprised and I thank you for your quick response.. It is so nice to know that someone will get back to us so quickly.....*smile*....I think you will be hearing from the rest of my family, .and you can count on me to be passing the word on your book/ lifestyle......I love it. Thanks again. – Kathy Keegan, USA

Dear Don, I just want to say your trio of books are very helpful to me in the battle against salt!! The recipe for soy sauce was amazing. Thanks for your help. – Nancy Milo, USA

Wonderful cookbook. The more people that can be touched by such an awesome cookbook the better Have a great day. – Diana Segal, USA

I think your Web site and cookbooks are wonderful - I was recently diagnosed with Meniere's disease and your site and books have been a huge help in adapting to a new eating lifestyle. – Kim McCann, USA

Good Morning, I have just received your June Newsletter and always look forward to reading them and your recipes. Since our no-salt lifestyle change, and your assistance, we have been doing very well. I find it quite amazing that the grocery stores offer so little in the way of no-salt or low-sodium items. Again, thanks for your good Newsletters and the best of summers to you. – Corinne J Walker, usa

Thank you so much for the uplifting encouragement. I was moved to tears.....I am a fighter and I am encouraged not to give up....I love your attitude....you sound like my hubby.....that's what he's been saying. I'm going to print this letter and read it often. And I will keep you tuned in....but not abuse the privilege. Thanks again, – Sunny Sterling, USA

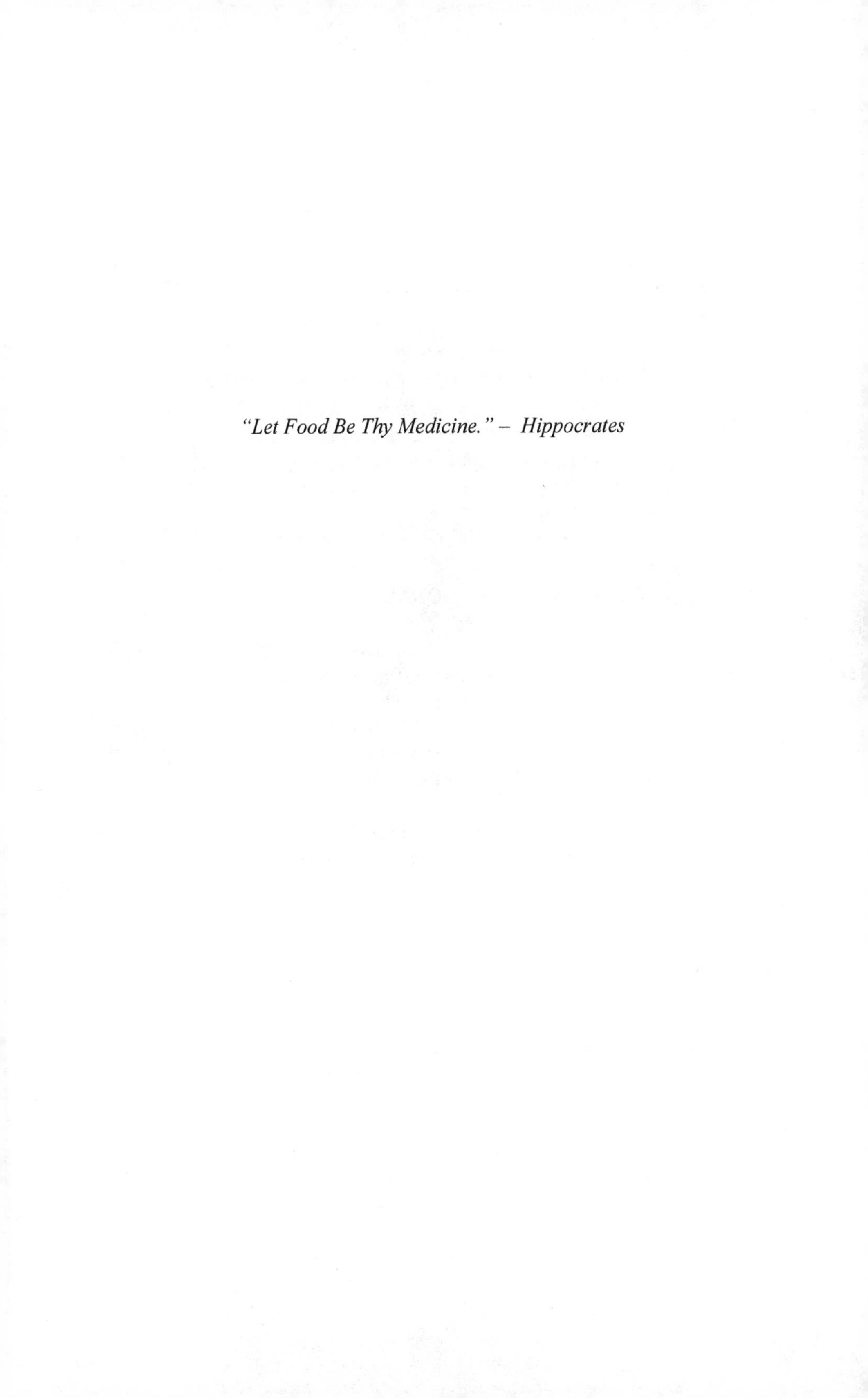

"Let Food Be Thy Medicine." – Hippocrates

ALSO BY DONALD A. GAZZANIGA & MAUREEN A GAZZANIGA

The No–Salt, Lowest–Sodium Light Meals Book
The No–Salt, Lowest–Sodium International Cookbook
The No–Salt, Lowest–Sodium Cookbook
The No–Salt, Lowest–Sodium Baking Book
The No-Salt, Lowest-Sodium Barbecue & Grilling Cookbook

OTHER BOOKS BY DONALD A GAZZANIGA

No Assembly Required
A Few Good Men, The Marines
Air France One
*G*A*M*E*S - X-TREME PAINTBALL*
War Hawks
Who Killed Rita Colleridge?

All titles above available in print and on Kindle and other e-readers. Visit www.smashwords.com for any e-reader downloads.

The

No-Salt, Lowest-Sodium

Living Well Without Salt

Cookbook

Donald A. Gazzaniga
and
Maureen A. Gazzaniga

Foreword by

Dr. Michael B. Fowler, M.B., F.R.C.P.
&
Chef Scott Leysath

THE NO–SALT, LOWEST–SODIUM
LIVING WELL WITHOUT SALT COOKBOOK

Visit: www.megaheart.com

Cover photo used with permission from Heart Healthy Living® Magazine, ©Copyright 2009 Meredith Corporation. All Rights Reserved
Visit: www.diabeticlivingonline.com
Cover design: William Karoly
Editor: Tony DiMarco, Becky Winch
Interior Design, Typesetting: The Graphics Company

Library of Congress Control Number: 2010903527

Gazzaniga, Donald A.
Living Well Without Salt / Donald A. Gazzaniga and Maureen A. Gazzaniga; foreword by Dr. Michael B. Fowler; introduction by Scott Leysath – 1st ed.

Includes index
ISBN-10: 188651-05-8
ISBN-13: 978-1-886571-05-1
Salt free lifestyle– Recipes 2. Research; Information
1. Gazzaniga, Maureen A. II Title

All of our books are available on Kindle. This book available on Kindle and all other e-readers. Visit www.smashwords.com/books/view/108455?ref=arrohead.

Books available in all bookstores.

Fourteenth Edition: November, 2016

Printed in the USA

A Special Thank You For . . .

. . . All who helped with this book and to my wife Maureen, without whom this book would not have been possible; to our patient children and grandchildren and to Scott Leysath our favorite professional chef, and especially to Dr. Michael Fowler and his wonderful staff at Stanford Medical Center, who have believed in our efforts since the beginning . . ..

Contents

Salt, Hypertension & Heart Failure

By Dr. Michael B. Fowler, MB, F.R.C.P.
Director, Heart Failure Program
Medical Director, Cardiomyopathy Center
Stanford University Medical Center

The amount of salt in food has a major influence on health. There is increasing awareness that excessive sodium in our diets is an important factor in the development of common diseases of the heart and circulation. It is also apparent that reducing the amount of sodium in the diet of patients with established disease, especially heart failure, can have a profound impact on symptoms and major clinical manifestations of illness.

The increased awareness of the importance of dietary sodium intake on the development of major cardiovascular diseases has resulted in the recommendations that the amount of sodium that should be consumed on a daily basis be 5.8 grams of salt (2300 mg of sodium), and a lower target of 3.7 grams of salt per day (1500 mg sodium) has been set in people over 40 years old, African Americans, and individuals with high blood pressure. The average American male consumes 10.4 grams per day, which is almost twice the advised amount. In patients with disease states characterized by sodium retention, especially heart failure, much lower levels of sodium intake are generally recommended and sodium restriction can have a profound impact on the clinical manifestations.

Salt And Hypertension and Heart Failure

Hypertension is the condition which is most closely linked to dietary sodium content. Currently 90% of all Americans will develop hypertension in their lifetime. Hypertension (or high blood pressure) is very closely linked to the risk of stroke, coronary artery disease (which causes heart attacks), and kidney failure. Hypertension is especially common and significant in patients with diabetes – itself linked closely to the modern American diet and relative inactivity. Many of the complications of diabetes, including heart attacks, stroke, and the risk of developing heart failure can be reduced by controlling blood pressure. Heart failure, a devastating condition that will occur in one in five Americans in their lifetime is also very closely linked to hypertension. Hypertension is the most common pre-existing condition in patients who develop heart failure, and reducing blood pressure has a profound effect in reducing the risk of developing heart failure. Reducing dietary sodium intake has a major role in the treatment and stabilization of patients with established conditions that are characterized by the retention of salt and water. The most common of these is heart failure. Sodium retention or the inability to remove excess sodium also plays a major role in kidney disease. Patients with end-stage renal disease on dialyses will routinely receive precise instructions on daily sodium restriction.

The relationship between dietary sodium intake and the development of hypertension (high blood pressure) is widely accepted. Most studies have shown that reducing average dietary sodium intake will result in a clinically significant reduction in blood pressure. Extrapolating these effects for populations with or without hypertension it has recently been estimated that reducing dietary salt by 3 gm per day could reduce new cases of coronary artery disease by 60,000 to 120,000 each year, stroke between 32,000 and 66,000 per year, and heart attacks between 54,000 to 99,000 each year in the United States.

Human development as hunter gatherers lasted for 6000 – 8000 years with the evolutionary influence of very low levels of sodium occurring naturally in their diets throughout this period. The human body appears to have developed specific mechanisms to retain appropriate levels of sodium in the body from the naturally low levels of salt present in the diet. It has been estimated that primitive man was probably eating 20-40 mmol sodium/day. The daily physiologic required is between 8-10 mmol/day. Modern man consumes 100 to 200 mmol [1]sodium/day![1]

It is striking that observations made in those primitive tribes still exist today, who are exposed to only low levels of salt in their diet show that hypertension is rarely found, and the progressive rise in blood pressure with aging is not observed. When members of these societies move and are exposed to processed foods and a high sodium diet, they develop all the common disease of modern man; hypertension, diseases of arteries causing strokes and heart attacks, as well as heart failure. Of course, those individuals who move from their traditional lifestyle are also exposed to excess calories, a sedentary lifestyle and cigarettes.

Conversely, in areas of the world where salt intake is especially

---

[1]To convert mmol to mg, multiply by 18

high, observed in some areas of Japan the risk of stroke is amongst the highest in the world. Strategies at reducing sodium intake in those areas have been shown to be effective in reducing risk of stroke. In the U.S. epidemiologists and policy makers are currently debating the potential impact of the health of Americans of developing more aggressive food policies which reduce the average daily consumption of salt by only 3 grams per day, with the potential to save between $10 to $24 billion in health care costs.

Salt and Heart Failure

For those patients who have developed heart failure (a lifetime risk of one in five for Americans over the age of 40) sodium restriction can have a profound effect on how well they feel and their ability to survive without hospital admissions. Sodium restriction is a key component of the strategy to prevent excess sodium and fluid retention in the body. The failing heart activates systems in the body which cause sodium retention. *Simplistically, the sodium regulatory system in patients with heart failure seems to misinterpret the reduced pumping performance of the heart as dehydration.* The consequent activation of nerves and hormones result in excess retention of fluid. The patient can recognize those changes when they become short of breath from the heavy water-logged lungs, when they develop swelling of the ankles and legs, and when they develop painful swelling of the abdomen. Some patients will wake up in the night with a sensation of drowning and being unable to breathe.

Diuretics are used to correct this retention of sodium (and fluid). They work by causing the kidney to remove more sodium (and with it water). The dose and requirement for diuretics are directly related to the salt intake in the diet and to the severity of heart failure. Patients who intermittently eat very high levels of sodium in a single meal – more than 10 grams with Chinese food for instance, will either fail their diuretic therapy and develop severe symptoms often precipitating an admission to the hospital or they may be required to take an excessive dose of diuretics, which have been associated with a higher risk of dying. High dose diuretics can also result in impairment of kidney function.

Patients with heart failure and other patients with conditions which require therapy with diuretics, such as some with kidney or liver disease are usually advised to restrict sodium intake. They are rarely given practical advice on how to do so.

In this book, Donald Gazzaniga takes his own personal experience surviving and thriving with heart failure since he adopted a very low sodium diet in early 1997. He has developed a practical primer of how to actually control the sodium intake in the diet.

The book will be an invaluable tool to help those who are trying to prevent cardiovascular disease – still the number one killer of men and women in modern societies. Adoption of this dietary policy to reduce salt in the daily diet will improve the quality of life of those with diseases requiring diuretics. In many of these individuals sodium restriction can make a difference between a comfortable quality of life spent outside the hospital as opposed to a shorter life with severe symptoms and pain characterized by recurrent hospitalization due to the retention of excess salt and water.

BY DONALD GAZZANIGA

"Just cut the salt down and you'll be okay." That advice was prescribed a half-dozen years before I was diagnosed with congestive heart failure (CHF). My blood pressure had risen slowly but steadily, and we wanted to lower it using a lower "salt" diet.

I should have suspected something back then, since I never used a saltshaker when I cooked, nor when I was served a meal. The prescription for cutting salt out of my life, however, presented new questions. What was I to cut down? Better yet, why would cutting something I hadn't added to my diet help? The answers to those questions and many more would come sooner than I would have expected.

My internist's "cut the salt down" prescription for blood pressure (bp) control was a few years before the FDA labeling act that required all food manufacturers to include the FDA nutrition label. In other words, we had no way of knowing just how much salt had been added to processed and "manufactured" foods. At best, we could only guess.

Besides, back then a controversy in the medical and science world concerning the ingestion of salt in regards to hypertension or high blood pressure existed and it confused. Little if any knowledge was openly discussed or exhibited concerning how sodium affected a variety of chronic ailments, each now known to be helped by cutting salt out. Back then, if public comment was made by any scientist or medical researcher about "salt" being a culprit in any of the above or with any other chronic illnesses, then lobbyists and propagandists from the salt industry would jump out front with an opposing statement.

"That's the only way to get iodine," was a pitch some of us might remember. And of course we still hear, "Your heart needs salt." Neither is true. Our heart needs some sodium, but never needs salt. As a matter of fact, recent research has indicated that salt/sodium is harmful to more than our blood pressure or heart. Hypertension also damages our brain, kidneys, and other organs. Salt itself is even linked to stomach cancer. Salt and the sodium it contains causes so much damage that the human costs and actual monetary costs exceed any need for salt in our food.

Fast forward to the present. Many researchers and foundations involved in health have declared that, "Everyone should reduce their salt intake appreciably."

Salt was used abundantly in family cooking not too long ago. Just pick up a popular cookbook and check out the recipes, past and present. My mother used to make lasagna with two tablespoons of salt. Other recipes from her records also show a large amount of salt even with fresh vegetables, which never really needed them. Deadly? Yes, however, I feel she wasn't alone. Has the world changed since then? Not much. The public at large is still assaulted with high doses of salt and sodium from fast foods, restaurants, and processed foods and yes, newspaper and magazine recipes, and cookbooks. And look out for those TV chefs. Wow, high fat and salt pour into recipes like there's no problem at all.

The good news is that based upon the letters we've received at *Megaheart.com* since early 1997, many of us have adapted to a no-salt lifestyle with terrific success. We've proved without question as well, that it works.

When will we learn?

Within weeks of my heart failure diagnosis, I did a lot of Internet research into heart failure. There weren't any sites "devoted" to heart failure or anything to do with cutting salt out to effect recovery. Some medical sites were up by that time but few of today's large sites were yet online. There was some controversy about whether or not lowering "salt" might help. Many stuck to the concept of going for the transplant or lo and behold, there was a new procedure out of Brazil from Dr. Randas J. V. Batista. He was taking tissue, or as some reports stated, "carving" out pieces of the heart. This procedure, he explained, would make room for it to pump more efficiently. This guy was all over the Net and featured in TV interviews. Large and famous heart clinics were going to test it and in fact some in the U.S. did.

Did I want to do this? More than one person suggested I should.

That was when my alleged and often absent intelligence returned. The answer was easy for me. No, I didn't! It was a good decision too, since at least sixty-percent of his patients died rather quickly. The procedure by the way, is no longer offered.

The lower-sodium approach was much more appealing. However, before I launched myself on a new course, I figured another medical opinion might offer me a new direction.

That's when my life and possibly yours changed. Without knowing it when I first met him, I was on a new course to recovery and all without a transplant. The "authority," Dr. Michael Fowler, enthusiastically believed in the salt reduction concept, but he also believed in it being reduced to as low a level as I could.

Macho me bragged, "I think I can get it down to 500 mg a day. Will that work?" I felt that it could be done. I had no clue as to where salt/sodium was coming from, but sure, let's go for it, I thought.

At that moment, my wife, Maureen, proved to be an important presence.

Dr. Fowler looked to her and asked, "Can he?"

She rolled her head and her eyes and said, "Oh yeah. If he says he'll do it, he'll do it."

Fowler became excited. "Good. My goal is to get you back to rowing. I think we can do this."

The rest is history. I got back into rowing shape, but unfortunately we moved too far away from the aquatic center where I rowed to make that a daily trip. Good rowing requires at least five days a week. Instead, I did do a lot of heavily physical things like lift and carry heavy objects such as eighty-pound planter-pots, shovel scores of yards of dirt and gravel, hike or walk long distances, and more. We even drove across the country for three weeks, meeting people, searching for low sodium in stores from California to New York, and south to Virginia and back. I was in great shape.

Dr. Fowler succeeded in his mission. In turn Maureen and I have worked hard to bring this success to you and others.

Five cookbooks and a major Web site later, thousands have written that they have recovered to a healthier life and scores have told us they avoided a heart transplant. As we learned later, there are thousands of others who have other chronic maladies who also needed to lower their sodium intake.

Diabetics are part of the no-salt, low-sodium challenge as well. If you have diabetes you are at least twice as likely as someone who does not have diabetes to develop heart disease or a stroke, and heart attacks are also a possibility. Unfortunately, many with heart disease also develop diabetes. Of the hundreds of thousands who have visited *Megaheart.com,* I would have to guess that a third have diabetes and heart failure, while another third have Meniere's Syndrome. The balance of visitors consist of those with heart failure, A-fib, hypertension, nephrotic disease, stomach and other maladies affected by salt/sodium.

When I had played macho-man with Dr. Fowler, I had absolutely no concept of how much salt food processors were dumping into our diet.

I learned quickly however that these processors weren't just feeding us beans or soup or frozen foods, they were literally poisoning us with an excessive amount of salt. And that answers my question at the beginning. The reason that just cutting the salt shaker out hadn't helped me avoid hypertension was because of the salt in bread, processed foods, and restaurants. (I traveled a lot back then.)

Right after diagnosis, and when I could move around on my own, I found myself in a large grocery store reading FDA labels.

It took me about three aisles of food to realize that the sodium level listed for each product was for the listed serving size and not for the whole container, and the serving sizes were nearly always smaller than what we consume. They also demonstrated that products marked, "Low Sodium," weren't low in sodium, but instead "lower" than the standard fare, and it hit me pretty hard when I realized that a half cup of beans or soup or other canned food had so much sodium in it that the levels for just one serving went over my target of 500 or fewer milligrams a day.

I checked all the cans of food we'd been using, and then the frozen food packages, only to realize that we were consuming thousands of milligrams of sodium a day, when we thought we'd been cutting back. Dairy products, especially cheese, butter, and milk contained much more sodium than I had ever considered.

I could find nothing acceptable in the store except for fresh fruit and vegetables, and I wasn't sure what levels of sodium they contained.

Meat and fish were a mystery as well since the stores at that time didn't have FDA ratings displayed or available. I also discovered the calories and saturated fats were much higher than I had figured.

After visiting several stores I found some no-salt-tomato products and a few other products that no longer are available. These included no-salt-added cheddar and Swiss cheese, pickles, and eggless mayonnaise, to name a few.

I mulled this over for a few days. I was going to have to learn how to prepare completely unsalted meals and do it with products or ingredients that weren't salted, brined or otherwise altered.

I spent a lot of time figuring out what to do. It was May of '97, and I decided the first thing I needed to do was put this challenge on the Web. I had played around with making a Web site for low-sodium eaters and now I felt I had to bring it to life. I had built Web sites before, mostly for business purposes, so the Internet wasn't new or foreign to me. (In 1997 it was just 5 years old. I had first dipped my Web toe into it in 1993.)

With the help of a friend, Bill Karoly, we put the first version of

Megaheart.com online, and I started getting hits within two weeks. The Web was still relatively primitive. Blogs had not been invented and search engines were rather poor. This was before Google as well.

No matter, I received visitors, and I started responding to E-mails.

By then I had pulled together all the recipes I had already created and some old family recipes, most of which I found useless because the salt had been so overpowering that that's all there was for flavor. Also, the high-fat content, which is often the flavor in some foods, was impossible to replace even with spices and herbs.

A few months later I found that I had a notebook full of recipes. Over three hundred of them. Some were handwritten, others were typed on my old Smith Corona and IBM Selectric, and a few were so tattered and had been used so much that reading through the often present food stains proved difficult.

A search of the Net produced no other sites that helped no-salt eaters with recipes or guidance. And no cookbooks that addressed heart disease or any of the other maladies that needed a no-salt lifestyle could be found in stores or online.

I began to look at my thick notebook of recipes with new thoughts. I had already successfully adapted many of them. New spices and other safer ingredients would make them very tasty and a lot healthier. Why not try to get these published and see if anyone else could use them?

I had already posted a half dozen daily meal plans and about fifty recipes online. They had become very popular. I thought that maybe I could put a small book together and make it available to anyone who needed the help.

I started to work again on all my recipes and testing them as well. The more often they were prepared, the better they would get. I first extracted those that would never be converted just because of what they contained. I also bought a book of USDA nutrient figures, and after looking up every ingredient for over 350 recipes I practically had the book memorized. I think I became a bit of a pain about then. We'd walk through a store and Maureen would point at a carrot. "35 milligrams," I'd respond. Celery? 85. Potato? 7. We would start to laugh, I had become a walking, talking encyclopedia of sodium content.

There's nothing like a wife who can cook up a storm also serving as your critic. She wasn't always happy, but sometimes she was quite pleased. The latter recipes definitely made it into the book. Her best compliment back then was, "You're really creative in the kitchen." She still says that.

We also had help from family and friends. One night Maureen's cousin, Susan, brought us chicken pot pies; all cooked without salt or salted ingredients. The recipe made it into our first no-salt cookbook.

The cookbook was coming together and my wife was on the road to recovery. Maybe, I began to think again, I could get a real publisher to produce my effort. Since I had worked for many years in Hollywood, I understood that nothing gets filmed, published, printed or sold unless you have an agent. Oh, maybe now and then someone penetrates that system, but generally forget it without a good agent.

Fortunately, I had a niece who had just moved from senior editor at a national magazine into a life as a literary agent. So, I contacted her and she asked to see the material when it was ready.

She called later and wanted to know if anyone else had ever published such a book; one specifically created for patients who had to cut salt out of their lives and had to figure out their daily nutrient values at the same time. The answer was, no.

"That's too bad," she said. "Publishers would prefer to understand the market and another book's sales would help out."

Go figure.

"What if I can prove a need for it?" I asked.

She agreed it was worth a try and I turned to *Megaheart.com* and sent out a newsletter to hundreds of people asking if anyone was interested in a good no-salt cookbook. (At that time we had a mailing list of over three thousand.)

The response was overwhelming.

Bingo! Ruth Cavin, senior editor at St. Martin's Press liked the support. Within a few weeks the first draft was sent off to New York.

We had to come up with a completely parsed book. The nutrient data was accurate, but my very early concept of a meal-planning guide needed to be built and parsed by a registered dietitian. The plan I had conceived in 1997 and tested with a few on the Net was about to come to life at the hands of a pro. It would grow to a 28-day meal-planning guide. All in the family was beginning to have more meaning to me than an old TV sitcom. Our eldest daughter Jeannie, is a registered dietitian, with a Ph.D. to boot. She jumped into the project and her contribution has turned out to be the most popular section of all four No-Salt, Lowest-Sodium Cookbooks.

As of this writing *The No-Salt, Lowest-Sodium Cookbook* remains a best-seller. We have received thousands upon thousands of E-mails thanking us and many of those notes are posted at *Megaheart.com/testimonialsbook.html.*

Doctors and cardio nurses have told us stories of patients on the transplant list who worked their way off. And we are always reminded of the thousands and thousands who have returned to a normal life. The biggest treat of all is that the books and plans have helped more than just heart patients. Nearly all chronic illnesses related to high sodium intake have reported major improvements.

Megaheart.com had turned into a huge family affair on a world-wide basis. We needed to redesign and expand it, a site with much better navigation and more sections of information. More help arrived in the person of our son, Dan. Dan works with computers. He designed Megaheart as you see it today. He and a friend put the html language together and turned over about ten pages to me. The site now has more than three hundred pages and plenty of information as well as recipes.

Since 1997, we have felt very lucky that we've been able to help so many and hope we can continue to do so for a long time.

We hope this book helps you as well.

\- Don

BY SCOTT LEYSATH

Author, "The Sporting Chef's Favorite Wild Game Recipes,"
and the host of the HuntFishCook.com TV show

Much has changed over the past few decades about the way we look at the things we eat and how we get it to the table. Long gone are the days when there were only a handful of TV chefs like Julia Child, Graham Kerr - The Galloping Gourmet and Justin Wilson ("*I gar-on-tee!*"). We now have entire networks devoted to making cooking and eating more complicated than it actually is. Seriously, how many times do we need to see someone show us how to smash garlic with a knife? Or tell us that "searing meat on the outside will seal in the juices" which, by the way, isn't true. TV cooking shows have changed the way we look and feel about food, and while it has clearly added a bit of mystique to those of us who cook for a living, preparing a great meal at home is actually very simple.

Having been raised on a steady diet of casseroles, TV dinners, canned vegetables and Jello, it's a miracle that I'm still alive today. When I think of mom's home cooking, it doesn't evoke the fond, warm memories that it does for others whose mothers' culinary skills excelled beyond Hamburger Helper. I'd say that my mother's cooking was just below average, but not by much. Our neighbors gorged themselves on pretty much the same level of fare. Mario Batali and Bobby Flay weren't on the television extolling the virtues of Italian and Southwestern cuisine. We had Spaghetti-O's and canned tamales.

As an active outdoorsman, I made it a point to make the most of my harvested fish and game, often hosting fish and game dinners for my college friends in Tucson, Arizona. Grilled quail, pan-seared duck and freshly caught fish were my specialty. Looking back on some of my early attempts at fine dining, I'd like to get in touch with some of my friends so that I could apologize. I didn't know that duck could be served medium-rare and, yes, it did taste like liver. Thanks to everyone for pretending to like it.

Growing up in Northern Virginia didn't afford me the chance to try many southwestern and Hispanic flavors. The closest we got to Mexican food were Jack-In-The-Box tacos. Tucson opened up a whole new world of bold, assertive flavors that I hadn't yet experienced, but soon came to be a large part of my cooking repertoire. I later moved to Northern California, right about the time "California Cuisine" was making waves across America. The emphasis was on fresh, local fruits, vegetables and proteins. Less cooking time, brighter and livelier tastes and vibrant, colorful plates. Cooking elements from various ethnicities were being fused into a single dish. No cans or frozen ingredients. Rules were being broken left and right. And then along came Emeril Lagasse and FoodTV.

Emeril's style of free and easy cooking – "You don't like garlic so much, use less garlic. Hey, it's your chicken!"- turned cooking into entertainment. Families would spend an hour every weeknight watching him banging away and kicking everything up a notch or two. Food became fun, but to many home chefs, food was and is still intimidating. How do you know how much seasoning is enough? How long should you cook your fish? You followed the recipe, but it was unfit to eat. Fortunately, with every failure in the kitchen, you learn something. Believe me, I've learned plenty through some memorable mistakes; like my goose loaf. You don't want to know.

Today's TV chefs are flipping pans, setting their food on fire and using ingredients not known by most normal people. I learned early on that cooking is much less complicated than the chefs on television often try and make it appear. There is still a bounty of ingredients that you *are* familiar with. Those are the ones you should use until you just can't think of anything else to do with them. When you're ready, start working new ingredients into your growing list of dishes you can prepare. Good, healthy cooking is actually not complicated.

My transition from restaurateur to professional chef was not a well-planned career path. While running a series of chain and independent restaurants, I spent a great deal of time in the kitchen, learning how to properly use a knife – the most important kitchen skill anyone will ever need, how to season anything and how to use your imagination to create your own signature dishes. My goal was to cook as well as the chefs who worked for me. Chefs can be an irritable lot, and I didn't want them to have leverage of threatening to walk out in the middle of a busy Friday night dinner. Go ahead and leave, I'll take your spot. At some point, people started calling *me* a chef.

Back to the knife. Let me state without hesitation that there is no better way to improve your kitchen mastery than by learning how to properly use a chef's knife. Gadgets that chop are not the answer and they rarely work at home like they do on TV. If you don't already own a decent chef's knife, get one. You can spend anywhere from $20 to $500. For most people, a good eight or ten-inch chef's knife that will last many years can be found for around forty bucks. If you use a sawing, rather than a chopping motion to cut through a carrot, it's time to move forward. Put the serrated Ginzu knife back in the drawer, grasp your new chef's knife firmly, and while keeping the front of the knife constantly in contact with the cutting surface, walk your sharpened blade through a carrot or two. At first it seems awkward. A new way of doing something usually does. The next time you're at the grocery store, pick up 10 pounds of carrots and spend 15 minutes or so each day, chopping, not sawing through them into assorted sizes. Slice, dice and make thousands of match-stick-sized morsels. Armed with your new knife, you will soon have the skill to speed through the most time-consuming part – getting your ingredients chopped and ready to cook. Now you can pack up the canned vegetables and drop them off at the local shelter.

The cooking part is where the fun begins. Once you are no longer at the mercy of prepared canned, frozen and otherwise processed ingredients, almost all very high in sodium, your food will taste better. While it may take awhile for your taste buds to adjust to natural foods if they are more familiar with over-salted, fatty foods with little nutritional value, the transition will happen as long as you stay the course and do not retreat to your past comfort zone. Of course, you won't sacrifice flavor by using fresh ingredients. A word of advice about shopping for a specific recipe; take advantage of seasonal produce, meats and fish. Although the global market has enabled us to get just about anything at anytime of the year, the best quality goods will come from within a few hundred miles of where you live, not from South America. Also, if you have your heart set on swordfish, for instance, and the fresh albacore looks and smells better than the swordfish, make the switch and go with the fresher choice. If the fish doesn't smell good, it's either old or has been mishandled. Don't buy it and try to cover up the aroma with a strong marinade, brine or buttermilk. Get the albacore.

If you are embarking on or continuing a weight loss or otherwise restricted diet, you don't have to substitute flavor, but you will have to forego processed and fast foods. Very often, adding chopped fresh herbs or a big squeeze of lime or lemon will awaken the flavors in a dish. Lemon and lime juice stimulates the palate and acts like a natural

MSG by making other ingredients come alive. After packing on "a few" extra pounds following a year of surgeries that I couldn't put off any longer, I decided that it was time to get rid of the excess baggage. It was time to either lose the weight or give in and get some bigger clothes. Just by eating lean meats and fresh vegetables, lots of fresh vegetables, I lost fifty pounds in four months and never went hungry. I ate when I was hungry, but it was often a head of steamed broccoli. Lucky for me, I like broccoli.

Preparing food like a professional doesn't require a great deal of skill. Don't be intimidated by high-priced cookware and cutlery. You can prepare a fabulous feast with a ten-dollar skillet from the discount store, a decent knife and a handful of fresh ingredients. Meal preparation shouldn't take all day. Most of your everyday meals shouldn't take more than 20 – 30 minutes to prepare from prep to plating.

Cooking really is all about having the confidence to throw a few compatible ingredients into a skillet or onto a grill and making them work together on the plate. It's not necessary to complicate a dish with obscure, often very expensive ingredients just because you saw it on TV. Start with simple dishes and get used to real cooking with real ingredients. In short order, you will be anxious to expand your culinary horizons to places you never imagined.

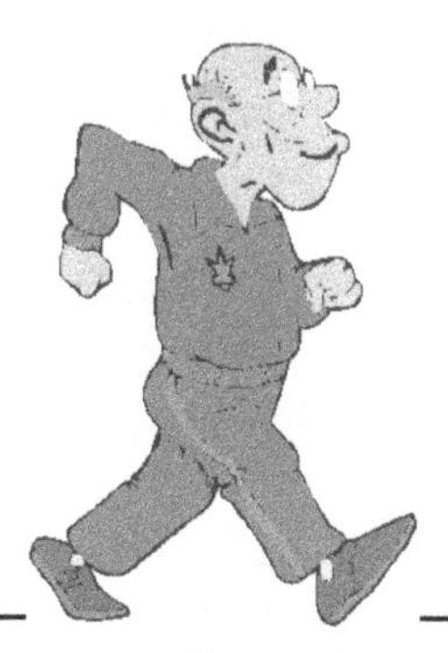

The Road Map Back To Good Health

When first diagnosed with a chronic and sometimes life threatening illness some of us wonder, "What happened?" "Why me?"

The truth is we feel violated, as though just mugged or robbed. Some of us fall into an immediate funk, an occurrence more natural than we might like to believe.

Our physical and spiritual being has been attacked and we are put into the position of having to solve a challenge that pills alone won't fix. We need help and we learn that the help must come from our own effort. It's not always easy to point out the solution to others, but here it is: We must face the reality that in order to recover, we must adapt to a new lifestyle. We must help to cure ourselves.

Let's consider for a few moments what happens after that initial and often shocking diagnosis. Generally we have a reaction so common that I'll assume that you, like me, were or are in denial.

In the world of psychiatry, the word denial refers to "denial of death," a concept that first came to public awareness with Sigmund Freud, Søren Kierkegaard, and one of Freud's understudies, Otto Rank. I'm pretty sure that when I heard the word terminal in my diagnosis that I went into complete denial. I had been misdiagnosed for a few years as having had "adult onset asthma," which made rowing quite difficult. However, after I "collapsed," the heart cath test was made and when I awoke I was told I had, "Terminal dilated cardiomyopathy among other things." My rapid arrival of denial showed when I asked, "Does that mean it's not asthma?"

When I speak of denial here, it's not deep depression nor mental anguish like those spoken of when referring to Freud and his peers. Our reactions are normal and acceptable, yet potentially a barrier we have to get through.

Certainly, a level of denial geared to rejecting serious ailments belongs in the human nature, especially when challenges could be life altering. It is amazing that no matter what some might think or say aloud about the end of life, the human spirit is such that it begs to hang on as long as it can.

We want to live.

But while we're being rolled into OR-1, we have to admit that thoughts of bolting or getting the heck out of there to avoid investigative surgery seems like a much better concept than what may lie ahead.

In Elisabeth Kubler-Ross's model of the five stages of grief, the end of the denial phase is noted by "heightened awareness" of the problem. That's a good thing. Once aware, we can deal with it.

Denial can be a seductive helper or a hostile adversary. In the beginning denial seemed to me like an anesthesia protecting me from the reality of that "terminal" diagnosis. It had become a hurdle to leap over if for no other reason than to get to the other side of wherever I thought I was at the time. How did I deal with it? Well, first I made sure our family records, assets, et al, were protected with a family trust. After that I bought a Tracker bass boat. My first boat ever. Why would I do that? The answer is easy now: The boat gave me hope, and that was the unrecognized-at-the-time reality.

Change Our Lifestyle – Cut the salt out

For heart patients during the period of my diagnosis, when our EF (ejection fraction) dropped too low, medical science generally called for a heart transplant. Initially, I fell into that group, but while being "worked up" for eligibility for the heart transplant list I began to improve. The doctors held off. Something good was happening. In fact, so good I never needed the transplant.

Cause, and the ultimate care for cure are not always married nor even cousins. But when it comes to salt, the relationship between disease and cure might be staring at us straight on.

I reversed my heart disease because I took salt out of my life. I believe you can get the same results if you really work at it. It's a good program, or as a doctor might refer to it: a good procedure.

Part of our effort is to also include medications, exercise, and a strong effort to put our brain to work, to keep active, to live forward and not to accept defeat or retreat. By the way, the best part of not eating any salt is being able to cut back on medications, especially the diuretic and potassium tablets.

We have been inundated with salt in every prepared meal ever eaten. However, that alone is not conclusive for any of us. Causal factors for CHF can also include genetics, viruses, and our working lifestyle, such as longer hours, stress, diet while working, sleep apnea, and the environment of our work place including noise or physical toxins.

Still not figuring out exactly what brought mine about, I looked back and realized that I had put in very long hours at work and longer hours of driving and flying. During the sixties and very early seventies I flew a few million miles in airlines and actually ate their meals. I also flew my own planes and stacked up quite a few thousand hours as pilot in command. Too often I took along all the wrong foods to nibble on.

That kind of lifestyle could challenge anyone's heart, and I'm certainly not alone in that uptight, workaholic, travel-a-lot-arena. Fortunately, I was not a smoker nor an alcohol drinker.

After a review of my lifestyle before diagnosis, I had to ask myself: Did that take a toll on my heart? Remember back then? Aerobic exercise was the big thing to help prevent heart disease.

In my case rowing was my best aerobic exercise. I had been a skier and on the National Ski Patrol, but that came to an abrupt ending with a rather vicious accident. Still, rowing and skiing served me well except when I traveled. To "solve" the loss of exercise I joined a gym in L.A., the city where I traveled to mostly.

So where does that lead us? Abuse of my diet, long hours of work and travel, strenuous exercise and I develop heart failure?

My response after diagnosis was to develop a balanced diet, get back to a good exercise and adopt a less stressful lifestyle.

Denial can be a Friend

Whichever chronic illness diagnosis you have received, whether congestive heart failure, hypertension, Meniere's Syndrome, or any of the myriad of other ailments that require cutting salt and sodium out of our diets, adopting a no-salt lifestyle generally produces the same result in nearly everyone:

Improvement. Impressive improvement.

Cutting salt out combined with prescribed medications and exercise is like a magic pill. It works.

Denial can potentially stop us from accepting the "cure," or steps to a cure. For instance, are you ready for a no-salt life? Do you deny that it will help you? If so, that form of denial is the one I call hostile denial, especially since many others have succeeded by cutting salt out.

Family and Friends Needed

Denial in any form is also a time when family love and help come into play. I have strong sympathy for those who don't have loving help during a time of need. I was lucky to have Maureen and our children. Her care when I was ill was and remains second to none. However, I have received E-mails and letters from Megaheart visitors and book users who were, "On my own." Some were married but their mates, "just would not help." Most, however, have much happier stories, some have been quite beautiful tales, and Maureen and I have met many such couples and even visited a few when they called us for help.

The best road to recovery is when it's paved smoothly and the bumps are removed, and that kind of help usually comes from family and friends.

Taking Stock

If you find it difficult to accept your doctor's diagnosis, or his or her plan for your recovery or survival (like cutting salt out of your life), then you might want to outline on paper where you are and just what you need to do to get control of your health again.

As much as I don't like to admit it, I realize that getting ourselves out of any level of denial is easier said than done. It's not a party. But it is necessary, and once we face that reality we can work our way to the next stage: our recovery. This is assuming your diagnosis is not in fact so harsh that the only way out is major surgery, which for some includes a transplant.

Transplants, however, do work for many. Pete Eiden, founder of healthyheartmarket.com, a primary source for low sodium foods online, had a heart transplant and is now living a healthy, fruitful life. He was in his thirties when he received his new heart, and is back ice fishing in Minnesota along with his wife and children.

We know of many who avoided a transplant, however, and they too are living fruitful and healthy lives. So, the good news is that there's an upside to cutting salt and trying your best to reverse your heart disease. My diagnosis was "harsh." Flat out I had six months to a year to live. A transplant was staring me in the face, yet here I am. A lifetime down the road from 1997, no transplant and an active life. I was determined, but also lucky since it was not known whether my plan would work or not. We now know that it does work so, I hope I can pass some of that determination and luck on to you.

To begin, we have to irrevocably get rid of the salt shaker. No excuses, no lapses, no kidding. Salt is dangerous, damaging, and not just to us, but to a large group of healthy people as well.

Why Not Just Use Salt Substitutes?

Most salt substitutes are pure potassium chloride or potassium carbonate. Some mix in other flavors or nutrients like lycopene, etc. We need potassium, but it seems that all no-salt-added food products are using potassium as a replacement. Large amounts of dietary potassium can create new problems, and if processors continue their program of replacing salt with potassium it's one we'll all have to deal with.

The alternatives for "salt" are not salt substitutes, but instead spices and herbs, and for the nutrient balance of our health, whole grains, fresh fruits and vegetables, fish, lean meat and some nonfat dairy products, and great recipes no matter how large or small. Non meat eaters generally know the dietary routine for getting enough protein, how-ever, they now face the challenge of having to do it without using salt to flavor their food.

If you're just getting started, there is much to learn about our no-salt life. What to eat, where to buy it, how to prepare it, and then there's that eating out challenge as well. I think we can help you with each, including eating out. Each recipe in this book is also rated for diabetic choices and whether it works for vegetarians. For those of you who aren't aware of diabetic needs, they count carbohydrate levels, not sugar.

So How Do We Do This?

First, let's remember that we need a balanced diet. The well-known food pyramid is a terrific guide and should be referred to. However, we must consider using it as a guide, not a bible.

This is where you can develop your personal health care. Now is the time. Make sure you know the calories you should eat and then develop a good meal plan.

My first plan was posted at our Web site in February, 1999. It was basic, but vital and successful. It was designed for a 1500 calorie daily plan and included:

Breakfast: Applesauce Oatmeal

Lunch: Quick Tacos

Dinner: Nasir's Curried Chicken, table queen squash, and spinach with mushrooms and onions.

Dessert: Strawberry Delight

Note that I didn't include snacks, which we did include later in the first of the no-salt, lowest-sodium cookbook series. Snacks include fresh fruits and vegetables, muffins, yogurt and more.

One reason we like a monthly plan is that we can then make sure the special no salt added foods we need are on hand.

When making a plan, why not apply the FDA pyramid, but without the salt? As Dr. Trevor Beard of the Salt Skip Program in Australia wrote:

"The random evolution of the universe has not provided all the nutritional requirements of every species in every corner of the globe. Yet no human population has ever been offered salt as a public health mea-sure, for the very good reason that we have no evidence that any human population needs it. Salt was offered only as a vehicle for iodine, but it is no longer needed."

Beard's statement above illustrates the advance in transporting foods around the world or from one geographical area to the next. For instance, if you lived in your current geographic area but had no means of transporting or accessing the large variety of food needed to obtain all the nutrients we need, would you be able to provide your family and yourself the required daily nutrients? Generally the answer will be no. But today we have overnight shipments of fresh food into most areas of the world and that provides us with the daily nutrients we need, including iodine.

Exercise.

Start with walking. Exercise is important for diabetics as well as heart and hypertension patients. When strength returns add other exercises to your routine from working in the yard to your favorite games or sport like rowing or fishing or hiking. If generally sedentary, then move around the house at least every half-hour. While sitting at a desk raise your legs up, reach for the space behind your desk, then raise and lower them straight out. Stretch your arms out and pretend you're lifting weights or lift a heavy book up, lower it, lift it, etc. Exercise, turns out, is as important as cutting salt and taking your meds. No matter which method of exercise you choose, do keep at it. It pays off.

Develop A Hobby or Volunteer

The first thing my daughters did was bring me some paint brushes and a few canvasses along with the paints needed to turn me into a second Rembrandt. They launched me in a new direction. They understood their dad. He always wanted to try his hand at painting. Nothing new there. My father had the same idea about me painting. When I was young I was tall, so he'd hand me a paint brush and a can of paint and say, "Here Don, you paint the ceilings."

The relaxation and positive control a hobby gives you is profound. If you already have a hobby, then you've got it made. Just keep at it. It will help you improve your health immensely and more quickly.

Become a volunteer. Volunteering offers huge benefits to you and to the group you help. Maureen volunteered us for work with a lighthouse in northern California (Point Cabrillo Light Station). The lighthouse work had proved to be one of the most enjoyable things I've ever done and I truly credit it for adding more years to my life. Just to get there you have to walk a mile round trip down a slope that quite suddenly becomes an up-slope when leaving. The exercise has been great. All good for the heart.

At this writing we have also volunteered to help a young group of Big Brothers, Big Sisters "at risk children," some of whom are homeless. They will learn how to cook and make a cookbook as a fund raiser.

You might want to find someone in your area who needs your talents. It's a win-win situation.

What lies ahead?

It will take personal motivation, determination and persistence to change your lifestyle. The effort is more than worth it, so don't let the "start-up" period discourage you. It can be life saving. Additionally, it can also help you cut the number of medications you're currently taking and in some cases, curtail the need for a heart transplant.

Maybe you've a great spouse who has done all the cooking for you and your family, but if she's the one affected, then it's going to be up to you to help her get back to good health.

From what I have gathered there are many men in my senior citizen category who need to learn how to prepare meals for themselves, and sometimes for a spouse or family. Importantly, to help your mate or yourself, you'll really have to dump the fast-food routine if that's been your lifestyle. "Take-out," will only exacerbate the problems already at hand. If you're waiting for the pizza man to arrive, forget it. Instead, head into the kitchen and make your own very low sodium pizza. It tastes better and it's a lot healthier. We have two dough recipes in this book.

The bottom line, however, is that a change in dietary lifestyle for one member of the family might mean change for all members; at least that's often true in the beginning. It may prove difficult to prepare two different meals, one with salt, one without, but the person needing to change needs the family to join in at least at the beginning of their recovery period. The patient eating a salt-free dish doesn't need to watch their spouse or family eat a giant Big Mac or salt laden pile of trans fatty, cholesterol-busting pizza. Also, nutrition must be taken into account. A salt-free balanced diet is what we need to achieve.

The end goal.

I believe you can get better and you can do a whole lot of that getting better on your own. Medical science alone isn't going to put you back on your feet as a whole person. It's a partnership. It takes a lot of what you have to offer as well. Doctors need willing partners to help their patients back to health.

Cutting salt out helps every single chronic illness that salt has either led to or aggravated and no amount of distorted viewpoints from the national and international salt organizations can change that.

Don't worry about the sodium that your heart and organs need. It's a very small amount, and we get plenty of sodium in fresh (natural) foods. Remember this: No food has salt in it unless it's added by humans.

Within a few months after adopting my plan, my heart began its journey back to normal size, or as Dr. Michael Fowler described it, "The heart remodeled." My ejection fraction climbed back to 48% from a low of 18%. My breathing improved remarkably.

We have heard from literally thousands of our book users that our no-salt plan has brought them back to good health.

Best of all, however, are the thirteen grandchildren I would not have known had I not improved. They make life wonderful and each visit is a pure joy. Including today's sojourn on the local lake with three of them aboard the bass boat.

Bottom Line

Look upon your change in lifestyle as a new beginning that will give your life back to you, not as a negative that is taking something away.

Grab a cup of hot green tea, comfy up for this read. This chapter will prove to be of value to you.

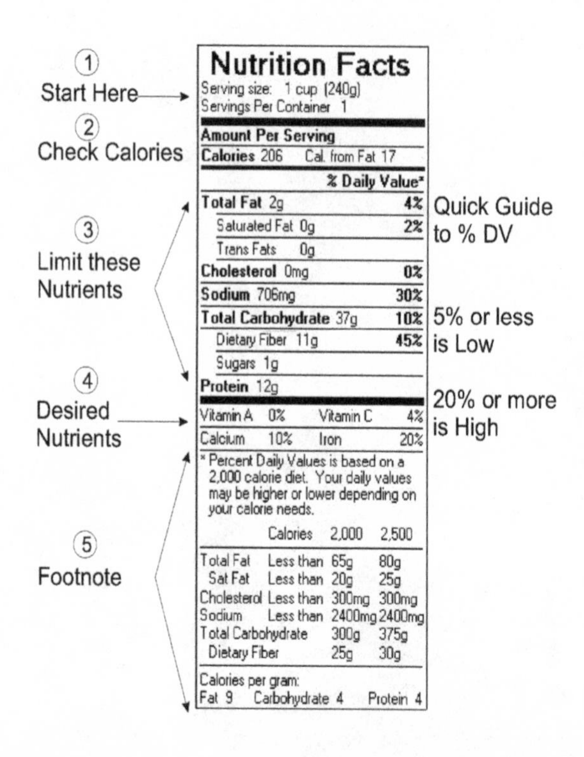

To help you determine FDA Food pyramid choices, check out the FDA's Food-a-pedia at:
http://www.myfoodapedia.gov/Default.aspx

The FDA Label

To help you determine FDA Food pyramid choices, check out the FDA's Food-a-pedia at: http://www.myfoodapedia.gov/Default.aspx

The sample FDA[1] label to the left is for one cup of commercially processed canned pinto beans with salt.

The information in the main or top section can vary with each food product. It contains product-specific information (serving size, calories, and nutrient information). The bottom section contains a footnote with Daily Values (DVs) for 2,000 and 2,500 calorie diets. This footnote provides recommended dietary information for important nutrients, including fats, sodium and fiber. The footnote is found only on larger packages and does not change from product to product. If you are eating a lower daily calorie plan, then for accuracy you'll have to do the math for all daily value figures.

It may seem complex, but it isn't. This may be a good time to learn how to read the FDA label. It has more information available to us than we might suspect.

1. The Serving Size

The first place to start when you look at the Nutrition Facts label is the serving size and the number of servings in the package. Serving sizes are standardized to make it easier to compare similar foods; they are provided in familiar units, such as cups or pieces, followed by the metric amount: the number of grams. Remember that 28 grams equals one-ounce.

The size of the serving on the food package influences the number of calories and all the nutrient amounts listed on the top part of the label. Note: As of 2010 the FDA is requesting that processors use realistic serving sizes on food labels instead of the very low serving sizes generally used. The FDA wants consumers to fully understand just what they are eating, believing that such meaningful numbers might raise a red flag or two before we dive into a bottle or can of cola or soup, etc.

When reading the serving size ask yourself, “How many servings will I consume?” (e.g., 1/2 serving, 1 serving, or more.) Especially be careful of juice or cola drink containers. In the sample label, one serving of pinto beans equals one-half cup. If you ate the whole can, you would eat three and a half servings, which means you’d have to multiply the listed numbers by three and half times. Since the serving size is a half-cup, eating one-cup that would double the calories and other nutrient numbers, including the percent of Daily Values as shown in the sample label. One-cup therefore would equal 706 milligrams of sodium.

2. Calories (and Calories from Fat)

Calories provide a measure of how much energy you get from a serving of this food. The calorie section of the label can help you manage your weight (i.e., gain, lose, or maintain.) Remember: the number of servings you consume determines the number of calories you actually eat (your portion amount).

In the example, there are 103 calories in one serving of pinto beans from this can. How many calories from fat are there in one serving? Answer: 9 calories. For some foods that you may have been eating however, calories from fat can be more than 50 percent of total calories. Double the serving and you’ve doubled the fat intake.

General FDA Guide to Calories

§ 40 Calories is low

§ 100 Calories is moderate

§ 400 Calories or more is high

The General Guide to Calories provides a general reference for calories when you look at a Nutrition Facts label. This guide is based on a 2,000 calorie diet. If you have a medical condition then you’ll want to pay as much attention to the calories/saturated-fat content as you will the sodium and carbohydrate content.

The General Guide to calories is also designed for healthy people. Most chronic diseases like heart disease require that we adjust the guide for our use to help lower numbers.

3. The Nutrients: How Much?

Look at the top of the nutrient section in the sample label. It shows you some key nutrients that impact your health. The nutrients listed first are the ones Americans generally eat in adequate amounts, or even too much. These include: Saturated Fat, Trans Fat, Carbohydrates, Cholesterol, and Sodium.

Eating too much of these may increase your risk of certain chronic diseases. You'll want to make sure these numbers are low.

4. What We're Looking For.

Most Americans don't get enough dietary fiber, vitamin A, vitamin C, vitamin D, calcium, and iron in their diets. Eating enough of these nutrients can improve your health and help reduce the risk of some diseases and conditions. For example, getting enough calcium may reduce the risk of osteoporosis, a condition that results in brittle bones as one ages. Eating a diet high in dietary fiber promotes healthy bowel function. Additionally, a diet rich in fruits, vegetables, and grain products that contain dietary fiber, particularly soluble fiber, and low in saturated fat and cholesterol may reduce the risk of heart disease. Combine these higher figures with low fat, cholesterol and sodium and you'll live a much healthier life.

Remember: You can use the Nutrition Facts label not only to help limit those nutrients you want to cut back on but also to increase those nutrients you need to consume in greater amounts.

5. Understanding the Footnote on the Bottom of the Nutrition Facts Label

Note the asterisk (*) used after the heading "Percent Daily Value" on the Nutrition Facts label. It refers to the Footnote in the lower part of the nutrition label, which tells you, "Percent DVs are based on a 2,000 calorie diet." This statement must be on all food labels. But the remaining information in the full footnote might not be on the package if the size of the label is too small. When the full footnote does appear, it will always be the same. It doesn't change from product to product because it shows recommended dietary advice for all Americans - it is not about a specific food product.

Look at the amounts under each heading of either 2,000 or 2,500- these are the Daily Values (DV) for each nutrient listed and are based on public health experts' advice. DVs are recommended levels of intakes. DVs in the footnote are based on a 2,000 or 2,500 calorie diet. Note how the DVs for some nutrients change, while others (for cholesterol and sodium) remain the same for both calorie amounts.

6. The Percent Daily Value (%DV):

The Percent Daily Values (%DVs) are based on the Daily Value recommendations for key nutrients but only for a 2,000 calorie daily diet. Most of us have gone our whole lives without knowing how many calories a day we consumed. Now, we need to know. We can use the %DV as a frame of reference for daily consumption of 2,000 calories or fewer.

The %DV helps us determine if a serving of food is high or low in a nutrient. Note: a few nutrients, like trans fat, do not have a %DV - they will be discussed later.

We don't need to know how to calculate percentages to use the %DV. The label (the %DV) does the math for us. It helps us interpret the numbers (grams and milligrams) by putting them all on the same scale for the day (0-100%DV). The %DV column doesn't add up vertically to 100%. Instead each nutrient is based on 100% of the daily requirements for that nutrient (for a 2,000 calorie diet). This way we can tell high from low and know which nutrients contribute a lot, or a little to our daily recommended allowance (upper or lower).

Quick Guide to %DV: 5 percent DV or less is low and 20 percent DV or more is high. This guide tells us that 5%DV or less is low for all nutrients, those you want to limit (e.g., fat, saturated fat, cholesterol, and sodium), or for those that you want to consume in greater amounts (fiber, calcium, etc.). As the Quick Guide shows, 20%DV or more is high for all nutrients.

Example: Look at the amount of Total Fat in one serving listed on the nutrition label of what you are buying. On our sample label it's 0%. But on other products it can be much higher. If it is higher check the Quick Guide to %DV. If your intended purchase is 18%DV, which is below 20%DV, then you're not yet high, but what if you ate two servings? Coming from just one food, that amount leaves you with as low as 64% of your fat allowance (100%-36%=64%) for all of the other foods you eat that day, snacks and drinks included.

Note: %DV for Sodium Levels Does Not Work With Quick Guide or FDA recommendations. If you have established your daily intake of sodium at 500 mg or 1,000 mg, then you will have to do the math for milligrams and not apply the percent daily value pertaining to whatever calorie target you set.

Comparisons: The %DV also makes it easy for you to make comparisons. You can compare one product or brand to a similar product. Just make sure the serving sizes are similar, especially the weight (e.g. gram, milligram, ounces) of each product. It's easy to see which foods are higher or lower in nutrients because the serving sizes are generally consistent for similar types of foods, except in a few cases like cereals.

Nutrient Content Claims: Use the %DV to help you quickly distinguish one claim from another, such as "reduced fat" vs. "light" or "nonfat." Just compare the %DVs for Total Fat in each food product to see which one is higher or lower in that nutrient - there is no need to memorize definitions. This works when comparing all nutrient content claims, e.g., less, light, low, free, more, high, etc.

Dietary Trade-Offs: You can use the %DV to help you make dietary trade-offs with other foods throughout the day. You don't have to give up a favorite food to eat a healthy diet. When a food you like is high in fat, balance it with foods that are low in fat at other times of the day. Also, pay attention to how much you eat so that the total amount of fat for the day stays below 100%DV.

Calcium: Look at the %DV for calcium on food packages so you know how much one serving contributes to the total amount you need per day. Remember, a food with 20%DV or more contributes a lot of calcium to your daily total, while one with 5%DV or less contributes a little.

Experts advise adult consumers to consume adequate amounts of calcium, that is, 1,000 mg or 100%DV in a daily 2,000 calorie diet. This advice is often given in milligrams (mg), but the Nutrition Facts label only lists a %DV for calcium. Our recipes give you the mg amount of calcium.

For certain populations, they advise that adolescents, especially girls, consume 1,300 mg (130%DV) and post-menopausal women consume 1,200 mg (120%DV) of calcium daily. The DV for calcium on food labels is 1,000 mg.

Don't be fooled - always check the label for calcium because you can't make assumptions about the amount of calcium in specific food categories. Example: the amount of calcium in milk, whether skim or whole, is generally the same per serving, however, the amount of calcium in the same size yogurt container (8 oz) can vary from 20 - 45 %DV (for calcium).

Note that Trans fat, Sugars and Protein do not list a %DV on the Nutrition Facts label.

Trans Fat: Experts could not provide a reference value for trans fat nor any other information that FDA believes is sufficient to establish a Daily Value or %DV. Scientific reports link trans fat (and saturated fat) with raising blood LDL ("bad") cholesterol levels, both of which increase your risk of coronary heart disease, a leading cause of death in the US and Great Britain.

Protein: A %DV is required to be listed if a claim is made for protein, such as "high in protein." Otherwise, unless the food is meant for use by infants and children under 4 years old, none is needed. Current scientific evidence indicates that protein intake is not a public health concern for adults and children over 4 years of age.

Sugars: No daily reference value has been established for sugars because no recommendations have been made for the total amount to eat in a day. Keep in mind, the sugars listed on the Nutrition Facts label include naturally occurring sugars (like those in fruit and milk) as well as those added to a food or drink. Check the ingredient list for specifics on added sugars.

Take a look at the Nutrition Facts label for the two yogurt examples. The plain yogurt on the left has 10 grams of sugars, while the fruit yogurt on the right has 44 grams of sugars in one serving.

Now look below at the ingredient lists for the two yogurts. Ingredients are listed in descending order of weight (from most to least). Note that no added sugars or sweeteners are in the list of ingredients for the plain yogurt, yet 10 grams of sugars were listed on the Nutrition Facts label. This is because there are no added sugars in plain yogurt, only naturally occurring sugars (lactose in the milk).

If you are concerned about your intake of carbohydrates (sugars), make sure that added sugars are not listed as one of the first few ingredients. Other names for added sugars include: corn syrup, high-fructose corn syrup, fruit juice concentrate, maltose, dextrose, sucrose, honey, and maple syrup.

To limit ingredients that have no %DV, like trans fat and sugars, compare the labels of similar products and choose the food with the lowest amount.

Below are two kinds of milk. One is "Reduced Fat," the other is "Nonfat" milk. Each serving size is one cup. Which one has more calories and more saturated fat? Which one has more calcium?

Answer: As you can see, they both have the same amount of calcium, but the nonfat milk has no saturated fat and has 40 fewer calories per serving than the reduced fat milk.

How Do I Know When I'm Buying Low-sodium Foods?

Nearly all fresh food may be considered low in sodium and generally high in nutrient values. Fruit, vegetables and some fish and meats are generally low in sodium (a few exceptions do exist). Unsalted packaged spices and herbs are low in sodium and again, high in nutrient values. However, most processed foods, those that are packaged, frozen, hermetically sealed, canned, jarred, etc. are usually high in sodium and often not as high in nutrient values as fresh food counterparts.

Processed food package labels may claim health benefits or nutrient benefits or they may state that the product is "low sodium," "lowered sodium," "no salt added," or they might allude to natural or "naturally flavored" among other claims. These are sometimes misleading.

To help clear the air, the FDA has posted a nutrient claim guide that processors must stick to. Here's the FDA list for claims concerning sodium that processors may use.

Sodium-free: fewer than 5 milligrams (mg) per serving.

Very low sodium: 35 mg or fewer per serving, or if the serving is 30 grams (g) or lower or 2 or fewer tablespoon, 35 mg or lower per 50 g of the food.

Low-sodium: 140 mg or fewer per serving, or if the serving is 30 g or fewer or 2 tablespoons or fewer, 140 mg or fewer per 50 g of the food.

Light in sodium: at least 50 percent less sodium per serving than average reference amount for same food with no sodium reduction.

BI at least 50 percent less sodium per serving than reference amount. (If the food is not "low in sodium," the statement "not a low-sodium food" must appear on the same panel as the "Nutrition Facts" panel.)

Reduced or less sodium: at least 25 percent less per serving than reference food.

Salt-free, Unsalted, without added salt, no salt added: each means no salt added during processing, and the food it resembles and for which it substitutes is normally processed with salt.

(If the food is not "sodium free," the statement "not a sodium-free food" or "not for control of sodium in the diet" must appear on the same panel as the Nutrition Facts panel.)

Serving size becomes important to us. Serving sizes listed on FDA labels on processed foods was supposed to be what we would normally eat. Well, that's not exactly what has happened. Often we purchase snacks or fruit drinks or other products and learn later that we consumed two or three times the values listed on the labels. If you see sodium is 40 mg on a fruit drink that sounds great. But actually, you may be consuming 80 or 120 mg. The FDA intended for this area to be what we normally consume or cook with or consume. Since that's not always the case it's best to read the labels and do the math.

Also you may want to check levels of potassium and calcium and magnesium. These often help lower blood pressure, so getting your share of these on a daily basis becomes as important as lowering sodium. Caution: Many no salt added products are using potassium in various forms. This could lead to getting too much potassium.

Although it's important to identify what is high-sodium, we also need to learn what is low-sodium. This is again where the FDA labels come in handy.

The FDA label examples to the right demonstrate the comparison method of figuring out which product is high in sodium and which is low.(Note: According to the Federal food-labeling guidelines, if a food contains less than 5 milligrams of sodium or .5 grams of fat per serving, the total value found on the Nutrition Facts label is rounded down to zero. If a product contains less than 2 milligrams of cholesterol per serving, this value will be rounded down to zero. This is the same rounding that occurs when a product might have 129 mg of sodium. The package may read 125 mg.)

Note too, that the sodium is 300 mg lower with the Spoon Size shredded wheat than with the Honey Graham Chex and protein is 3 grams higher. Also, note that appreciable differences occur with the fiber and calories from fat. Remember, neither of these add in the milk that you'll add to your cereal. The label on the left is for Honey Graham Chex cereal. The label on the right is for Spoon Size shredded wheat.

What About Restaurant Food?

Many restaurants today are providing this important data in store and on the Net. Just "Google" your restaurant and you'll probably find it quickly along with complete nutrient data for their entire menu. If you find a great restaurant where they provide a no salt service, let us know at megaheart.com/restaurants.html. We'll post it to help others.

Eating out is not easy for those of us who must cut down on sodium and trans fats or saturated fats. The move by many fast-food chains to rid themselves of trans fats has been slow but working. Still, the fat and sodium delivered to consumers is exceptionally high when the servings are mostly pre-salted and fried, such as French fries, batter coated fish, or chicken.

Another tidbit for us concerns French fries in restaurants. You can order them without the chef adding salt, but in all but a few restaurants the fries come to the chef frozen, pre-salted, and ready to just plunk them into the deep-fat fryer. (French fries are not healthy even without salt. Deep-fat frying of any food in overheated oil or oil that's been used over and over is considered carcinogenic.)

I had an experience once while filming a famous Chinese restaurant. I watched while a chef put an order together. The guest for that dish was about to consume 216 grams of fat (high trans fats type of oil) and nearly 2,000 calories just from the oil. Add about 350 to 400 calories

Nutrition Facts

Serving Size 1 Cup (240 mL)
Servings Per Container about 8

Amount Per Serving	
Calories 90	Calories from Fat 0
	% Daily Value*
Total Fat 0g	**0%**
Saturated Fat 0g	**0%**
Trans Fat 0g	
Cholesterol Less than 5mg	**1%**
Sodium 130mg	**5%**
Total Carbohydrate 12g	**4%**
Dietary Fiber 0g	**0%**
Sugars 12g	
Protein 9g	**18%**

Vitamin A 10% • Vitamin C 2%
Calcium 30% • Iron 0%
Vitamin D 25%

*Percent Daily Values are based on a 2,000 calorie diet. Your daily values may be higher or lower depending on your calorie needs:

	Calories:	2,000	2,500
Total Fat	Less Than	65g	80g
Saturated Fat	Less Than	20g	25g
Cholesterol	Less Than	300mg	300mg
Sodium	Less Than	2,400mg	2,400mg
Total Carbohydrate		300g	375g
Dietary Fiber		25g	30g
Protein		50g	65g

Calories per gram:
Fat 9 • Carbohydrate 4 • Protein 4

Nutrition Facts

Serving Size 1 Cup (240 mL)
Servings Per Container about 8

Amount Per Serving	
Calories 122	Calories from Fat 0
	% Daily Value*
Total Fat 0g	**0%**
Saturated Fat 3g	**0%**
Trans Fat 0g	
Cholesterol Less than 5mg	**1%**
Sodium 100mg	**5%**
Total Carbohydrate 12g	**4%**
Dietary Fiber 0g	**0%**
Sugars 12g	
Protein 9g	**18%**

Vitamin A 10% • Vitamin C 2%
Calcium 30% • Iron 0%
Vitamin D 25%

*Percent Daily Values are based on a 2,000 calorie diet. Your daily values may be higher or lower depending on your calorie needs:

	Calories:	2,000	2,500
Total Fat	Less Than	65g	80g
Saturated Fat	Less Than	20g	25g
Cholesterol	Less Than	300mg	300mg
Sodium	Less Than	2,400mg	2,400mg
Total Carbohydrate		300g	375g
Dietary Fiber		25g	30g
Protein		50g	65g

Calories per gram:
Fat 9 • Carbohydrate 4 • Protein 4

from the rice and more for the meat in the dish and you've got a heart busting dinner. I had no way of measuring the sodium back then since the man had poured salt in along with other spices and a dose of MSG[2].

Are There Any Low-sodium Foods We Can Trust?

There are. Vegetarians have the best of all worlds. They eat high fiber foods with higher overall nutrient levels, and they are consuming naturally unsalted and low-sodium food. If we all ate vegetarian diets without added salt, we'd be much better off when it comes to lowering sodium and saturated fats. (Both fats and high sodium contribute to heart disease and other illnesses.) Fruit and vegetables have enough sodium in them to fill the actual daily requirements for all humans. We need never add salt to these foods. Instead, spices and herbs will help with enhancing flavors.

Also, never overcook vegetables. Boiling them for long periods boils out the nutrients and the flavors. You can bake, broil, grill, sauté lightly, or you can steam or drop them into boiling water for a minute or two. Vegetables should have a bit of a crunch when you serve them. You'll find they have more flavor that way and you'll receive the benefits of the nutrients[3]. When we were children, I remember everyone salting melons, lemons, and tomatoes. Now we've learned to enjoy the natural flavors of these fruits.

When it comes to adding meat to your diet, all non-brined meats, including fish, are relatively low in sodium except for shellfish, which are usually too high. Small to medium fresh shrimp, although low enough in sodium for us to consume three or four, are almost never without having been salted. Shrimp in your local store may now come from other parts of the world like Vietnam, Bangladesh, and other countries in which case they have all been salted before shipping. Fresh shrimp off the boat might be available locally if you live near a shrimp area, but in other parts of the country, even the "fresh" shrimp in your store's showcase is probably straight out of a container that states the shrimp were salted before packaging. The original packaging will list salt, but may not have an FDA label.

Fresh lobster tails (known sometimes as rock or spiny) are edible if fresh and the serving size is small or within reason. The sodium is higher than other meats, but acceptable if we hold our lobster down to under 4 or 5-ounces and if it was not salted or cooked with salt.

Crab meat ranges from around 300 mg for 3-ounces of Dungeness crabs, to around 710 mg for 3-ounces of Alaskan King Crab, and that's unsalted. Unsalted crab cakes, sometimes served in restaurants are generally around 434 mg per each crab cake (about 4-ounces). If salted, they will be at least triple that amount.

What About Lowered Sodium Items?

We have to be careful about products that state they contain "lower" or "lowered" sodium. The FDA doesn't display lower or lowered in their nutrient guide. But we have learned that lower and lowered mean only that the sodium from salt levels are a bit lower than the standard product.

Remember to always check the FDA label for what the serving size is and then do the math. There are some lower-sodium chicken noodle soups available that list more sodium per serving than I consume in a day.

Have you ever bought a bottle of pop at the gas station mini-mart and read the label? It might say 40 to 80 mg of sodium per serving, but the bottle may contain as many as 3 servings. In other words, that "low sodium" soda really has 120 to 240 mg of sodium. If you're really serious about adapting to a very low sodium lifestyle for heart or other health reasons, then you may have just consumed a big hunk of your day's allowed sodium intake. By the way, most fruit juice bottles you might purchase with a lunch in a sandwich shop or other location will have twice the sodium level in the bottle than you see on the label.

The bottle will probably contain two servings instead of just one and be overloaded with high fructose corn syrup[4] as well.

Lowered or lower simply means the food processor just cut out a little of the salt. No-salt-added (NSA) means that the sodium you see listed on the FDA label is naturally found in the food in the package or can. If the package or can has "concentrated" food then the sodium levels will read higher. For instance, tomato paste is a concentrated product. So, even though a single tomato might have only 11 mg of sodium for the whole tomato, the paste might have upwards of 30 mg per tablespoon, the natural result of reducing many fresh tomatoes that have been converted to paste. Those that have added ingredients such as Garlic Tomato Paste will usually be higher in sodium. It's better to buy plain paste and make your own flavored version.

Will My Grocery Store Have All The Products I Need?

Unfortunately, we haven't yet found a grocery store that carries more than just a few no-salt-added products. In some parts of the U.S., Canada and Great Britain, NSA products are not available at all[5]. They may have some, but no-salt and low-sodium products are hard to find in most local stores and in small or medium size towns. During our nationwide tour I mention later, we found middle America to be a wide open country with very little support for no-salt lifestyles. That's one reason locating low-sodium food support on the Net is important. We like healthyheartmarket.com but you can also find a list of suppliers at megaheart.com/wheretobuy.html.

Healthyheartmarket.com has a terrific "starter kit" that will supply you with basic ingredients and help you get started making soups, breads and generally getting to know the no-salt, low-sodium world.

See the chapter in this book for the "Top Twenty No-Salt-Added Products You Can't Live Without."

(Footnotes)

[1] All FDA information based on FDA provided materials with their permission. The FDA history for labels can be found at the FDA Web site. It reads: 1990: Nutrition Labeling and Education Act requires all packaged foods to bear nutrition labeling and all health claims for foods to be consistent with terms defined by the Secretary of Health and Human Services. The law preempts state requirements about food standards, nutrition labeling, and health claims and, for the first time, authorizes some health claims for foods. The food ingredient panel, serving sizes, and terms such as "low fat" and "light" are standardized.

[2] Accent is 100% MSG

[3] Note about nonfat diets: Recent research has shown that the BMI is too imprecise and that being overweight just a little is healthier than being "too thin." Research data

is from the American Medical Association and the Centers for Disease Control and Prevention.

[4] High fructose corn syrup has become the devil of the food industry for the past few years. Slowly processors are replacing high fructose corn syrup with sucrose (sugar or honey).

5 You can find no salt added and unsalted products from various suppliers at megaheart.com/wheretobuy.html

High Blood Pressure
&
Where's The Salt?

In 1904, two French doctors discovered that some of their patients with high blood pressure showed enough recovery after removing salt from their diet that they pursued what became historic research. Using salt, they first reintroduced increased sodium levels to the same patients. Just as they had suspected, their blood pressure rose again. When they took away all salt the blood pressure of each patient dropped appreciably.

Since then, the realization that dietary sodium levels can affect our blood pressure has become strong within the medical community. High blood pressure contributes to a myriad of health problems as well as a loss of calcium, which some scientists suspect leads to osteoporosis.

Dietary sodium levels do matter.

Defining Salt & Sodium

We write of sodium here, although much of the world speaks of salt when they actually are referring to sodium. Salt is not the real culprit. Sodium is. Salt just has a lot of sodium in it. And therein lies the secret to success in lowering our dietary sodium. Stop the salt. In fact, cutting any amount of salt from our diet will lower our sodium intake.

Get rid of the saltshaker and stop eating processed foods that list salt in their ingredients. Admittedly this is a tall order, but one that has been successfully proven beneficial. It is now accepted knowledge that over 80% of the salt we ingest comes either from processed foods or restaurants. The rest it is assumed, comes from the saltshaker in our kitchen.[1]

But Everything Has Salt In It, Right?

No. Most everything has some level of sodium, but only processed foods have added salt.

Don't We Need Salt?

We humans need some sodium but not a drop of salt. Five hundred milligrams of sodium a day is more than enough for our bodies. Some researchers believe we can live with 180 mg a day[2]. I don't believe 180 mg a day is doable with a balanced die, which means getting all the nutrients we need in a day.

We need some sodium. Sodium is important for transmitting electrical impulses through our nerves. It also helps with muscle contraction and it monitors fluid distribution in our bodies. The sodium for these important tasks is known as "essential sodium." Five-hundred milligrams a day has stopped my dizziness and helped many Meniere's patients reduce or stop their dizziness. It has subdued my tinnitus that I have experienced for a long period.

Whole societies that do not eat salt whatsoever still exist in this world, and they are much healthier than those of us who have been stuck with a "salt diet." According to Dr. Trevor C. Beard[2], a salt researcher and Senior Research Fellow at the Menzies Research Institute at the University of Tasmania, an Australian medical expedition measured the stamina of the Tukisenta people (Papua, New Guinea). The Tukisenta used absolutely no-salt or salt derivatives in any of their diet. They were tested with the Harvard Pack Fitness Test. The Tukisenta produced higher scores than the fit young men in an Australian air force unit stationed at the same district[3]. Dr. Beard's lifelong research into salt and sodium has backed this study many times with other research as well.

We need some sodium. Sodium is important for transmitting electrical impulses through our nerves. It also helps with muscle contraction and it monitors fluid distribution in our bodies. The sodium for these important tasks is known as "essential sodium."

Whole societies that do not eat salt whatsoever still exist in this world, and they are much healthier than those of us who have been stuck with a "salt diet." According to Dr. Trevor C. Beard[2], a salt researcher and Senior Research Fellow at the Menzies Research Institute at the University of Tasmania, an Australian medical research expedition measured the stamina of the Tukisenta people (Papua, New Guinea). The Tukisenta used absolutely no-salt or salt derivatives in any of their diet. They were tested with the Harvard Pack Fitness Test. The Tukisenta produced higher scores than the fit young men in an Australian air force unit stationed at the same district[3]. Dr. Beard's lifelong research into salt and sodium has backed this study many times with other research as well.

So, What's Happening Here?

Humans have adapted to the foreign taste of salt to such a degree that all foods "must have salt in them" in order to meet that one and only flavor salt eaters recognize. Take salt away and in a few weeks you'll begin to discover the true flavors of foods especially vegetables, and you'll actually begin to enjoy them a lot more. Stick to the no-salt program for about 3-months and after that period you'll learn just how bitter and harsh salt is. You'll wonder how you ever ate it. I have been off salt for more than a decade. If I bite into anything with salt, I know it instantly and just that one bite will leave a bitter aftertaste in my mouth for hours. And by the way, so do "salt substitutes," and baking soda.

It takes about three months for our palate to repair itself from the damage salt has done to it. That's why I offer the three month taste challenge. Once the palate is cured, it will rebel at the taste of salt.

So, Why Do We Eat It?

Salt was first discovered to preserve food between five and six thousand years ago. It later became a large trade item, was taxed more than anything else on the planet at that time, and it became a customary although biting flavor for humans that masked poor quality food. It also began to shorten human lives rather than extend them.

Is It Safe To Stop Eating All Salt?

My 500 mg a day plan reflected an arbitrary guess at the time. Today, I recognize it as a level of daily sodium intake easier to meet than the actual daily required amount. Remember, we need only about 8-10 mmol/day of sodium for physiologic health[2]. Without even trying, you'll get enough sodium in your diet through a variety of unsalted foods.

What about iodine? Is salt the only way to get it?

Sources of iodine include seaweed or products made with seaweed, cow's milk, yogurt, meat, fruit, vegetables (unless produced in iodine deficient areas), strawberries, and some multivitamins.

Many salt producers have not added iodine to their salt for years. Another point to make here is that the salt added to processed foods does not now nor did it ever have iodine added to it. Of course, some salt products do contain iodine, but at least in the western world the inclusion of iodine with salt is more a hangover from the past than a necessity. We can get too much iodine so let's not go overboard. The RDA for iodine is 150 micrograms (mcg) a day except for pregnant women who should get 175 mcg per day.

So, How Can I Tell Where The Salt Is?

When you start reading the ingredients of the packaged, frozen, bagged, canned, shrink-wrapped foods you buy, you'll find that salt has been added to nearly everything including many items you might not suspect. From juices to cheese, breakfast cereal, vegetables, soups, and salad dressings, candy, pizza, pies, junk food, snacks, ice cream; wherever we turn, salt is the single most used ingredient along with MSG. (See: MSG, in the glossary for a more complete description of MSG and ingredient words or phrases often used to disguise it.)

What about hot weather?

According to Dr. Trevor C. Beard and other researchers, "The amount of salt lost in sweat is variable. Aboriginal Australians in their tribal state used no added salt in their diet, yet were well adapted to strenuous exercise in very hot climates. Paradoxically, it is better for athletes and travelers to the tropics to skip salt, so that they lose less sodium through sweating."[5] Ironically, a salty sweat is one of the results of eating salty food (a vicious cycle). Beard makes one other point that's interesting. The salty taste that drips onto the tongue of sweating athletes disappears when they stop adding salt to their diet. They sweat the same amount, but it's goodbye to the biting salt. "Sports drinks" by the way, are contraindicated for hard workouts. These high sodium drinks actually help to drain energy from the user. Water would work better[2].

What about those salt tablets we took in the Navy?

Dr. Beard helps us with this question as well. You won't find those tablets on ships or elsewhere in the U.S. Military today. Actually, I'm surprised they ever handed them out. In the past, when doctors felt a patient should be made to vomit, they used salt as an emetic. That didn't always work. Sometimes the patients got too much salt and died. Salt pills were loaded with too much sodium, a major reason many of us who took them while aboard navy ships became ill . It was thought that the salt was needed to "replace" the fluids lost through sweat. They couldn't have been any more wrong.

How can I tell if I'm eating too much sodium?

The first thing you should do is keep track of your sodium intake for a week. Then try to reduce this number to recommended levels. This will help give you a clearer picture of where you are starting and what you need to do.

As to the level you should be at: In 2006, the American Medical Association announced that the daily intake of sodium for healthy people should range between 1300 milligrams to 1800 milligrams a day depending on activity. This author feels that's too high for those of us with ailments. We need to help ourselves with a low-sodium lifestyle, and to do so we need to get lower than the recommended levels recommended for "healthy" people.

I am familiar with the difficulty of preparing meals, snacks, and desserts within the lower recommended range. That's why in 1997 our eldest daughter Jeannie, who is an R.D., PhD., developed and parsed a plan that has proved successful. It is the guide in the back of *The No-Salt, Lowest-Sodium Cookbook.* The plan is a good guide designed to help you make up your own plan. In this way, you can be prepared for the low sodium ingredients and foods you'll need. The plan has been used by thousands of people successfully and is recommended by many hospitals, registered dietitians, nurses and doctors. Diabetics can also plan their low sodium and low carbohydrate intake this way. Others who must cut their potassium levels can also use this plan while inputting their specific needs. You don't have to use the recipes in the plan since our books are all designed with recipes you can fit into the plan and still end up with the same levels of sodium, carbohydrates, etc.

The low sodium intake was most recently validated in April of 2007 with the release by a research team at Boston's Brigham and Women's Hospital. According to Doctor Nancy R. Cook, ScD., "Results of our follow-up study reinforce recommendations to lower dietary sodium intake as a means of preventing cardiovascular disease in the general population and should dispel any residual concern that sodium reduction might be harmful."

Hypertension is not the only ailment exacerbated by high levels of sodium chloride. High levels of sodium cause high levels of fluid retention in a great number of humans. This retention can cause swollen ankles in any weather, but especially in hot weather, and it can cause edema if you sit for a long time such as while traveling. And here's a surprise for you: a low-sodium intake will often relieve carpal tunnel syndrome[2]. Another benefit is that PMS or premenstrual syndrome can be relieved with a lowered sodium lifestyle.

Probably the most dangerous of all foods are those completely preserved with salt. These may include some seafood as well as luncheon meats, bacon, most ham products, and jerky topping the list. Ingredient lists may include a multiple array of sodium items like sodium nitrate, sodium nitrite, sodium benzoate, other preservatives that begin with the word sodium, and of course don't forget salt.

Another challenge for us is that too many chicken and pork processors are now brining many of their products. This bounces the natural sodium levels from around 80 milligrams of sodium per 4-ounces to nearly 500 mg per 4-ounces. Make sure you are not buying brined meat. If the FDA label states that the sodium level is over 100 mg per 4-ounce serving then chances are the product has been brined or mislabeled.

What about my Meniere's Syndrome and salt?

Meniere's is directly affected by a high sodium intake. Too much "salt" is often blamed for the dizziness and vertigo with Meniere's patients but it's really the high level of sodium that concerns us. Thousands of visitors to Megaheart.com are patients with Meniere's Syndrome, and letters to the site from these patients praise our help with each writer's success at stopping vertigo problems after cutting salt out and lowering their sodium intake.

So how do we count sodium levels?

In the U.S. the federal government has "established" recommended dietary allowances for us to follow. The USDA laboratories provide nutrient data and the FDA controls the labeling of foods inspects processor plants or foods that enter the country. The FDA uses the USDA data. Manufacturers (food processors and marketers) publish the labels on their products. Nearly always we use more than the size the processor has chosen for the label. (See: FDA Food Labels chapter.)[7,12]

Confusion sometimes arises from recipes published in the print media and elsewhere including with food products. Even our *No-Salt, Lowest-Sodium Cookbooks* might have nutrient data variations from one book to another, simply because the USDA is constantly changing their database. One that seems to change often and upwards is the egg. When I first started working with these numbers a large egg had 63 mg. At this writing it's 70 mg. Olive oil was listed with zero milligrams by the USDA just a couple years ago, today one list shows it has .27 mg sodium per tablespoon while another list from the same USDA source shows zero. As you can see, the adjustments to recipes aren't huge, but they do occur and sometimes with confusion.

The reason given by the USDA for their many changes is that the food they test actually changes. Their figures are based on an average of what they test. The soil where food and animal feed grows has a lot to do with the changes. The USDA will take an average off these readings and post the results as the official data. Sodium in animal feed can change the sodium level in the meats we eat. These changes aren't usually large enough to notice in a single serving size, but sometimes they may be noticeable in a per item calculation. When the *No-salt, Lowest Sodium International Cookbook* was written, the current USDA Release was #16. Two years later (at this writing) we are using Release #21. Milk with added vitamin A for instance, was changed in 2005 from 126 mg of sodium per cup, to 102.9 mg for all types of cow's milk. Two years later all that was changed to 107.4 mg per cup for 1% low fat or 100 mg for reduced fat, but kept the 102.9 mg per cup for nonfat milk that contains added Vitamin A. In just a few years, they have changed from one reading (126 mg) for all milks, to specific ratings for each type of milk. No reason is offered for this and most dairies have not changed their sodium levels on their printed cartons.

How could they possibly keep up?

At Megaheart.com, and in our No-Salt, Lowest-Sodium Cookbooks we stick with official USDA figures that are current while we create our recipes.

Here's what a cereal breakfast would look like if you took the numbers off the cartons or packages. For a fruit on the cereal we have used a medium size banana.

For this demonstration, sodium levels for each ingredient are in parenthesis alongside the food.

Breakfast Using Food Manufacturer's Published Nutrient Data

1 cup Nabisco Spoon Size Shredded Wheat (0 mg)
1/2 cup nonfat milk with Vitamin A added (65 mg)
1 medium banana (0 mg)
1 8-ounce glass orange juice not from concentrate (0 mg)

With the above figures the total sodium based on manufacturer/ processor numbers would be: 65 mg.

Breakfast Using actual USDA Nutrient Data

1 cup Nabisco Spoon Size Shredded Wheat (3.43 mg)
1/2 cup nonfat milk with Vitamin A added (51.5 mg)
1 medium banana (1.18 mg)
1 8-ounce fresh orange juice (2.48 mg)

With the above figures the total is 58.5 mg.

This points out three items were listed by processors as zero but in fact they do have sodium. The difference between these two doesn't seem like much, but appreciable differences do occur when we get into highly processed salt added foods for breakfast, lunch, or dinner and sometimes with snacks. Here are two samples of the ever popular (basic) hamburger, one with the food producer's USDA data, followed by the same lunch with USDA figures for our homemade version.

By the way, we don't recommend a 1/4-pound burger. We use 2-ounces, flattened and charbroiled or barbecued. It's plenty of meat and has the right amount of protein and fewer calories. We use the 1/4-pound of meat in this demonstration because we couldn't find a USDA figure for a commercial 2-ounce hamburger.

Commercial Cheeseburger with Bun, lettuce, ketchup/sauce and onion.
1 Wendy's cheeseburger, ¼ pound beef (1240 mg)

No-salt Cheeseburger with Homemade Bun
1 homemade Ciabatta bun (1.982 mg)
¼ pound 95% lean ground beef (73.9 mg)
1 slice low-sodium cheddar cheese[2] (5.954 mg)
1 tablespoon no-salt-added ketchup (3 mg)
1 slice medium onion (.56 mg)
1 leaf of iceberg lettuce (1.5 mg)

Total sodium for a basic home prepared quarter pounder cheeseburger (86.9 mg)

[2] Cheese is one-ounce. A low-sodium cheese package may show 5 mg or 10 mg sodium. Data here is official USDA rating.

Make that a two-ounce burger and you have a burger with about 36.9 mg sodium. Make it a lettuce wrap and you cut calories and sodium down even more.

We see a difference of more than 1,100 mg between these two cheeseburgers. The commercial burger has a lot of sodium (salt) in the bun and additional salt is nearly always mixed into commercial burger meat before the restaurant or fast food eatery receives it. The salt is added ostensibly to add "shelf life." After that, many cooks sprinkle enough salt on a patty to practically reach our daily limit just with that one shake. For those of you who are In-N-Out fans, just watch the meat chef, which you can do. His generous saltshaker is nearly upside down when he/she first starts to cook the meat. Yes, they'll make one without salt for you and wipe the grill clean, but you have to ask for it. Take your own bun, sliced, order a lettuce wrap and place it into your bun. If that's too inconvenient then use their bun and allow about 250 mg sodium or better yet.

What about salt substitutes?

We don't recommend salt substitutes. One reason is that most are either pure potassium chloride or some are half potassium chloride and sometimes half salt. Too much potassium in our systems can be just as harmful as not enough. Some substitute producers attempt to offset the bitter taste of potassium with L-lysine or Lycopene. Some use natural spices, but often with a lot of additional pepper, the combination of which subdues natural flavors extensively.

Salt substitutes do not behave like salt in cooking or baking and they become just another taste crutch, often one that overpowers the great natural flavors of food just like salt does. Some salt substitutes use onion powder, which we believe is good to use, but why pay an exotic price for something that's really inexpensive in a spice jar?

You can make your own flavor enhancer with spices and herbs you probably have on hand now. Spices and herbs are nutritious additions for most dishes but especially for soups and stews.

Where Can I Buy No Salt Added Foods?

There are a few good selections of NSA products in some parts of the USA, but unfortunately not enough nationwide nor worldwide to make shopping for no-salt, lowest-sodium meals easy. Fortunately, most of the no-salt-added foods that do exist are available online. Visit: megaheart.com/wheretobuy.html. This page lists a wide variety of foods and providers. Megaheart does not sell products but will guide you to the sellers.

Since 1997 we have seen the discontinuance of quite a few good no-salt, low-sodium products including no-salt bread.[8] At this writing we just learned that Grandma's Chili Powder is no longer available as Grandma's but is available as Williams Chili Seasoning. (Visit: megaheart.com/wheretobuy.html and click on Healthy Heart Market)

Heluva Good made a good unsalted cheese but in 2010 they added salt to it, raising the sodium level per ounce from 5 mg to 25 mg.

Other former unsalted cheese producers include Tillamook, Alpine Lace[9], Safeway Stores, and Rumiano. Check our no salt food section in this book for other unsalted cheese makers.

Product	Standard	No Salt Added
Tomatoes are canned		
Tomato Sauce 1-cup	1284 mg	16.8 mg
Whole Tomatoes, 1-cup	307.2 mg	24 mg
Tomato Paste, 6-0z can	1343 mg	166.6 mg
Cheddar Cheese, 1-oz	176.1 mg	10 mg
Swiss Cheese 1-oz	54.4 mg	5 to 10 mg
Jack Cheese 1-oz	159.7 mg	30 mg
Pinto Beans 1-cup	705.6 mg	30 mg
Cornflakes, 1-cup	254.7 mg	2.5 mg
Frozen peas 1/2-cup	80 mg	1.6 mg

Doesn't Cutting Table Salt Out At Home Do The Trick?

Our long experience at Megaheart.com has demonstrated to us that many home-cooks believe they have cut sodium way down because they don't add salt to recipes when preparing meals. Others who eat out tell us that they don't add salt to their food in restaurants. All of this is good, but it's not enough.

Take a look at the list of foods in the chart above and the difference in sodium levels in processed products (using USDA nutrient data) and the same products with no-salt added.

The reason there is a difference in the sodium in the listed products is that the food processors have added a great deal of salt to what is currently considered "standard." They also add salt and MSG to food containers (canned, bottled, packaged, frozen) even though containers often boast that the product inside is "all natural."

In the group shown above, standard Swiss cheese is the only reasonable product with added salt. The difference is between 54.4 mg of sodium compared to about 5 to 10 mg for low sodium cheese. If you don't have scales in your kitchen, remember that 1-cubic inch of cheese will often equal one-ounce.

A note about low sodium cheese: It's not easy to find. However, some local brands are occasionally available. If you can't find a low sodium cheese, try making our easy recipe for "Yo Cheese." It makes a good sandwich spread that can be flavored. It can be used with Italian dishes, or as a mayonnaise (after adding some dill weed and a dash of Splenda or sugar), and it can be enhanced with dehydrated onion/garden mix or with spice mixes or from a few no-salt added spice-mix companies like Nutrifit, Nantucket Offshore, Frontier, or Mrs. Dash. These suppliers make spice mixes without adding salt. If you do find a brand of low sodium (no-salt) cheese, please E-mail us at our Web site contact page, and we'll post the brand and source on our *Where To Buy* page.

The no-salt-added (NSA) tomatoes and the Eden Organic NSA beans are available nationally in most grocery and health food stores, from edenfoods.com, or at healthyheartmarket.com. Other products are available regionally. Make sure that you read the ingredients label before buying - some may not be as low in sodium as you'd like.

You are invited to submit any supplier of no-salt added or unsalted products to megaheart for listing there. We'll check them out and if they fit into our format, we'll happily add them along with the merchant who sells via the Net or mail or in local grocery stores. Just click on the contact button at megaheart.com, provide the information and we'll do the rest. Your effort can prove to be a great help for others. (We don't post fad diets, fad foods, etc.) We list only foods that do not contain any salt or high-sodium solutions such as soy sauce.

What about meat? Does it have a lot of sodium?

Normally, not a lot, but once again, it's the processed meats that are too high in sodium. Non-processed turkey is higher than chicken and beef by a few milligrams; various pork cuts are similar at around 18 mg per ounce but processed ham is too high to eat. Fish is generally low unless it's shellfish, making king and Dungeness crab the meat with the highest sodium level of any of them.

However, as stated before and as of this writing, many meat processors are now brining their fowl and pork mechanically. Meat moves along a belt through a large machine that punctures the meat with "needles" that inject salty fluids, and then the meat is hermetically sealed or wrapped for shipping to the store or restaurant suppliers. This is a dangerous practice for the general health of the public, and even more dangerous for us. Some claim they are doing it to "add flavor," but they mostly tell us they do it to "preserve" the meat for a longer period of time. You will find hermetically sealed meats more and more at your meat counter since they last upwards of two weeks longer for selling than fresh cuts. Watch out for those Thanksgiving turkeys. Fresh is best.

Most canned meats are out of the question for a no-salt lifestyle and so are seasoned meats. Some canned tuna (albacore) is acceptable[10]. There are several brands available and each is quite good. (Check FDA labels and ingredients.)

Meat and fish handling become very important to us as well. Today's grocery chain butchers aren't the butchers of yesterday. Today, most chain-grocery-store meat is processed in a central warehouse. It's then shipped to the local grocer either already packaged or cut. With large grocery chains some have "traveling butchers" who visit the various stores to cut meat into that store's needs. That meat is then wrapped in a shrink wrap package with a Styrofoam container or placed into the "fresh" meat display case. If they don't attach an FDA label[11], ask for a list of nutrients. They should have them available for you.

(Footnotes)

[1] If you're taking supplements, you might want to check with your supplier for the sodium level. For instance, we have found one brand of Glucosamine/Chondroitin that contained 2,000 mg of sodium per capsule. All gel capsules contain some MSG as well.

[2] Beard, Trevor C, Salt in Medical Practice, 2000; Salt Matters, 2004;1;2; Fowler, Michael, Living Without Salt, 2010, page 2

[3] Simnett PF, Whyte HM. Epidemiological studies in a total highland population, Takkisenta, New Guinea. Journal of Chronic Disease 1973;26;265-90.

5 Beard, Trevor C., Salt Matters, 2004;1;5

6 In-N-Out is a west coast chain.

7 Pages 35, 36

8 Alvarado bakery in California still produces a No-Salt bread under their label and under the Trader Joe's label. Safeway still sells their Mrs. Wright's Very Low Sodium bread as well.

9 We like Merino's Unsalted Pole Caught Albacore Tuna (canned) for its freshness and excellent flavor. Whole Foods has a few no-salt added brands as well.

10 Information about nutrition labels provided by FDA.

11 Processed foods from other countries can often mislabel their FDA numbers. I have a can of Italian tomatoes here that states a 1/2 cup serving has zero sodium. In fact, it probably has from 35 to 50 mg of sodium since the tomatoes themselves contain enough sodium to reach that level.

12 Google "salt we ingest percentage from" for a long list of substantiation.

SALT MYTHS

Salt is comprised mostly of chloride and sodium ions. There are 6-grams weight of salt per teaspoon and sodium comprises 40% of that or 2,350 mg per teaspoon. Sodium is usually listed in the FDA nutritional information on food labels. Salt is usually listed in the ingredient lists of most manufactured or processed foods. The sodium on the FDA label can come from both the food itself and added salt. You will not find salt listed in the FDA panel when products are "No Salt Added," but you will usually find sodium levels in the FDA nutrient panel.

For instance, a 6-ounce can of unsalted tomato paste will list ingredients as: Tomatoes. However, the FDA label will show 20 mg sodium per serving size, which will be listed as 2-tablespoons. The can will have 5 servings, which should mean that the whole can has 100 mg of sodium even though no salt was added. But wait, the confusing part hasn't been explained yet. The USDA's posted figures for a 6-ounce can of no salt added tomato paste equals 166 mg of sodium per can. How could this be? Well, for one thing the USDA does the lab work, the FDA only regulates the labels and the manufacturer is responsible for its labels with the margin of error mentioned in the previous chapter.

We stick with the USDA numbers when using ingredients since it's our health at risk, and not the food processor's. It is rare in most grocery stores to find fresh fruits, vegetables, and meats/fish with FDA figures. You can always check the USDA numbers for any food you want to use by visiting Megaheart.com and clicking on the USDA Nutrient Database at the bottom.

What we have found that isn't too rare, are myths concerning salt. These myths are sometimes like hoax E-mails.

Myth: Salt your meat before cooking it.

Wrong. An old myth that was truly dreamed up by someone who wasn't a good cook or who hadn't "tested" their mythology. Salting meat before it is cooked changes the flavor, but doesn't necessarily improve it. Here's what happens: salt pulls the meat's moisture out. If you salt meat before cooking, say for a few days, it will dehydrate the surface and change its texture before and during cooking. Consequently, it has never been a good practice to salt meat before cooking. In line with that, marinades using spices and herbs and no salt actually work better for flavoring than marinades with salt.

Myth: Cutting Out The Salt Shaker Alone Will Do It, Right?

No. About eighty to ninety-percent of the sodium many us of consume before we changed our lifestyle was in the food we ate, whether from the grocery store or in a restaurant. The balance was probably from our saltshaker, either at the table or while preparing meals.

Originally salt was added as a preservative, but newer packaging technology allows them to make the same products without a drop of salt, which they have. (See the list we gathered for you in chapter 16). The myth here is that they "need to add salt." They don't, in fact they add it only to satisfy the biting taste they have trained our palates to accept.

Myth: Adding salt to boiling water speeds the process.

The truth is that salt will increase the boiling temperature, which in turn decreases boiling time, usually by about one millionth of a second. In other words, it's a myth. What it might do is make your food taste salty, but cooking time will remain the same.

Myth: All Food Has Salt In It.

This incorrect assumption is heard often. All foods do not have salt in them. But most all foods contain some sodium.

Myth: Food needs salt for flavoring.

Our palates have been "damaged" by salt. It takes about three months for them to recover. During that time you might think you need something to give your meals a kick. If so, start using spices and herbs you might not have used before. Start with spices like unsalted garlic powder or the garlic itself. Onion powder, a good salt replacement, plus cardamom, mace, thyme, marjoram, cloves, cinnamon, curry, cumin, cayenne pepper, sage, etc.

Our palates will heal after we cut out the salt. You'll find that you enjoy the natural flavors of foods and the flavors spices offer. And remember this, many spices go beyond just the flavor element. Many are antioxidants and offer other health benefits as well.

Myth: Kosher salt is blessed by a Rabbi and comes from the Dead Sea.

It is also claimed by some that kosher salt contains no additives. None of the above are true. Kosher salt is any coarse-grain mineral salt, taken from any salt source (mine or surface), and it's a salt that is used to make meat kosher. Most kosher salt, like all other salt packages uses an anti-caking additive.

Myth: Only over-salted foods taste salty.

This myth is really referring to sodium and not just salt. We can't taste sodium but we can taste the chloride. If you find a processed food that is listed high in salt but doesn't taste salty, the odds are it's overweight with sugar, such as breakfast cereals and some cookies or crackers, which generally have both the salt and sugar at high levels.

There's another, more inconvenient answer to this myth as well. Taste buds, often damaged by too much salt, might actually seek the flavor of salt. After you stop eating salt for a while, you'll soon discover that you can taste salt in any salted product, and it may surprise you to learn you don't like the bite. Often the salt used in restaurant prepared foods will taste overwhelmed with salt.

Myth: Only the elderly and sick should worry about their level of sodium intake per day.

This myth has been around a long time. It's way off target. It became obvious to us at Megaheart.com that a lot of young people were also affected by too much sodium. Young people as well as elderly need to cut down their sodium levels. At times the draw down will seem radical to younger people. Additionally, elderly people have been trained to believe that many of their "ills" are part of the natural aging process and that it's all inevitable. If that's so, I know a few in their mid-nineties who are still out exercising every day and are sharp as a tack. Two of them go to work every day of the week. I also know they eat right, don't smoke or drink and live with their spirits high.

Remember what Hippocrates said: "Let food be thy medicine." Eat right, exercise and right now, cut the salt out of your diet. Bottom line is that if you have high blood pressure when you're young, you're at greater risk than others of the same age to develop one or more chronic illnesses or more severely, a stroke.

Myth: Artisanal Salts are better for you than table salt. (In some countries these are known as "posh" salts.)

This rather new myth created by marketing companies to pedal "natural artisanal salts," often "designed" in a rainbow of different packaging, is as false as any myth could be. They might taste a bit differently, but salt is salt and sodium lies waiting in each crystal at the same level.

Myth: We need more salt in hot climates because we sweat so much.

It is well known that heavy sweating can increase the need for water. But those who increase their salt intake in hot weather are merely increasing their salt/sodium loss when they sweat and lowering their physical endurance. Fluid volume does not change.

Myth: If we cut down on salt our bodies won't get enough sodium.

It's actually difficult if not impossible to eat too little sodium. We have to work at it even without using or ingesting salt. Cutting salt out altogether, including from processed foods, will not reduce the sodium levels below what our body needs if you eat a nutritionally balanced diet of fresh foods.

Myth: I will feel it when I have high blood pressure.

Most of us don't have symptoms for high blood pressure. About thirty percent of the population may have hypertension and not know it. It's important to find out, however, since the results can be congestive heart failure, stroke, heart attack, kidney failure or blindness. Either have yours tested or if you need to take your blood pressure (bp) on a daily basis, buy a blood pressure device that will automatically give you an accurate read.

Myth: Sea salt is better for us than table salt.

Sea salt and table salt have exactly the same level of sodium. The only possible differences between table and sea salt might be in their texture. Some sea salt processors add lycopene or other "nutrients" to their salt to cut the sodium level in half or at least down per equal measurement. Actually, sea salt may be considered more dangerous than regular table salt since it is sold as "healthy," "safe," etc. Although the USDA lists all salt with sodium levels at 2,350 mg per teaspoon, research with islanders in the South Pacific found that sea salt users had higher blood pressure than table salt users in the same society.[1]

Myth: Our bodies rid themselves of extra sodium.

Not true at all. However, when we eat natural foods and add no salt to our diets - either with a shaker or via processed foods - our bodies do manage sodium well. Our body's system just can't handle all the excess sodium in what has become standard fare. The primary effect of all this overabundance of sodium usually ends with one or more complications including Meniere's, kidney and liver ailments, higher blood pressure, heart attack or heart failure, a stroke, and unfortunately an early death.

Myth: Whole societies and cultures that consume high levels of sodium from salt live longer than the rest of us. The argument therefore is that salt is good for us.

Not true. Cultures that consume high levels of sodium actually live much shorter lives. Studies point to one of the most obvious areas of our world. Northern China, where salt ingestion is very high. The death rate from high blood pressure alone is off the charts.[1]

Myth: There's no real evidence that salt is a major contributor to high blood pressure.

This myth shouldn't even be around anymore, but it is. There have been endless controlled studies to prove that salt (high sodium) does, in fact, cause high blood pressure. Bottom line is that research has proved that even a "modest" reduction in sodium intake for just a few months will significantly reduce blood pressure. However, that reduction in sodium must be maintained since increasing the sodium levels again, also increases blood pressure.

Myth: Don't we still have to drink 8-glasses of water a day?

No. We never did. That has been a long standing myth that truly needs to be corrected or stopped. We get most of the fluids we need from the foods we eat and the liquids we consume. The fruit and vegetables you eat during the day also contain appreciable levels of fluids as well as the lettuce in that sandwich and the bread itself. Sure, have a glass or two of water, but best to do it when your thirst calls for it.

(Footnotes)

1 Dr. Trevor Beard, Salt Skip Program, Australia.

2 Salt Matters, Page 42, 108, Dr. Trevor Beard, Senior Research Fellow, Menzies Research Institute, University of Tasmania.

Diabetes, Meniere's Syndrome & Other Chronic Illnesses

Requiring a No-Salt, Lowest Sodium Lifestyle

At Megaheart.com we have learned that the salt-free lifestyle is needed by millions of patients with chronic illnesses such as heart failure, diabetes, hypertension, cardiovascular disease, Meniere's Syndrome, Nephrotic Syndrome, stomach cancer, Lupus, and other diseases.

Statistics show that three out of five diabetic patients will develop congestive heart failure. Let's face it, that's a double whammy. Diabetics have to watch more than just sodium intake, they have to account for carbohydrate, fiber, fat and protein to manage their blood glucose. Diabetics also work with food exchanges or carb choices, but at any rate must keep track of the grams of carbohydrates they consume each day and continue to ingest all the other needed nutrients. The USDA has constructed a food pyramid for healthy eaters, but there is also a special food pyramid to guide diabetics. This pyramid takes into account the daily carbohydrate allowance and other needed nutrients. What we want to discuss here are the basics of diabetes when applying a no salt, lowest sodium equation into the mix. For instance, one slice of homemade unsalted bread might work for most of us without taking into consideration the levels of carbohydrates, potassium, or other nutrients, but for a diabetic it will affect their daily carb choices as well as their level of sodium intake. Let's say we want to exchange that bread with something else since we need to adjust our day for other nutrients as well. So what can we choose to replace that low sodium item that doesn't have high sodium? Therein lies just one of the challenges.

About Diabetes

There are two types of diabetes: Type 1 and Type 2. Type 1 occurs initially mostly in children and is an autoimmune disease. About 20% of diabetics have Type 1. Type 2 usually develops in adults over the age of 40. Unfortunately, too many young people are now developing Type 2. Type 2 is when our cells reject or resist insulin action and our glucose doesn't get into the cells very well. Glucose is what provides our body its energy.

As to the cause it all depends on whether or not you fall into one of a few groups. Today, childhood obesity combined with a sedentary lifestyle is believed to be causing Type 2 diabetes in a frightening number of young people. For adults, however, the top cause is "genetics." If you've had or have a family member with diabetes, especially Type 2 diabetes, then you are predisposed to possibly being diagnosed sometime in your life with diabetes. Other reasons include women who might have had a baby weighing in at more than nine-pounds, or had gestational diabetes. Another cause can be if you've led a sedentary or very inactive life. Additionally, there are cultural reasons. It seems that diabetes is common among African Americans, Hispanic Americans, Native Americans, Southeast Asian or Pacific Islanders.

If you know you're family is susceptible to diabetes, you will want to lose weight or maintain a low weight (this helps your insulin work better) and to maintain a healthy, well-balanced diet.

Q. If sugar isn't what a diabetic has to watch, what is?

A. For years sugar was blamed for causing diabetes and it was blamed for making a diabetic's life a real challenge. We know today, however, that none of that was true. Sugar was not the cause nor the culprit in daily maintenance. Instead, carbohydrates are.

This doesn't mean you can run out to the candy store and have a party. We don't want to get into the chemistry of all this so we're going to stick with counting dietary points and what we can and can't eat.

You might be surprised at what diabetics can eat. Most of the recipes in this book fit into a diabetic lifestyle, although a few might present a challenge to adapt. If so, they are marked as such.

Not unlike a no-salt lifestyle or a medication procedure, diabetics don't want to skip a meal or even a snack if that helps them get through the day. Also, maintaining a healthy daily intake of nutrients is important and so are choices with such things as fat or nonfat, low or high calorie, etc. In other words, diabetics pretty much can eat the way we all eat, except that some foods need to be adjusted or portions resized to help keep carbs within a daily point schedule.

Diabetics, however, will want to eat lean meats and smaller portions to obtain the needed protein and other nutrients in meat. Diabetic Vegans understand how to do this without meat.

A registered dietitian specializing in diabetes diets can be a big help if you aren't quite able to put all this together. If you don't know where to look for one, visit www.eatright.org. That's the American Dietitian Web site. They have a section where you can locate a local dietitian (R.D.). We also recommend a terrific magazine called Diabetic Living, from the same company that produces *Better Homes & Garden*.

In this book we list Carb Choices for diabetics. CHO exchanges are calculated by dividing a servings total carbohydrates by 15. We list total carbohydrates in the nutrient date of each recipe in each of our books. If you are using "carb choices" or are exchanging then the carbohydrate data in this book are the latest USDA figures as of this writing. Next to each banner you'll also find that we've done the math for you by listing the carb choices calculation:

0-5 grams = 0 Carb Choices
6-10 grams = ½ Carb Choices
11 –20 grams = 1 Carb Choices
21 – 25 grams = 1½ Carb Choices
26 – 35 grams = 2 Carb Choices
36 –40 grams = 2½ Carb Choices
41 – 50 grams = 3 Carb Choices

If you want to cut the carbs in a recipe down even more, then a half portion will work. If you want to adapt a recipe, we make suggestions of how to do that but in any case you can E-mail us, and we'll try our best to get the job done. If a recipe states that it cannot be adapted or we can't lower its carbohydrate level enough (there aren't many in here like that), then we might suggest a lower or at least a half serving. We have also tried to keep calories within range for each of our recipe recommendations. As most diabetics know, the "food pyramid" for diabetics is not like the food pyramid for the rest of us.

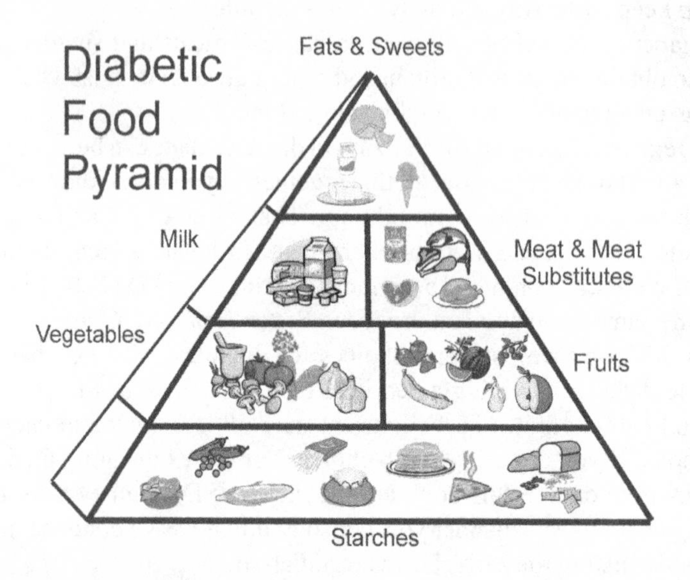

So, how do we adapt a recipe?

The most difficult to adapt are often the bread recipes. That's because we use sugar or honey and flour in bread and therein lie most of the carbs and calories. Surprisingly, our bread recipes often meet diabetic needs (per serving) on the low side for carbs, but cutting calories is more often related to portion sizing - that is, sometimes it's better to enjoy only half the serving. Specialties like Danish, or other similar treats may prove pretty much out of range for carbs and calories without some serious changes. The above by the way, applies to all the bread recipes in each of our five books.

We do have guidance offered in some of the bread recipes and a few notes throughout the section. But let's cover most of them here as well. Also you can find a few links at megaheart.com both on our site map page and at the links at the bottom of every page. Online calculators are available for calculating CHO exchanges and carb choices. If you have problems find these, please E-mail us through our megaheart.com/contact.html page and we'll gladly help you.

Some flour products are lower in carbohydrates than white or whole wheat flour. We like to use Soy Flour as an exchange for part of a bread recipe to help lower carbs. We use Bob's Red Mill Soy Flour, which is ground from dried soy beans. It works very well when adjusting carbs.

We recommend, however, that you exchange only 30% of the flour in a recipe with soy flour. The downside is that soy flour is just as high in calories per measurement as is white unbleached flour, but it is lower in carbohydrates. One more point: estrogen positive breast cancer patients are still being advised to limit soy in their diet.

We also find Splenda sugar substitute a good choice for altering carbs. But please understand that contrary to the readings on the FDA label of Splenda, the product does have calories and does have complex carbohydrates and sugars although it is claimed by the Splenda processor that these will not "cause a glucose spike." Splenda also has a trace of potassium. You can read more about Splenda in our Glossary. Briefly though, Splenda (McNeil Nutritionals) has produced a small variety of Splenda products. The small yellow packet has three ingredients while the Splenda Granulated has only two. Then there's also the sugar/Splenda mix. Granulated Splenda is for baking. The packet is for coffee, tea or salad dressings, etc. It's third ingredient is Dextrose, which is in fact, sugar and not in the granulated variety. Splenda alone will not work in bread recipes so we recommend Splenda Blend when trying to lower calories and carbohydrates.

Here are the carbohydrate readings for Splenda Granulated that you can use to help lower carbs in a bread recipe if you find it necessary.

1 cup = 24 g carbs, 79.4 calories
3/4 cup = 18 g carbs, 59.6 calories
2/3 cup = 16 g carbs, 53 calories
1/2 cup = 12 g carbs, 39.7 calories
1/3 cup = 8 g carbs, 26.5 calories
1/4 cup = 6 g carbs, 19.9 calories
1 tablespoon = 1.5 g carbs, 4.97 calories
1 teaspoon = .5 g carbs. 1.655 calories

To help understand the benefit of this, one cup of white granulated sugar contains 200 grams of carbohydrates. The differences of sugars are appreciable at any measurement and therefore helpful when attempting to adapt a bread recipe.

White, unbleached flour contains 95.4 grams of carbohydrates per cup while Bob's Red Mill Soy flour contains 32 grams of carbohydrates. If you combine an exchange of the flour and sugar in a bread recipe, then you'll often find that you lower the carbs enough to shave off a carb point or at least a half point per serving.

Another addition to bread you can make that will help is Flaxseed Meal. Two tablespoons equal 4 grams. This addition will change the texture of your bread, so we don't recommend more than one tablespoon per each 2½ cups of flour.

Most diabetics reading this will already know about points and exchanges and the use of "choices" and understand the importance of fiber in their recipes/food. For instance, if any of our recipes have five (5) or more grams of fiber, then you'll subtract the total grams of fiber from the total carbohydrate number before establishing your carbohydrate points or choices.

Other fiber food we use in this book include beans (either dried or Eden No Salt Added Organic canned beans) and legumes. Eden by the way has a variety of no salt added beans, including kidney, pinto, garbanzos (otherwise known as chick peas), white beans, and navy beans and more.

Good fiber is also available in fruits and vegetables. For many we leave the skin (the fiber) on when eating or cooking such as beans, apples, potatoes, etc. You can also get fiber from whole wheat products like cereals, however finding a low sodium commercial cereal is difficult. We stick to Spoon Size, however the carbs are a bit over the top. Of course a whole grain unsalted bread is excellent. Commercial bread sometimes contains a good amount of whole grains, but make sure when reading the ingredients label that you see Whole Grain or Whole Wheat and not simply "Wheat flour."

This book does not contain specific help for those who can't consume potassium, but if you visit megaheart.com/sodium_all_about.html and click on the potassium button at the left you can learn more about which foods and substitutes contain the most potassium. (Understand that like sodium, nearly all foods have some potassium.)

What about Desserts, Snacks, Sweets?

Counting points is important and it matters each day. We recommend a daily meal planning guide where you plan ahead and that way know exactly what you're going to eat all day, including snacks and desserts.

We recommend that everyone on a no-salt diet, especially those with diabetes, simply split a dessert (that stays within point range) for more than one reason. Keeping the sodium level down is important, but so is keeping the calorie count down. Of course you could choose lower calorie desserts like fresh fruit or a sugar-free sherbet or sorbet low in both sodium and carbs. (See page 271)

We enjoy dried fruit for snacks (but keep track of the higher calories, they're often four and five times more than fresh fruit). Fresh fruit works best, especially apples, pears, oranges, berries, and bananas.

If you're a coffee or tea drinker, stick with the artificial sweeteners. If you're not a Splenda fan try one of the following:

Saccharin - Sweet 'N Low and Sugar Twin . Not acceptable if pregnant or breast-feeding.

Stevia - No caloric intake. Stevia doesn't adversely affect blood glucose levels and may be used freely by diabetics. (Per Stevia site.) More information about this product is available on-line. Search: Stevia Sweetener.

Aspartame - NutraSweet and Equal . Loses sweetness at high temperatures, therefore not good for baking. Not recommended for patients with phenylketonuria.

All artificial sweeteners have some side effects.

Artificial sweeteners in prepared foods are not always the same as the sweetener you buy in packets or packages. Diabetics, like no-salters, have to read labels very carefully. The ingredients aren't always what they say they are. You'll find claims like "no sugar," "no added sugar," "sugar-free," "all natural." No sugar should mean no sugar at all but you might find alcohol sugar or one of the above artificial sweeteners. No-added-sugar, like no-added-salt means that no sugar or salt was added during processing. There may be sugar, however, from the original source just as there is sodium. Sugar-free means pretty much what "no sugar" means. "All Natural" means no artificial anything but it could contain sugar, sugar alcohol, MSG, or sea salt.

Meniere's Syndrome

Meniere's disease, known generally as Meniere's Syndrome impacts lives rather severely. Serious episodes of Meniere's are possibly the most debilitating experiences among those who survive any chronic illness[1].

Our inner ear normally functions independently of the rest of our body's fluid and blood management system. With a healthy inner ear, fluid remains at a constant volume with specific levels of sodium, potassium, and other electrolytes all on its own. This uniquely maintained fluid level keeps our inner ear cleansed and allows our sensory cells to function normally.

Meniere's Syndrome is when degeneration or damage of the inner ear loses its independence from the rest of the body causing a fluctuation of inner ear fluids. This fluctuation causes symptoms of pressure in the ears. The best known result is tinnitus, known because so many of us at later stages of life develop this symptom. Meniere's patients, however, develop severe dizziness, vertigo, hearing loss and debilitating imbalance.

Some Meniere's information states that a 2,000 mg a day of salt diet (they mean sodium) is doable for Meniere's, that it's not the salt (sodium) that's important but keeping it balanced.

We can get it lower, and we should. It can be done safely while still consuming all the other nutrients that we must eat every day to achieve a healthy body and system. And it goes without saying that I have proved since 1997 that it's safe and extremely effective to get down to 500 mg a day of dietary sodium. I should think that anything under 1,000 mg would be an immense help.

Meniere's patients visiting Megaheart.com have told us that our cookbooks have played a big part in relieving their symptoms and helping them get through life without dizziness, imbalance and other challenges they face. Cutting sodium way down makes sense to them, and because of all the notes in support of this effort, we suggest you at least give it a try. It makes sense that if our inner ear can no longer control the sodium, then our diet can. That alone will help ease the pressure (hydrops) on our inner ear mechanism. You can find some of these notes at megaheart.com/testimonialsbook.html.

Still, keeping the amount at a steady level will also help greatly. So whether you choose 300 mg, 500 mg a day, 750 or a thousand, that's what you want to keep your daily diet at. Fluctuations are not only a poor idea for the heart and other ailments, they definitely aren't what a Meniere's patient wants. Once you feel better, stick with your plan.

And when it begins to work for you, please let us know at Megaheart.com. We're there for help and we love to hear success stories.

Nephrotic Syndrome

Nephrotic syndrome has a list of symptoms such as low blood protein levels, high cholesterol and high triglyceride levels, swelling and protein in urine[2].

Nephrotic syndrome is caused by various disorders that damage the kidneys, particularly the basement membrane of the glomerulus. This immediately causes abnormal excretion of protein in the urine.

Nephrotic syndrome can affect all age groups. In children, it is most common from age 2 to 6. This disorder occurs slightly more often in males than females.

The goals of treatment are to relieve symptoms, prevent complications and delay progressive kidney damage. Treatment of the disorder that causes the condition is necessary to control nephrotic syndrome.

The goal is to keep blood pressure at or below 130/80 mmHg. Your doctor may also prescribe meds not unlike those prescribed for hypertension and heart-failure patients.

According to the NIH: "Angiotensin-converting enzyme (ACE) inhibitors or angiotensin receptor blockers (ARBs) are the medicines most often used for Nephrotic syndrome. ACE inhibitors may also help decrease the amount of protein loss in the urine. Corticosteroids and other drugs that suppress or quiet the immune system may be used. High cholesterol and levels should be treated to reduce the risk of heart and blood vessel problems. However, a low-fat, low-cholesterol diet is usually not as helpful for people with nephrotic syndrome. Medications to reduce cholesterol and triglycerides may be needed, most commonly statins.

A low salt diet may help with swelling in the hands and legs. Water pills (diuretics) may also help with this problem.

Low protein diets may or may not be helpful. A moderate-protein diet (1 gram of protein per kilogram of body weight per day) may be suggested.

Vitamin D may need to be replaced if nephrotic syndrome is chronic and unresponsive to therapy.

Blood thinners may be required to treat or prevent clot formation.

Again, we recommend a good daily plan to help you keep a body-balance of nutrients, meds and fluids.

For renal patients we have put a page online at megaheart.com/renal-diet.html. We will add to this page in the future and also build pages for patients with other specific challenges that require more than just cutting salt out. Renal patients must also safeguard against potassium and phosphorous. The potassium exclusion makes a no-salt life more challenging since food processors who make no salt added products have exchanged potassium for salt. A dietitian specializing in renal dietary needs is of course the preferred way to deal with your dietary needs, but in the meantime we hope the above Megaheart page will help.

(Footnotes)

[1] Anderson JP, Harris JP. Impact of Meniere's disease on quality of life. Otol Neurotol 22:888-894,2001

[2]A protein urine test measures the amount of proteins, such as albumin, found in a urine sample.

Anti-inflammatory Foods In a No-Salt World

While there are many anti-inflammatory drugs on the market, some issues can be helped via diet including low-sodium and anti-inflammatory foods. This chapter will discuss the relationship between diet and inflammation.

What we shouldn't eat

The best way to mitigate inflammatory problems is to not eat inflammatory causing foods. These include baked goods using hydrogenated oils, margarine, potato chips, the ubiquitous French fries, most junk food, trans fats and saturated fats. Saturated fats are mostly from animal products. With beef or fowl we want to cut all visible fat from the meat before cooking. If you like ground meat, purchase the 95% or higher fat-free beef. Same with lean ground turkey and chicken.

Refrain from deli meats like luncheon meats and hot dogs, sausages and bacon, any meat with sodium nitrites in them or meats otherwise commercially processed may also be inflammatory. Other inflammatory foods often include saturated fats in dairy products. Try to get nonfat or at least low-fat dairy. Other culprits include lots of sugar, or soft drinks, pastries, candy, sugar-laced or coated cereals and other sugar laden processed or packaged foods.

Here's what we can eat

Grain should be in our diets. One-hundred percent whole grain breads, cereals, and pasta are each anti-inflammatory foods. If you don't care for this type of grain then why not add flaxseed meal to your morning cereal or into your bread recipes? It works well. Also good to eat are green leafy vegetables and brightly colored vegetables and fruits. Nutritionists tell us to eat at least five or more fruits and vegetables a day (combined count), a good idea that encompasses many benefits. Visit www.5aday.gov to figure out exactly what five a day means for you.

Additionally, Omega-3 essential fatty acids such as unsalted walnuts, almonds and hazelnuts, oily cold water fish (wild salmon is an example), flax seeds or flax seed meal, extra virgin olive oil, pumpkin seeds, peppers (capsicum), and walnut and olive oils are good anti-inflammatory foods.

Beverages should include water, herbal tea, pure vegetable or fruit juices (not those with high fructose corn syrup). Most of what we eat contains a lot of water, especially fruit, vegetables, juices, and even meat or fish. While on a no-salt low-sodium diet, you'll dispense with those fluids after they've done their job for you.

Wild Salmon - Contains anti-inflammatory fats called omega-3s. Wild salmon has more of these super-healthy fats than does farmed salmon otherwise known in super markets as Atlantic salmon (Salmon salar). Farmed salmon often contains high levels of pesticides. Wild Atlantic salmon is not the same as farmed, but instead is from the northern Atlantic. It's much healthier but not as high in Omega-3 levels as Wild Alaskan salmon. Farmed salmon is generally grown in pens alongside rivers that flow to the ocean and has generated a fear that many have escaped from the pens and may be endangering wild ocean salmon.

All salmon from Alaska is wild. Unsalted albacore tuna also contains omega-3s. Other seafood with Omega-3 fatty acids include trout, unsalted canned, or fresh tuna and sablefish. Low in sodium. Salmon oil capsules are mostly free of the mercury we find in ocean fish. Visit *www.megaheart.com/supplements* to find at least one supplier who verifies mercury free salmon oil capsules. See the next chapter for more information concerning salmon.

Animal foods - Cattle and sheep raised on free-range grasslands contain anti-inflammatory omega-3s, but in lower concentrations than cold water fish. Stockyard grain-fed animals have virtually no omega-3s but instead higher levels of saturated fat. Free-range, grass-fed beef is generally tougher. Cook free range slower than usual. Works well in crock-pot where the process will tenderize the meat. Generally average around 20 mg of sodium per ounce. Do not buy brined or marinated meats.

Extra virgin Olive Oil - Olive oil is a great source of oleic acid, another anti-inflammatory oil. In company with olive oil is avocado oil, which is one of many reasons we list avocados under fruits here, and use them in salads and sandwiches in our books. Very low in sodium.

Salads. Lettuce - (the darker the leaf the better), spinach, toma*toes,* celery, berries, avocado, mandarins, pineapple, lemon juice, and other salad fruits and vegetables are rich in vitamin C and other antioxidants and nutrients that ward off inflammation. Fruit is generally very low in sodium. Vegetables are generally low in sodium.

Vegetables - Bok choy, bell peppers, broccoli, Brussels sprouts, cabbage, cauliflower, chard, collards, fennel bulb, garlic, green (string) beans, green onions, spinach, sweet potatoes, turnip greens, and kale, are loaded with antioxidants. All are generally low in sodium.

Blueberries - Beneficial for more than a few reasons. They reduce inflammation and help protect the human brain from the affects of aging. Frozen blueberries work just as well as fresh. Very low in sodium.

Herbs and Spices - Include turmeric, which contains an active and efficiently effective anti-inflammatory compound. Other effective herbs and spices include cayenne and chili peppers, cinnamon, ground cloves, oregano, parsley, rosemary, and thyme. (A mix of oregano, rosemary, sage and thyme make a wonderful rub for barbecued and baked chicken or as a mix in lean ground turkey or beef patties.) Curry spice usually contains some turmeric and also makes excellent seasoning with chicken.

Gingerroot - Gingerroot is closely related to turmeric and is known worldwide for its anti-inflammatory benefits. Some suggest making a ginger tea by removing the skin from gingerroot and then putting a piece or very thin slice or two into a cup of hot water. Steep for up to five minutes and Voila! Ginger tea. Very low in sodium.

Green tea - Promoted worldwide as a natural anti-inflammatory. Some researchers feel it might reduce the risk of heart disease and cancer. A cup a day is recommended. Iced green tea is just as effective. Traces of sodium.

Another way to remember what to eat is to use the acronym GYRO (as in a spinning top or a classic Greek sandwich). Green, Yellow, Red and Orange fruits and vegetables are generally excellent for anti-inflammatory effectiveness.

Testimonial note: For a long time my finger joints flared painfully with what was diagnosed as rheumatoid arthritis. The only solution involved two different medications and cortisone shots. I balked and decided to try adding cinnamon to my diet every day. Surprise! It worked. For quite a few years now I have had no inflammation or pain. It's something you may want to try.

What We Can Eat

No matter whether we are perfect or imperfect, salt carries a potential for being a negative in each of our lives no matter what we hear from "salt boosters." Some of us get hit early with that problem, others later. Some of the lucky among us never get hit at all, or at least never show it. Do I need scientific studies to prove salt affects me? No. If I get a dose of salt now, my system reacts quickly. Before restricting my sodium intake I used to "sweat" after eating a high sodium meal and become flushed and somewhat ill. I always thought it was the heat in the room or that maybe I ate too much, but no, it was a high sodium reaction.

We learn when first entering the no-salt, low-sodium world that the best tasting and the best healthy unsalted food has been with us much longer than processed foods. Fresh fruits and vegetables are the key components to a much healthier life.

Realistically, our eating patterns don't have to change much unless we've been on a high-fat, high-sodium diet.

We should try to include unprocessed and whole grains such as barley, flaxseed meal, oats, brown rice, wheat germ, and more; each of which provides us adequate fiber. We want to eat legumes such as lentils, beans, and unsalted peanuts for protein. Other sources of protein include fish, fowl, eggs, and lean red meat. Also healthy is a bit of unsalted peanut butter (almond and walnut butter also work).

If you're already making a sandwich with unsalted peanut butter or with meat and vegetables, then make sure you use homemade or commercial unsalted bread. We suggest adding flaxseed meal to your favorite bread recipe. We usually add flaxseed meal to all our bread from cinnamon rolls to baguettes or burger buns. This increases the fiber content and adds an enticing nutty flavor. Another addition to bread can be raw oats or Quaker Quick Oats.

You can find nutrient data tables in the back of *The No-Salt, Lowest-Sodium International Cookbook* or at megaheart.com/ sodium_all_about.html. The online version is printable. Read through these files, learn which foods have the nutrients you are most interested in and apply the data to your daily count.

Instead of cooking white rice, why not try brown or wild rice, which are no more difficult to prepare than white. Wild rice contains the highest level of fiber at 9.92 grams per cup and it's highest in protein at 23.6 grams. Brown rice is a third less than that but it beats white rice by a lot. White rice does provide 12.9 grams of protein, however.

We can enjoy snacks and desserts as well. When preparing either of these, just apply all your current information and abilities to help add nutrients and fiber. Accept the challenge and "think out of the box," as they say. Need a dip for a party? Want to use it with raw vegetables like carrots or other veggies? Then prepare a healthy base such as our Yo Cheese recipe (See Page: 233) and a packet of "Toasted Onion Dip Mix" from HealthyHeartMarket.com (HHM). If you're in a hurry then mix in onion powder, minced garlic and maybe a dash of salt-free chili powder and little chopped onion. The dip works well with veggies and unsalted potato chips and your guests will think they're eating cream cheese with a fresh and tasty mix.

Desserts or snacks can often include the addition of fiber or be made with less fat, especially less saturated fat.

Tofu (soy) can be found without added salt. You might want to investigate adapting this for some of your recipes as we have done in our No-Salt, Lowest-Sodium Cookbook. Soy provides Vitamins B1, B12, D, and protein as well as calcium, folate, magnesium, zinc and potassium.

In each of our *No-Salt, Lowest-Sodium Cookbooks*, we recommend using the best fresh fruits and vegetables available. We have included a list of recommended foods here, each one found either in our cookbooks or in recipes on Megaheart.com. These are not only salt-free, they are heart-healthy and I believe that anything that is heart-healthy, is also healthy for the rest of your body.

Vegetables We Can Enjoy

The following are average sodium counts in vegetables based on one-half cup for sliced, diced, shredded or chopped, unless otherwise noted. For frozen varieties, make sure to check the package for sodium count. You can find some No-Salt-Added canned goods from Del Monte, S&W and Contadina (All the same company.) Visit www.delmonte.com

for more information. They do have no salt added corn, creamed corn, string beans, tomatoes, etc.

Acorn squash, 2 mg

Artichokes, 1/2 medium 62 mg Banana Squash, per ounce 3 mg Beets, 1 raw 59 mg

Broccoli, 12 mg

Buttercup squash, 3 mg

Butternut squash, 3 mg

Cabbage, 6 mg

Carrots, 1 medium 7" 25 mg

Cauliflower, 7 mg

Chives, 1 tablespoon trace

Cucumbers, 1/2 cup 1 mg

Endive, 6 mg

Garlic clove, 1 mg

Green beans ,3 mg

Green peas, 3 mg

Hubbard squash, 4 mg

Iceberg Lettuce, 1 leaf 2 mg

Leeks, 10 mg Mushrooms, 1 mg

Mustard Greens, 7 mg

Onions, 2 mg

Parsley, 1 2 mg

Parsnips, 7 mg

Peas, Snow, Pod Pumpkin, 1 mg

Peppers, Sweet, Bell, all colors 2 mg

Radishes ,14 mg Red cabbage, 4 mg

Romaine lettuce, 2 mg

Scallions, 8 mg

Shiitake Mushrooms, 3 mg

Snap beans, 3 mg Spinach, 1/2 cup, 22 mg

Summer Squash, 1 mg

Turnips, 44 mg Turnip greens, 11 mg

Watercress, 7 mg

Zucchini, 5.65 mg

The complete nutrient data for the above vegetables is listed at megaheart.com/sodium_all_about.html. Click on the vegetable on the left to find other nutrient levels such as vitamin K, potassium, calories, etc.

When you consider the variety of nutrients the above vegetables contain, it's no wonder we refer to them as health food. Nutrients include

Vitamins A, B1, B2, B6, C, E, K1, folate, phytochemicals, copper, fiber, calcium, magnesium zinc, potassium, lycopene, carotenoids (carrots), and more. (Learn more about nutrients in our Glossary at the back of this book.)

To ensure you don't cook the nutrients out of your vegetables, we suggest you don't boil them. It's best to sauté, steam, barbecue, or roast with very little oil, but no matter which way you choose, don't overcook them. Keep all fresh vegetables sealed in zipper lock bags in your refrigerator's vegetable bin prior to cooking. Vegetables used in making stock or stews will leave their nutrients in the stock.

Some Of The Fruit That We Can Eat

The list of fresh fruit is long, however, heart patients may want to avoid grapefruit.[2] Sodium levels below are based on either 1/2 cup or a whole fruit, such as the apple.

Apples, all varieties, 1 mg
Apricots, fresh and dried, 1 mg
Avocados, 21 mg
Banana, 1 mg
Blackberries, 1 mg
Cantaloupe, 1/2 of a 5" melon 23 mg
Cherries, Fresh, 3 mg
Dates, 0 mg
Grapes, 1 mg
Gooseberries, 1 mg
Honeydew, cubed 1/2 cup melon 9 mg
Lemons, 3 mg
Loganberries, 1 mg
Mandarins, Satsuma, 1 mg
Mango, 1.65 mg
Mulberries ,7 mg
Orange, 0 mg
Papaya, 1/2 cup 2 mg
Peaches, 1 mg
Pears, 1 mg
Persimmons, 1 medium 3 mg
Pineapple, Fresh 3 ounces 1 mg
Plums pitted, 1/2 cup 1 mg
Prunes, Dried, Pitted 4 mg
Raisins, black and golden, seedless 10 mg
Raspberries, trace

Strawberries, 1 mg
Tangerine, 1 mg
Watermelon, diced, 1/2 cup 2 mg
Wild berries, all varieties, 1 mg

The complete data for the above fruits is listed at megaheart. com/ sodium_all_about.html. Click on the fruits button on the left to find other nutrient levels such as vitamin K, potassium, carbohydrates, calories, etc.

Most fruit contains vitamin C, but many also contain vitamins A, E, B6. Fruit is generally high in fiber while some yellow fruit like apricots contain carotenoids. Oranges additionally provide bioflavonoids[3]. Generous amounts of potassium are found in bananas, berries, oranges, peaches and cantaloupe. If you are on a potassium restricted diet you'll want to check with your R.D. or doctor about bananas, peaches, papaya, oranges, cantaloupe, berries and a few other fruits.

Other benefits we get from fruit are the antioxidants. Antioxidants are highest in a few berries. Leading the pack are blueberries and cranberries, but other berries and ripe fruit also contain antioxidants.

So, what are Antioxidants?

Briefly, antioxidants help neutralize harmful by-products called "free radicals." Free radicals can lead to cancer, heart disease, diabetes, and perhaps brain degeneration. Some research has shown that antioxidants like those found in berries can neutralize free radicals. Research has also shown that getting these antioxidants in fresh fruit is superior to taking supplements that allegedly provide the same antioxidants.

Meat We Can Eat

All meats, including wild game, have an appreciable but generally acceptable amount of sodium. Although wild game has close to the same sodium levels as domestic meats, it is much lower in fat and cholesterol, making it much more desirable for human consumption. Farmed wild game can be found in many specialty markets. If domestic beef is your choice, then look for the leanest you can find. You may want to change old habits and cut your meat intake to a lower level. Visiting with an R.D. who specializes in your particular needs is a good idea when attempting to figure out your food intake. The below listings are based on domestic beef, retail trimmed meat only. Data based on 4-ounces per serving.

Beef that we can eat (based on sodium levels only).

The general rule of thumb is to choose lean pieces and then trim more fat off before cooking. All figures below assume non-brined and non-marinated meats, 4-ounce weight.

Brisket, whole, all grades 74 mg
Chuck, 70 mg
Flank, 0" trim, 79 mg
Ground, raw, extra lean 56 mg
Ground, baked, well done 73 mg
Ground, pan-fried 79 mg
Ground, raw, lean 64 mg
Ground, lean, baked, 81 mg
Ground, lean, broiled 101 mg
Ground, lean, pan-fried 87 mg
Porterhouse steak 69 mg
Ribs, whole 70 mg
Rib eye, 73 mg
Round, full cut 69 mg
Shank crosscuts 69 mg
Short loin T-Bone, Top Loin, 65.8 mg
Sirloin, top broiled, 70 mg
Tenderloin 71 mg

Meats We Should Avoid

Corned Beef 1286 mg (not used in our cookbooks)

Beef jerky, Hickory Farms 1360 mg, 1-ounce (not in our cookbooks)

Brined or marinated beef.

All processed meats such as luncheon, ham, turkey, sausage, hot dogs, etc. are off limits when it comes to sodium levels.

You'll want to make your own sausage with help from spices, lean ground pork, and lean turkey burger or with just lean turkey burger. Check out our "Don's Mock Sausage" as published in various national magazines such as Today's Diet & Nutrition magazine, February, 2009, and in healthy-heart Living magazine, Spring, 2009 (article is available at Megaheart.com). Recipe is also in *The No-Salt, Lowest-Sodium International Cookbook*, page 106.

Chicken and Turkey (not brined)

Chicken and Turkey are favorites and generally offer a variety of uses from entrées, to sandwiches, soups and salads. This list demonstrates the low sodium levels for most fowl. With fowl, a great deal of sodium is in the skin and fat. By cooking with lean, skinless and sometimes boneless chicken, you'll find your sodium levels down around 16 mg per ounce. Thighs have the highest sodium content of fowl, but by removing the skin before cooking, you lower the total sodium level of a chicken thigh by about 20 mg per thigh.

This list pertains only to fresh, unsalted (non-brined) fowl. Read the FDA nutrition label first. Ingredient labels don't always state "brined," or "salt added;" instead some may state "Natural Flavors," or "Natural Flavorings," which is also used for added MSG. There should be no more than 80 mg of sodium per 4-ounce serving listed for chicken. Turkey may be a bit higher up to 100 mg. Watch out for large packages of loose, frozen chicken parts like legs and breasts. Even from the finest processors these may have been brined before freezing. As of 2010 Foster Farms non brined chicken will state: Salt Not Added.

If you like chicken or turkey burger, we urge you to purchase lean unsalted and non-brined meat[4]. Cook over grill or on nonstick pan with just a dash of extra virgin olive oil. I like to add in a good spice mix. Look for brands that do not include salt or make up your own. We have some in this book and also in *The No Salt, Lowest Sodium Light Meals Book.*

When purchasing a Thanksgiving turkey, be cautious about how the bird has been treated or processed. We purchase only farm fresh or range free turkeys. Processed turkeys can be injected with lots of sodium-laced water or "other flavors," which are often salt, or MSG.

Be cautious with all fowl and pork. Many processors now brine fowl and pork. With pork, try to find very lean cuts. We do have recipes for ribs, but we buy only very lean baby-back ribs. The saturated fat in most other ribs is excessively high. If you must have ribs (we admit they are tasty with a great spice rub), then choose very lean unseasoned ribs. Sodium per ounce of rib meat is about 21.5 mg. Baby Back ribs tend to be the leanest, however, meat on one lean rib can add up to about 7 grams of total fat. If you use an oil-based sauce, more calories and fats will be added.

The following sodium data is based on bone-in, skinned, 4 ounces chicken - broiler or fryer.

Chicken

Light meat, 71.8 mg Dark meat, 92.7 mg

Turkey, Young Hen Light meat, 75.6 mg Dark meat, 91.5 mg

Pork (4-ounces) Raw
Back rib, lean, 85.1 mg
Loin, whole, lean, 59 mg
Loin, blade, lean, 61.2 mg
Loin, center, lean, 74.8 mg
Loin, center rib, lean, 47.6 mg
Loin, sirloin, lean, 57.8 mg
Shoulder, whole, lean, 73.7 mg
Shoulder, arm, lean, 93 mg
Shoulder cut, lean, 86.2 mg
Spareribs, lean & fat, 86.2 mg
Spareribs, country, lean 76 mg
Tenderloin, lean, 56.7 mg

Note: Meat trimmed to 0" or 1/4" fat refers to the amount of fat present during cooking. For "lean only" listings, all visible fat is trimmed before cooking. Bear in mind that some fat is always present.

Fish is recommended twice a week.

Many medical practitioners and nutritionists suggest we eat fish twice a week. Pink fish is the best for us, while we also like unsalted or fresh albacore tuna, which provides Vitamins B12 and D, and a good portion of our daily protein and omega-3 fatty acids. Vitamin is vitally important to your health. There are few ways to get it through food, it's mostly sunshine. There are also vitamin D tablets.

You can find canned unsalted tuna in some stores but always online. Otherwise we recommend fresh pole caught albacore tuna[5].

When it comes to salmon, we need to know where it came from. For instance, fresh wild caught Alaskan salmon has been the "safe" choice for years. Wild salmon off the coasts of Washington and California should not be eaten more than once or twice a month (due to pollutants including minute levels of mercury). When searching for true Alaskan salmon, look for wild Alaskan or sockeye. You might also find Alaskan pink or Alaskan chum, which are good choices as well.[6]

Eating Out Tips: Ask your waiter where the fish came from, and if it has been marinated, processed or pre-salted? In a restaurant it's best to ask for broiled or poached fish cooked without butter. Extra virgin olive oil is okay.

Most seafood contains no fiber, sugars, Omega-6, or Folic Acid. If you can't get fresh fish when you need it, then taking a fish oil or salmon oil capsule is recommended by many nutritionists and doctors. However, some research has shown that some fish oil capsules may have high concentrations of toxins. This factor makes it a difficult choice for many, including this writer. I have found only one supplement maker who has been willing to put into writing that their "fish oil" capsules are toxin free. That company is listed at megaheart.com/supplements.html. If we find more, we'll add them to the list. At any rate, ask your doctor before starting any supplements.

Here are the fish we use in our books and the fish we enjoy at home.
Seafood below is based on 3-ounces, raw
Catfish, Wild Channel, 36.5
Catfish, Farmed, 45.1 Clam, 47.6
Cod, Pacific, 60.4
Cod, Ling, 50.2
Cod, Atlantic, 45.9
Cod, Alaskan, Wild, 50.2 Flounder, Flatfish, Sol, 68.8
Haddock, 45.9
Halibut, Atlantic, 45.9
Halibut, Greenland, 68
Halibut, Sole, Turbot, 68
Mackerel, Atlantic, 76.5
Mackerel, Pacific, 73.1 mg
Orange Roughy, 53.6
Pollock, Walleye, 84.2
Rainbow Trout, Wild, 26.4
Rockfish, Pacific, 51
Salmon, Atlantic/Coho, 39.1
Salmon, Alaska/King, 40
Salmon, Pink, 57
Swordfish, 76.5
Tuna, Yellowfin, 31.5
Tuna, Ahi, Aku, Bonito, 31.1

Shellfish

Shellfish can be a delightful meal, and is often on the menu at restaurants. However, shellfish that is acceptable at home will probably be inedible in the restaurant because of preparation and sometimes because they have been doused with too much salt for marinating or storage. The following list shows shellfish that are okay at home, and shellfish we need to avoid. Sodium data for each is based on 3-ounces, raw. Shrimp is nearly always salted by packers before shipping, even the shrimp often listed as "fresh" in your local grocery store. Ask the counter help for the bag it came in. If it was packed with salt then the sodium levels will be very high.

Lowest Sodium, assume no salt added, 3-ounce servings
Clams, 47.6
Crayfish, Farmed, 52.7 mg
Crayfish, Wild, 49.3 mg
Oyster, Pacific, 90.1 mg
Scallops, 136.9 mg
Oyster, Pacific 90.1
Shrimp, 125.8 mg
Lobster, Spiny 150.4

Shellfish we should avoid even though not salted, 3-ounce servings Abalone, 255.9 mg

Crab, Alaskan King, 710.6 mg
Crab Blue, 249.1
Crab, Dungeness, 250.8 mg
Lobster, Northern 251.6
Mussel, Blue, 243.1 mg
Oyster, Eastern, Farmed, 151.3 mg

Olive Oil

We recommend extra virgin olive oil for baking, making salads, grilling and other cooking. All other oils pale compared to olive oil's health benefits. Olive oil, by the way, is the only freshly-pressed-from the-fruit vegetable oil that can be consumed by humans.

Extra virgin olive oil is the juice from the first pressing of olives and is directly bottled and placed into shipping vats for bottlers after the pressing making extra virgin olive oil the least processed of cooking oils. Extra virgin olive oil is accepted by all chefs and users as the best because it is the least processed.

Expeller pressed refers to oil extracted from nuts (olives in this case) or seeds by crushing them with a screw drive machine. Expeller processing does not remove all the oil (or juice) from the raw olive (often referred to by olive growers as a nut or seed). As much as sixty-percent remains inside of the cake that appears after pressing.

Some processors take the first expeller pressing for their prime product and then the "cake" is treated with chemicals like Hexane to extract the remaining oil from the source. That is why you'll see us refer in our cookbooks to "expeller pressed canola oil" as the best canola oil to buy.

Olive oil can be found in four different categories depending upon the processing involved.

Extra virgin olive oil is extracted using a process known as cold pressing. No chemicals are used and therefore the oil has no foreign flavors. Extra virgin is the closest of the categories to its natural state and is therefore the better of the four varieties.

Virgin olive oil is generated from the second pressing of the cake.

Olive Oil is the oil consisting of a blend of refined olive oil and virgin olive oil fit for consumption as they are. The cheaper refined oil is mixed with more flavorful virgin oil. Some countries require a more specific designation. Most of the olive oil sold in the world falls into this category. Different blends are made, with more or less virgin oil, to achieve different tastes at different prices.

Note that with refined olive oil no solvents have been used to extract the oil, but it has been refined with the use of charcoal and other chemical and physical filters. An obsolete equivalent is "pure olive oil." Refined oil is generally tasteless, odorless, and colorless. Many countries deem it unfit for human consumption due to poor flavor, not due to safety concerns.[1]

Light or Extra Light undergoes considerable processing, is not always just olive oil but instead mostly refined olive oil (see above). Light/Extra Light olive oil is mostly a marketing effort for an oil that has no classification within olive oil grades. It is unregulated by any certification organization. There are no precedents as to what its content should be.

All cooking oils contain 14 grams of fat per tablespoon.

Health Benefits of Olive Oil

Olive oil is mainly comprised of monounsaturated fatty acids. A healthier type of fat, it reduces total and low-density lipoprotein (LDL or "bad") cholesterol levels in the bloodstream, while raising high-density lipoprotein (HDL or "good") cholesterol levels. High quality extra virgin olive oil, in particular, provides a high content of antioxidants, like polyphenols, vitamins E & K, chlorophyll and carotenoids. Antioxidants are key to strengthening the immune system and protecting the body from the damaging effects of free-radical molecules. Olive oil contains anti-inflammatory agents, like oleocanthal, that act as a natural ibuprofen-like substance.[1]

No other naturally produced oil has the same level of monounsaturated fats as olive oil.

What about Canola oil?

Canola oil is a relatively recent development and the oil is promoted strongly as being high in monounsaturated fats. It was originally produced from rapeseed with a eurcic acid level of 69%. Eurcic acid it turned out is harmful to humans, so scientists went to work and in the 1970s they introduced the canola plant, which replaced the rapeseed plant. Even though the canola plant was developed from the rapeseed plant, the eurcic acid level dropped to below an acceptable 2 percent level set by the FDA as safe.

If you don't like the flavor of extra virgin olive oil, then expeller pressed canola oil is a good alternative. However, olive oil beats it for health because of its higher content of monounsaturated fatty acids and its higher content of antioxidative substances.

We have used various oils in our kitchen while testing recipes; corn, sesame, peanut, and olive oils. After all our testing and samples we settled years ago on Extra Virgin Olive Oil for its extensive health benefits and the flavor it offered no-salt cooking, and for salad dressing.

Expeller pressed organic canola oil is our best choice for canola. There are a few national brands such as Hain, the makers of Featherweight Baking Powder, and Spectrum (ConAgra). If you can find it locally, you'll want organic expeller pressed canola oil in order to minimize ingestion of pesticides, many of which are fat soluble. You can find the Spectrum brand at www.spectrumorganics.com/. Spectrum also produces a trans-fat-free shortening comparable to Crisco.

Eating Out Tip: When ordering a salad, ask the waiter to bring you some balsamic and extra virgin olive oil or expeller pressed canola oil, and a little sugar or Splenda. Make your own dressing at the table and enjoy the salad knowing it's going to be heart-healthy. Leave the sugar out if you want, it's still an excellent dressing without it, or sometimes I like to add a squeeze of fresh lemon juice.

Store It In The Dark

Researchers have learned that both interior and exterior light destroys many of the antioxidants found in olive oil. Even with this information, many manufacturers still bottle olive oil in clear glass or plastic bottles. We buy only extra virgin olive oil in dark bottles or cans and then store the oil in a closed cupboard or dark pantry area. We should consider this research when purchasing olive oil in a store. How long has it been there, and is the bottle dark or transparent? Clear (not dark) bottles stored in a grocery store for more than a month or so will have lost about 30 to 50 per cent of their Tocopherol and carotenoids, the two antioxidants in olive oil. Also, research has shown that it takes only one to two months under "grocery store" lighting for the peroxide levels to rise enough to alter the classification of extra virgin olive oil to just olive oil.

We suggest that to prevent the loss of quality over time you buy smaller bottles and store your oil in a dark place. Storing oil that has been exposed to oxygen too long can result in a rancid oil.

Tips for Using Olive Oil: Sauté with olive oil instead of unsalted butter or another oil. Drizzle olive oil over fish while broiling. Mix with your favorite vinegar for your salad. Dip homemade, no-salt bread into small dish with extra virgin olive oil and some balsamic vinegar for a delicious flavor. You can add minced garlic or onion powder or basil, cilantro, rosemary, oregano or any desired herbs for more flavor.

Steam vegetables and then toss with a small amount of olive oil. Brush bread very lightly with olive oil before making your panini. Use olive oil when making unsalted bread instead of butter or other oils. (It's the oil that will make your bread soft.)

Add olive oil to your homemade barbecue sauce.

Brush insides of burger buns and set on grill for a minute or two before making your burger or other sandwiches.

Have an old wooden cutting board you'd like to protect? Just rub it with a light coating of olive oil.

Desserts Can Be Enjoyable

Desserts can be enjoyed without a high-salt or high-sodium content. However, most desserts we make at home will more than likely need alterations or the use of specially created and tested recipes like our Lemon Cheesecake and some of our pies.

We use fresh or frozen fruit with all fruit desserts, but sometimes we find we need to use frozen berries. Frozen blackberries, strawberries, peaches, and frozen raspberries are generally as good as fresh when it comes to making berry pies, cobblers or for making sorbets or smoothies.

Wild berries in season are about the best for flavor and nutrients.

Apples, apricots, pears, and delicate fruits don't freeze as well as berries. However, with worldwide supplies now available, we often find "out of season" fruits and vegetables at our grocery stores. It is a good idea when this happens to make sure you're not buying food that comes from another part of the world where free-wheeling pesticide use is a standard. You produce grocer should be able to answer to this.

Fast food restaurants usually offer ice cream, slices of pie or milkshakes. Ice Cream can range from about 50 mg sodium per scoop to over 550 mg. Fried or baked pie slices can range from 285 mg per slice to over 500 mg (depending on size of slice and source of fruit and how it was made.) Sherbet averages 44 mg sodium per scoop. Sorbet ranges from 8 to 16 mg sodium per scoop or half-cup.

Brownies are an example of a dessert with something chocolate - sometimes with a small scoop of vanilla ice cream. The Little Debby brownie (the only commercial brownie listed by the USDA) contains 174 mg of sodium. A homemade brownie with salt and baking powder can range from 85 mg upwards to 200 mg. Don's Brownies contain 11.1 mg of sodium. Now we see why we want to prepare our own desserts.

Eating Out Tip: When eating out, desserts are often very high in sodium. The only dessert I allow myself in a restaurant is either a sorbet or sherbet. Pies, puddings, cheesecakes, cakes, coconut filled, milk based, whipped cream topped, and those incredibly chocolate covered things with various names possibly have more sodium than the meal you may have just consumed.

What About Snacks?

Gone are the cheese and crackers, the cookies from a vending machine or that small bag of salted peanuts.

Today, your best decision for a snack will once again be fresh fruit or fresh vegetables like a carrot or slices of red bell pepper. Since we should eat at least five servings of fruits and vegetables a day, this is a good way to get one or two of those servings. I often choose a banana for my mid-morning snack. If I feel like I need a little protein I enjoy it with a tablespoon of unsalted peanut butter (4 g protein).

The 28-day meal-planning guide in the back of *The No-Salt, Lowest-Sodium Cookbook* takes good care to keep us on track with snacks. Snacks are beneficial for many of us. If we eat a healthy snack between meals, we are less likely to overeat during meal times, and we keep our energy up. Choose your favorites and fit them in by looking up their nutrient values and applying them to your daily plan. Mine include bananas, unsalted walnuts or peanuts and occasionally a piece of homemade bread toasted lightly with a light coat of unsalted peanut butter or my favorite, homemade wild blackberry jelly.

For a long time I used to "graze." Grazing is when we don't eat a "meal" but instead eat as we go along during the day. That worked well during my working years, and it was necessary since I put in very long days where sit-down meals just didn't exist. Necessary nutrient balances could not possibly have been met back then. Now that I don't expend a lot of the same levels of energy, I don't need to graze. However, light snacks keep me going between meals and that's proved to be the best program for my general health as well as my heart and waistline. Maybe it will work for you, too. Controlling my sodium level and sticking to the food pyramid pretty much keeps me trim and hopefully healthier.[10]

Which Foods Should I Avoid or Not Eat?

First, list all the foods you like or love to eat. Then look up their nutrient data and write down the sodium level per serving. If you're a diabetic, include the carbohydrate choices or your exchanges. Then make a new list with 2-columns, on the left the foods you can eat, on the right the foods you'll have to avoid, usually because of unacceptable levels of sodium, carbohydrates or other nutrients that affect your health.

You can search the USDA database for nutrient information or use the data on megaheart.com/sodium_all_about.html. Just click on the food list at the left. Megaheart's nutrient database is printable.

After your list is built, return to the database and search for the saturated fats, trans fatty acids, and if you have to because of your condition, the potassium and Vitamin K (If taking blood thinner see Vitamin K in the glossary). If the sodium is too high in a particular food item to include in a day's planning, then list that one in the right hand column. Then applying your own needs, such as diabetic, hypertension, Meniere's, etc. re-evaluate the left column and either keep them or move them over to the right column.

At least you now know which foods you believe you can eat. By the way, the above may sound confusing at first, but once you begin your list and open the database, it will flow quickly and easily.

Now for a reality check. The obvious grocery store foods that we should avoid are the processed, canned, packaged, and frozen food products that are overloaded with salt. Chances are you've already walked through a few food aisles of your local grocery store and discovered excessive levels of salt you've been eating. And it's not just salt that's been added to your food, but that too many packaged and processed foods are loaded with MSG and too often high fructose corn syrup.

Since we can't eat or cook with the high-sodium levels of standard processed tomato cans, we have to search for No-Salt-Added labels or unsalted labels. Again, always check the FDA Panel and Ingredients labels for an assessment of any packaged or canned food. We suggest you make your tomato based sauces and soups. Marinara for instance is easy or if you are "cooking challenged" just use our simple Marinara sauce in the sauce section of this book.

Cheese is another product we'll have to avoid. Most cheese is very high in sodium as are most dairy products. Although we use dairy products, we recommend nonfat milk and nonfat or low-fat or reduced-fat dairy products such as yogurt and sour cream. Actually, sodium is lower in standard yogurt and sour cream but higher in fat.

A few eggs a week aren't bad for us, actually the protein in them is good. But cholesterol should be counted for those of us who need to cut it down. (See: Cholesterol in the glossary.)

Butter, margarine, or spreads. When we bake we use extra virgin olive oil, depending that is, on what we are baking. We never use butter as a spread or to fry, or sauté. However, some recipes, like pie shells, cakes, and sometimes muffins demand solid shortening. Spectrum and Crisco offer a non-trans fatty acid shortening that works well and of course unsalted butter is also without trans fatty acid.

For healthy choices we find ourselves mostly in the produce section of grocery stores or local farmers markets, and I think you will, too.

Remember, too, the recommendations in this book are generally based on a dietary lifestyle of 500 or fewer milligrams of sodium per day.

If you elect to consume a higher level than that then life gets just that much easier. However, we have discovered that after a few months on a 500 mg a day it became an acceptable and rather easy achievement and it certainly has contributed to a longer life for me.

A popular place where you'll want to check the nutrients before stepping through the front door is Baskin Robbins (BR) and other ice cream shops. If you insist on having this treat (we do it once in a while), then please refrain from BR's Chocolate Blast with whip cream (Sodium 230 mg, Calories, 520). Their lowest sodium items include Daiquiri Ice (0 mg), Peachy Keen Sorbet (10 mg), Rainbow Sherbet (35 mg), Vanilla Ice Cream 60 mg) and Very Berry Strawberry Ice Cream (45 mg). Their smoothies are over 150 mg per serving except for the Very Strawberry Smoothie (70 mg) and their yogurt servings are 125 mg plus per serving. You can find many fast food nutrition ratings on the Web at *http://www.fastfoodnutrition.org*

Eating out Tip: If you make your own bread, you can enjoy vegetarian sandwiches at shops like Subway, Quiznos, Togo's and others. However, the meat in these places is loaded with sodium so stick with the vegetarian sandwich. Leave off the peppers, olives, and other marinated offerings. And definitely forego the cheese unless it's a Fresh Mozzarella (unsalted, or very low sodium mozzarella is available in some areas). Take your own bun or sandwich roll and Voila! Another good meal. I like to ask for extra avocado or tomato. Also, oil and vinegar make a nice dressing in lieu of mustard and mayo. If you're uncomfortable taking your bread into a sandwich shop, just leave it in your car, purchase the sandwich and then move the ingredients into your own roll.

(Footnotes)

[1] Information provided by and with the permission of the Olive Oil Source (http://www.oliveoilsource.com)

[1] Vitamin K can affect blood thinner levels. Some doctors recommend that if you like vitamin K foods then maintain a steady diet of them, instead of sudden bursts. This will help keep your ProTime stable (INR). Some doctors ask that we avoid vitamin K altogether, but that's a tough call since quite a few foods contain vitamin K. If your doctor recommends no Vitamin K, suggest you'd like to try to keep a dietary balance

Products Mentioned In This Book

All products mentioned in this book are considered registered ® or trademarked ™. Products include:

Accent
Alberto's All-Clad
Alpine Lace
Alvarado Bakery
Applebee's
Arrowhead Mills
B'rer Rabbit
Barbara's
Baskin Robbins
Beritos
Better Homes & Garden
Blue Diamond
Bob's Red Mill
Braun
Breadman
Campbell's
Conagra
Contadina
Cook's
Costco
Crisco
Crown Prince
Dan-D Pak
Dash
Del Monte
Denny's
Devonsheer
Diabetic Living
East Shore
Eden Foods
El Macero
Ener-G
Enrico's
Erewhon
Ezekiel
Featherweight
Francesco Rinaldi
Frontier
Garden of Eatin
Genisoy
Glenny's
Good Sense
Grandma's
Guiltless Gourmet
Hain
Health Valley
Heinz
Heluva Good
Hodgson Mills
Hormel
Hunt's
IHOP
In-N-Out
Ka-Ma

Keenan Farms Kelin's
Kellogg's
Kettle
King Arthur
Kirkland
Kitchenaid
Laura Scudder's
Libby's
Little Bear
Lundberg
Manishewitz
Maraatha
Marie Calenders
Mauna Loa
McCormick
McDonald's
McNeil Nutritionals
Melissa's

Mendocino Mustard
Meredith
Merino's
Michael's
Mickey T's
Morga
Mrs. Wrights
Muir Glen
Nantucket Offshore
Natural Sea
Natural Value
Nestle
Newman's
Nordic
Now Foods
Nutrifit
Old London

OXO
Padrino
Panasonic Planers
Post
Quaker
Quiznos
Rapunzel
Royal Oak
Ruby Tuesdays
Rumiano
S&W
Safeway
Salton
Shibolim
Snack Master
Williams
Wayzata Bay

Planning Ahead Is Healthy

By planning ahead, even as much as a month at a time, we will be prepared with enough unsalted and no-salt-added (NSA) ingredients and foods that we might need. This can also help us make meals a more enjoyable experience, as opposed to "the same old boring thing everyday."

Planning ahead is also necessary if you're still working and need to plan a sack lunch or an evening meal away from home. Since deli meats and other high-sodium foods are now out of our lives, a healthy alternate will have to be planned to ensure nutrients and low-sodium.

We find that planning into the future also saves money. When no salt-added canned tomatoes, sauces and paste are on sale, Maureen and I stock up. We know that we'll be making soups, sauces and other tomato dishes so why not cash in on the savings? The same policy is good for other unsalted or no-salt-added products. There is a caveat here, though. Make sure you don't buy products that will stay on your shelf past the "Use By" date printed on the product. Unfortunately, some products go on sale because those dates are catching up to the store's inventory.

We have also learned, that some stores just don't carry no-salt-added processed foods. Costco and Wal-Mart for instance cater to the "general" crowd and do not carry health-niche food products except for some fresh vegetables and fruits. Whole Foods, however, has some unsalted and no-salt-added items as does Trader Joe's, while large chains often carry national brands and in-house labels of NSA tomato products and various other NSA products like unsalted peanut butter and sometimes frozen unsalted corn and peas. Some very excellent products like *Eden Organic No Salt Added Beans* can prove difficult to find locally although not impossible. However, you can find them at the company's Web site *www.edenfoods.com*, at *healthyheartmarket.com* and occasionally at some health food stores. Specialty items like Ener-G and other baking goods are found more easily online. Again we suggest you visit *megaheart.com/wheretobuy.html* for the latest updates of what is available and who the sellers are. And remember, if you find a great no-salt-added product and a source for it, send us a note via *megaheart.com*, and we'll post your info so that others might enjoy it. You might also let *healthyheartmarket.com* know about it.

Planning ahead while also saving you money will provide you with the nutrition you need on a regular basis, simply because you won't find yourself eating a "quick" meal or being tempted to visit the local fast-food or worse, ordering in a pizza.

To help with having the right foods on hand when you want them, why not make up an inventory list for your pantry or cabinet and check off what you've used? Or you can use this list to write down what you need on your next grocery store trip or on-line visit to suppliers. We usually make sure that we always have:

Pantry

- All-purpose flour
- Apple cider, red wine, rice vinegar
- Ascorbic acid
- Balsamic vinegar (gourmet balsamic for meats & other dishes)
- Bread flour
- Brown Rice
- Decaf green tea
- Ener-G Baking Powder (or Featherweight)
- Ener-G Baking Soda
- Expeller pressed canola oil
- Extra virgin olive oil
- Flaxseed meal, vital wheat gluten, malted barley flour
- Fresh fruit
- Fresh vegetables
- Honey Mustard, low-sodium like Mendocino or East Shore
- No Salt Added canned tomatoes, paste, sauce, and ketchup
- No Salt Added Eden Organic Beans
- Oatmeal
- Low Sodium dry cereal like: Shredded wheat or Spoon Size

- Spices & Herbs
- Sugar and Splenda
- Unsalted canned tuna
- Unsalted peanut butter
- Unsalted potato and tortilla chips
- Unsalted walnuts, pecans, peanuts
- Whole wheat pasta

Fresh Fruits & Vegetables
- Fruits in season
- Onions
- Potatoes (Russet, Yukon Gold, New)
- Root vegetables
- Winter Squash
- Yams

Fridge
- Corn tortillas
- Eggs
- Low-sodium cheese
- Non-fat milk
- Unsalted butter
- Yo Cheese (you make from plain nonfat yogurt)

More Reasons To Plan

There are other reasons to prepare ahead as well. I remember well the beginning stages of heart failure. I was without strength and had little energy. I could barely move around without stopping to gasp for air, so conserving my physical energy was a must. Good planning was necessary.

However, after cutting my sodium to 500 mg a day and lower, the positive results kicked in after a few months, and I started to steadily improve. I add here that I also stuck to my medication program, which enabled me to start walking longer distances. I was getting stronger and stronger.

To add to the simple life in the kitchen, Maureen likes to make soups often, especially during the winter. We can get about eight to ten servings from each pot of soup, so that computes to a few meals, which helps to bring the cost of healthy eating way down. I make a special bread for each soup and together we end up with several meals and lots of nutrients. I usually make a grain bread, or something unique like Ethiopian Spice Bread, or French baguettes[1]. I confess to enjoying a flaxseed white-bread as well. Toasted with a light spread of our Yo Cheese with some tasty pepper jelly and served with soup makes for an enjoyable taste treat.

Enter our good planning and preparation. One trip a week to the grocery store can often save time, money and energy. The secret is to keep a list. Have the right things on hand. Organize, prepare, cook and serve.

We will do all the chopping, cutting, slicing, measuring, and mixing. I do like to clean up while working. If prepping is done and cooking or baking is in progress, I use the time to put unused ingredients away and clean up. Often when Maureen and I exchange kitchen duties, one cooks and the other cleans up after dinner. Volunteers are always welcomed.

I make two weeks worth of bread or buns or rolls and freeze them. If I know they are going to be used within a few days I bag them in zipper lock bags and store them in a bread box.

Other meals that we hold in the freezer include soups, stews, veggie burger patties, sliced bread or homemade tortillas with wax paper between the slices so we can pull one out at a time. We also will freeze pint or quart jars of broth we make. We use wide mouth jars by the way so that when used, they slip out much easier after a little warm water treatment to help thaw them. Then into the soup pan and quickly thawed into a stew or soup that we're making.

Within a few months of Megaheart.com going on-line, a new low-sodium food service introduced itself to the world via the Internet. Pete Eiden created Healthy Heart Market[2], and it became an "overnight" success. His store was the pioneer for low-sodium foods. Pete later received a transplant and returned to a happier family life including ice-fishing on the lakes of Minnesota. HHM is now owned by Lisa McComas and her husband, and they are doing well with it. HHM is up close and personal, too. Lisa will help you directly if you call (1-800- 753-0310).[3]

Help Is Also Available

There are more than a few ways for us to adapt and plan. One is to visit with an experienced registered dietitian (R.D.) who specializes in the field of your concern. There are R.D.s who specialize in practically every known area of health challenges we have. If you can't locate one through the phone book or your doctor's office, visit www.eatright.org and click on the "Find a Nutrition Professional" button. You'll find a good selection of registered dietitians near you.

Do It Yourself A Good Option

If you plan to do this by yourself, that's okay, too. Actually it's fun to play with a monthly plan. We have one in the back of our first cookbook that you can use as a guide to make up your own. It displays the calories per day (which should be adjusted to your needs) and other necessary nutrients. With experience you'll find it's easy to figure out nutrients, sodium levels, calories and more without even having to refer to a book or guide. It will become second nature.

The daily meal planner guide includes:

- Breakfast
- Midmorning Snack
- Lunch
- Mid afternoon Snack
- Dinner

One of the things I learned to appreciate with meal planning is that I could have a variety of foods for meals and enjoy each of them without adding salt or fats. Getting into a rut of eating the same thing over and over can get awfully old, boring, and not necessarily healthy. I confess my breakfast is pretty much the same from day to day, but the rest of the day often offers up gastronomic wonders, especially when Maureen gets into a soup, stew, casserole mood and produces dishes that are without salt, but always with tasty spices and herbs. For Maureen's chicken broth, used as a base for many soups and sauces, see page 231.

When you plan your meals, also plan for guests and other family members when they visit. If they are willing to try your unsalted food, then make enough for them. One of the things that became apparent to me right from the beginning was not wanting to have my meal different from others.

I remember a "bring your own pizza" dinner gathering while I was creating and testing our no-salt very low sodium pizza recipe. I made a large pizza just for me figuring that curiosity might necessitate more than just a small one. When the party started and pizzas were due to be served, I set the delivered pizzas out and put mine alongside. One of the guests wanted to try my "very low sodium pizza." The unexpected praise brought others to sample and gave a lift to my spirits as well. It can be done. Having others recognize and praise your efforts is helpful.

I tell this story to point out that no-salt meals can and do taste very good. The flavors are more natural than the overwhelming flavor of salt alone, and they are always healthier. I believe that every one should cut their sodium and saturated fat intake way down. Everyone. Even the giants of good health. Why wait until we are diagnosed with a serious illness to start? Why not start now? A good diet, good exercise and no medications seem a lot healthier than waiting for the inevitable, which include expensive medications. Medications all have side-effects, some of them seriously dangerous. Do you remember the song in the movie Paint Your Wagon? "Cured of what we suffered from, and sufferin' from the cure."

Why take a chance? I believe this idea of healthy people lowering their sodium and saturated fat intake is part of planning ahead.

Several of our low-sodium meals have proved to be acceptable to salt eaters as well. This past Thanksgiving we had about forty family and friends over. The food was set out in a large area and buffet service was expected. A few years ago I would ask, which one is no-salt and Maureen would point the few choices. This year, those who brought dinner selections with them like yams, cranberries, salads, etc. brought them made without salt. Everyone around here has come to realize that there's just too much salt in our diets and getting it out makes life much healthier for each of them.

I have noticed that those around us now eat less fat, use less sugar and no longer deep-fat-fry foods. Baking, sautéing, barbecuing, broiling and some grilling done mostly with nonstick cookware, are a much healthier choice. Life is just getting healthier and healthier around here.

Maureen will often cook a week's worth of evening meals in one day and put them into the refrigerator or freezer. Our low-sodium lasagna is a good one to keep in the fridge as well as soups, stews and other casseroles. We think that reheated soups and casserole dishes often taste better than they do the first day. Lasagna tastes particularly more flavorful after resting a day in the fridge and then reheated for a meal. For single servings we cut casserole dishes into serving sizes, wrap in freezer paper then place into zipper-lock freezer bags or containers and store them for later meals. Most will freeze well for up to a month and more.

Our experience has been that top allies for all this planning and cooking are the freezer and the microwave. The freezer will allow you to make next week's meals or even a few for the whole month. You can freeze practically anything you've cooked and thaw them quickly, then reheat them. It's kind of like making your own TV dinners. Add fresh veggies as a side dish when serving.

We often get a bit hungry between meals. In the previous chapter we discussed snacking. Now we need to plan ahead for that as well.

Unless you're in a unique location where fresh fruit is available from a machine, just putting a coin into a "snack" dispenser will not bring you a healthy choice. And grabbing a bite out of the coffee shop's bakery selections will not provide you anything more than some fat, sugars and, of course, lots of sodium, carbs, and added calories. (Diabetics have an especially tough time when "on the road.") But understanding the level of carbohydrates in many foods helps a whole lot when counting carb choices or making exchanges.

I've seen some snacks that would have contained enough calories and sodium to have been a whole meal for me. If you catch yourself eating that much, then you really do need to plan ahead. I don't think that will happen to you if adhere to a no-salt or diabetic diet. The only fresh food snacks I can find out there that don't have added salt in them are fresh fruits and vegetables. A banana, an apple, orange, or a few washed and peeled carrots prepared for your day make excellent snacks. For snacking packaged food however, I have found unsalted peanuts in most grocery stores, but I tend instead to eat a fresh fruit like the banana or a peach or an apple. At home you could have some unsalted Healthy Heart Market popcorn. Right after popping it, sprinkle it lightly with granulated onion powder. Or sprinkle it with a mixture of a sweetener and cinnamon. The cinnamon offers great antioxidant and anti-inflammation properties and the Splenda[4] replaces the unneeded sugar calories and carbohydrates yet helps sweeten the snack. In the long run your snacks can be used to answer that call of hunger and add vitamins and minerals.

Whatever we eat for a snack, we should make sure we aren't stacking up unusable calories. Remember, the theory for maintaining a healthy weight is calories in, calories out. That simply means that we want to burn what we eat or it begins to stack up on the body and are indicated on the scales as weight. (See: BMI in the glossary)

Desserts Are Okay, Too

At home you can make your own low-sodium desserts from pies to puddings to our very best lemon poppy seed pound cake[5]. Another special dessert might be a light scoop of ice cream with fresh sliced strawberries and a mix of balsamic vinegar and Splenda or sugar drizzled over the ice cream. (Don't reject this recipe yet. Give it a try. The excellent flavors will really surprise you.)

Planning ahead for desserts takes a little effort. Many desserts melt, spoil, or are packaged and probably not low in sodium.

If you like puddings, you won't be able to use commercial pudding mixes. Each is very high in sodium. But you can make your own. There are two excellent pudding recipes in *our No-Salt, Lowest-Sodium International Cookbook* on pages 19 and 26. We have added a chocolate pudding recipe in this book. (My apologies for referencing recipes in our other books, but we aren't permitted to reproduce more than just a few in this book.)

Now and then, a spontaneous treat is going to make its presence before you - usually at a friend's house or while eating out. With a good planning system in place, you can enjoy those treats, because you'll know exactly what to exchange them for during your dietary day.

I like a good fresh-apple pie. Some pies we can make with a single crust only, which helps cut down fat and calories, but apple pies need a topping of some kind. To help cut the calories and fat, I make a lattice top crust. That at least cuts about 25% of the extra carbs, fat and calories from the pie and it makes a nice presentation. My crusts do not have salt in them and neither will yours. Restaurant pies and those at your friend's house most likely will.

No matter your health challenge, food is necessary and planning ahead will make life a lot easier.

(Footnotes)

[1] Bread recipes in *The No-Salt, Lowest-Sodium International Cookbook* include Ethiopian Spice bread.

[2] www.healthyheartmarket.com

[3] Megaheart's wheretobuy.html page lists products and sellers and one of them is Amazon.com.

[4] Sucralose. There is also Stevia, however test it before you buy it.

[5] *The No Salt, Lowest Sodium International Cookbook*, Pages 27-28

[6] Adapted from USDA recommendations

Prep Chef For Yourself

Ever wonder who prepares all the ingredients that go into a meal you order in a restaurant? You've probably heard about K.P. duty in the military. KP stands for "Kitchen Police." In reality we are KPs serving as both prep chefs and clean up crew.

On those marvelous TV cooking shows the prep chefs wash, scrape, peel, cut, chop, slice and dice everything from onions to the main course. Some shows feature their prep kitchens, some don't. With professional chefs the rule is that the prep chef does not do any of the cooking, they only prepare what is to be cooked.

In the world of restaurant cooking and TV shows, the prep chefs are also responsible for keeping foods refrigerated or covered when necessary prior to being used. They are responsible for making sure food is properly stored.

One of the more important prep chef jobs is to make sure all the ingredients of an entrée about to be cooked are easily accessible, hygienically clean, and at the right temperature. We home chefs also have to shop for food and ingredients and believe it or not, food safety is part of what we should guard for. A few key points to remember while shopping:

· Purchase refrigerated or frozen items after selecting your nonperishables. (So they don't thaw before you get out of the store.)

· On warm days, carry a cooler in your car with some ice to store perishables while driving.

· Never choose meat or poultry in packaging that is torn or leaking.

· Do not buy food beyond the "Sell-By," "Use-By," or other expiration dates. Often markets will mark down meat products with one day left for a "sell-by" date. If you want to buy them to save money, which we do, but you aren't ready to prepare them in the next few days, then wrap them in foil, write the current date on the wrapper and freeze them. By writing the date on the wrapper you'll be reminded later when you thaw it that you have but a few days before you must cook it.

The Process of Cooking

In preparing your meals you'll also want to set out your planned cooking utensils including pots, pans, racks, oven ware, etc.

If you're new to cooking, then prepping for each meal will be a huge help during the process of learning. If you've been cooking all your life, then chances are you're already prepping without thinking about it.

Some recipes are easy to make, others a bit more complicated or time intensive. Either way, setting out ingredients and cookware will help things go along efficiently and in the end it will save you a lot of time.

For instance, let's say we're going to make a loaf of bread. We'll use the bread machine, which is supposed to be an easy process. But when making excellent no-salt-added bread you'll need a few more ingredients than just flour, water and yeast. Remember, too, that we can never use one of the prepackaged bread mixes, since they are usually high in sodium. So, let's put all the ingredients for our homemade bread on the counter top next to the bread pan. Let's work with a white bread recipe. We'll need water, extra virgin olive oil, vinegar, flour, sugar, ascorbic acid, vital wheat gluten, granulated onion powder and yeast and optionally potato flour, granulated soy lecithin, malted barley flour.[2]

We now have our ingredients ready, and we're about to save a lot of time and not forget anything. I place mine in the order I'm going to use them. Then one at a time they are measured and put into the bread pan. Bingo, the mix is complete. Pan goes into the bread machine and all the ingredients are stowed back where they belong. Total time? About five to six minutes.

Let's say that for lunch you want a burger. Set out the pan, meat, unsalted bun[3], no-salt-added ketchup, lettuce, onion, low sodium cheddar, and tomato. Then set out whatever you plan to serve with it like possibly unsalted chips or a Julienne sliced red pepper or some mini-carrots. Bingo again! Cooking time for 2 ounces of turkey burger about 6 to 8 minutes at the most. Prep time about 5. You've set out basically what you need and the burger goes together rapidly. You'll actually get to eat it while it's still hot.

Same goes for salads, soups, stews, sandwiches, and everything else you cook. Set each meal item out ahead of time and meal prep just sails along.

Dinners around here are a little more involved than just that, however. But the prep work is still the best way to go about it. Prep, cook and wash. Then clean the kitchen if things fly around you like they do around me. Compared to my style, Julia Child was Mrs. Neatnik.

Food Handling Is Important

When we eat out we trust restaurants to handle our food with near perfect cleanliness. The question for us is, do we do the same at home? Would you eat in a restaurant if you knew the owner's dog or cat had been on the counter top or sniffing the food in the fridge when they opened the door? How about setting raw chicken on your counter top, prepping it and then coming back later with a head of lettuce and putting it right where the raw chicken had been? Hands clean? Cookware clean? Utensils clean? Counter top cleaned?

I'm pretty particular about such things, and I believe you should be, too. If I want it done right in the restaurant, then I certainly want it done perfectly at home. When we handle food, hygiene is as important to our health as what we eat. For those of us with chronic ailments, adding another serious illness or disease could prove downright dangerous. The extra few moments to wash our hands and cookware during meal prep time is well worth it.

Food Preparation and Safety

You may have heard or read all this before, but we believe safety tips can never be overstated.

1. Always wash hands with soap and warm water before handling food and if handling beef, pork, poultry or fish, always wash hands after handling them and before handling other foods.

2. After using cutting boards and utensils with any meat or fish wash and scrub them with soap. Never place fresh vegetables on a surface that has not been completely scrubbed with soap and warm water. We use separate cutting boards, one for meats and one for vegetables and fruits. Possibly, for your health and that of others, you might like to adopt that policy.

3. Separate cooked foods from raw meat, poultry, or seafood in your refrigerator and on the counter top. Avoid purchasing meats that have been openly (unwrapped) displayed alongside each other in a grocery store or meat market. That is, poultry and beef and pork should not be in the same case, and fresh fish should always be in a separate case. Watch the meat handler to make sure they don't move from poultry to meat to fish without changing gloves or washing their hands. Apply the same rules to your own refrigerator.

4. Thaw all frozen meet in the refrigerator (sometimes you can thaw them in sealed bags or wrappings under cold water). Thaw cooked foods in the fridge or in the microwave using the defrost setting or other setting recommended by the microwave manufacturer. Always completely thaw meat and poultry before grilling so that it cooks more evenly. You can defrost beef in your microwave if the food will be placed immediately on the grill. Definitely thaw that Thanksgiving turkey in the refrigerator for up to three days before cooking. Keep other exposed foods away from it, even if the turkey is in a hermetically sealed wrap. (It is possible to thaw a packaged turkey under cold water as long as the whole bird is under water. This takes monitoring, however.)

5. When making one of our marinades, remember to let the meat marinate in the refrigerator and not on the counter top. The USDA states that you can marinate poultry, stew meat and cubed meat up to two days in a refrigerator. Lamb, beef, pork, veal, chops and steaks up to 5- days. Each should be covered.

6. *Very important.* Before serving, keep all cold foods cold and hot foods hot. It sounds easy, but sometimes we forget. Especially don't let salads containing dairy products sit out long.

7. Perishable foods should not sit out of the refrigerator for long periods of time. If you are going to freeze leftovers, do it right away.

8. Cook raw meats and fish as well as eggs thoroughly. Use a good clean thermometer to ensure that your meats are cooked to the recommended temperatures. It is difficult to use a thermometer with fish, so we simply make sure it's cooked all the way through (never overdone) before serving. It always cooks more quickly than you expect.

9. Be sure to bake casseroles for the recommended time or use a thermometer if necessary to determine if it's cooked thoroughly. Casseroles should be cooked to at least 140° F.

10. Some bread recipes have raw eggs in them. To make sure the bread is baked all the way through, use a long skewer to measure for moisture. Experienced bakers will snap their finger on the crust and listen for a hollow sound, which tells them the bread is baked through.

11. If you choose to stuff your turkey fill the cavities loosely. Cook the turkey immediately. Use a food thermometer to make sure the center of the stuffing reaches a safe minimum internal temperature of 165°F. (Tip provided by USDA)

12. Climate conditions can matter with food safety especially during hot summers. During warm season always have a cooler in the back of your vehicle when shopping for groceries, especially meat. Keep all meat, poultry and fish cold when transporting.

13. When reheating leftovers, before serving try to get them up to about 165° F or if no thermometer is available, steaming hot.

14. The USDA recommends throwing out cooked food that has been left out of the refrigerator for two hours or more, one hour if the temperature of the food has climbed higher than 89° F.

15. When barbecuing, before cooking meats or vegetables clean the grill thoroughly first and then heat the grill with flames.

16. When barbecuing we recommend convection cooking. Direct flame may char meats, and it is the charring that some researchers consider carcinogenic. You can cut charring down by removing most of the fat from your meat before cooking.

17. Pit roasting requires a thermometer. Pit roasting usually takes about ten or more hours depending on size of meat and its thickness. Be safe. Use the thermometer. (I filmed a pit-roasted wild pig in Tahiti in the seventies. There were no rules there other than dig the hole, line it with rocks, firewood, and coconut tree leaves, put the pig in, light the fire, cover the hole, and come back in eight hours. No thermometer, no particularly noticeable hygiene, just one roasted pig lifted out, placed on a wagon of sorts and taken over to the area where we would "enjoy" it, which we did. Leftovers were cut up and stored in a standing cabinet that was lined with "fly screen" material - and left out in the open to store like we might store cooked pork in a refrigerator. They ate the leftovers for a week and no one got sick. I didn't eat any of the leftovers but one of my crew members did, and he became awfully sick. "Maybe," our film biologist who also avoided the leftovers, said, "Americans live too cleanly and no longer can fight off some of this bacteria.[1]

A few more important points for our hygiene practices to remember include:

1. Cook everything to a proper temperature especially meats.

· Beef, veal, and lamb steaks, roasts, and chops may be cooked to 145° F.

· All cuts of pork, 160° F.

· Ground beef, veal and lamb to 160° F.

· All poultry should reach a safe minimum internal temperature of 165° F (We ensure this one with 170° F).

2. Cutting boards, utensils, and counter tops can be sanitized by using a solution of 1 tablespoon of unscented liquid chlorine bleach in 1 gallon of water.

3. Marinate meat and poultry in a covered dish in the refrigerator.

4. While Serving:

· Hot food should be held at 140°F or warmer.

· Cold food should be held at 40°F or colder.

· When serving food at a buffet, keep food hot with chafing dishes, slow cookers, and warming trays. Keep food cold by nesting dishes in bowls of ice or use small serving trays and replace them often.

· Place food into shallow containers and immediately put in the refrigerator or freezer for rapid cooling.

· Use cooked leftovers within 4 days.

(Footnotes)

[1]Our biologist in the Tahiti story noted to me later that he and I didn't get sick drinking the water either, although other crew members had contracted diarrhea. In the U.S., the biologist and I lived near each other in a rural area. We were used to drinking untreated water from our wells. It was his theory that we'd developed protection against certain bacteria that might be present in other water and food, but that those who became ill weren't protected because they drank treated city water. Today, after having moved from that country location, Maureen and I use filtered city water. Our filter cleanses the city-water of sodium and chlorine, which can kill bread yeast. We also like the non-chlorine flavor much better. We remember the well water as having tasted much better.

[2]Actually, you can make bread with fewer items than these, but these offer you freshness, flavor and longer shelf-life. The recipes in our *No-Salt, Lowest-Sodium Baking Book* are simpler and work just fine, but later in our experiments we tested mixes until we came to just the right combination of the above for a bread that could be stored in airtight containers outside of the freezer for up to a week.

[3]Defrost in microwave if it's frozen.

Eating Out In America

Restaurant sodium levels are much higher than anything you've ever eaten at home. If you eat out a lot, you'll find cutting salt out of your diet especially difficult.. This section walks us through a few specific subjects and a few different styles of restaurants. That said, here's a bottom line right at the beginning of this chapter concerning nearly all restaurants world wide:

- Ask your waiter what they can do to make a no salt, low sodium meal.
- Their meats may be brined even before they get them, but ask. Especially concerning chicken, pork, and ground beef may be salted or seasoned.
- Their fresh veggies should be steamed in unsalted water and not buttered.
- Very little butter, if any, should be used and it should be unsalted. Ask them to cook with extra virgin olive oil instead.
- For salad dressings try to get an extra virgin olive oil and vinegar mix (maybe a dash of sugar in it).
- Stick to fresh foods. If they use canned foods the sodium levels will be overboard.

Say No To Fried Foods

Restaurants and fast-food joints love to fry food. It's quick, easy and let's face it, tasty. However, we've learned the problems with a fried-food lifestyle. Frying adds more fats than when we broil, bake, or sauté. Up until recently, all restaurant fryers used partially hydrogenated oils, which were and remain a prime source of harmful trans fatty acids. Today many restaurants use non trans fat oils, but still, even with that we're adding more fat and possibly more carcinogens when we eat fried-food. Instead, ask waiters if they can bake or broil something for you rather than frying it.

Avoid Sauces and Cheese

Take a pass on food prepared with sauces and cheese. Sauces are usually loaded with salt and/or MSG, and commercial cheese is always high in sodium. Pass on gravy as well since it's high in sodium and usually saturated fat. (Nearly all recipes for gravy use pan drippings from meat, which of course are mostly saturated fat.) Sauces are generally made with salt, cream and other high sodium or saturated fat ingredients. Not too surprising for us, chicken and turkey skin with fat attached, contains about twenty-percent of the listed sodium. However, if we remove the skin and most of the visible fat we will have removed most of that sodium. Our cookbooks take this into account when we list sodium for various recipes with chicken in them.[1]

Avoid marinated and brined meats

Let's chat again about the brining challenge. Nearly all restaurants serve brined chicken and some even brine pork and shellfish. The chicken may have been brined during processing before delivery to the restaurant . Some chefs brine meat under the belief it "cooks better," or that it makes various meat cuts juicier. The only thing they do for sure, however, is increase the dietary sodium level by four to six times. Ask before you order. Has the meat been marinated or brined either by the chef or before it got to the restaurant? Either way, too much sodium has been added for our health. I usually end up with a fresh wild salmon dinner or sometimes a very small non-marinated steak with the fat cut off before it's cooked.

Check Kitchen Preparation (Oil, Salt, Spices, MSG)

We might want to take care of most of these questions by telephone before we show up at a restaurant, but if that isn't possible then ask your waiter or the Maître d' for answers and or exchanges. For instance, if a meal is made with butter or oil, ask them to use extra virgin olive oil (See Index: Olive Oil). If they don't have extra virgin olive oil, ask for expeller pressed canola oil. If they don't have that, then ask them if they can bake or steam or even sauté the dish without butter or any other cooking oil or fat. The less saturated fat you get, the better. Also, stay away from dishes prepared with cream or cheese. Many restaurants thrive on these. And if they state that all they add is Accent or "spices," ask them to hold off unless they name specific spices. Accent is pure MSG, and the words "other spices," used in the ingredients part of the FDA label often means MSG. In other words, if a processor uses "thyme" for instance, the ingredient label will say so. Unfortunately some spice makers use the wording *other spices* so as to not give away their total formula. The FDA by the way, permits this.

Size Matters

As to entrée size, we know we don't have to eat everything on our plates, but alas we are each human, and we generally do. Best bet: Take the leftovers home for the next day's lunch. Either split an entree with your spouse or friend or take half of it home. Weight Watcher advocates even ask for a ToGo box before their meal is served.

Eat A Snack Before Going Out

Never shop for food while you're hungry. I believe this applies to a couple of situations. I have found that eating a light snack of veggies or fruit or unsalted walnuts or almonds before going out often cuts my appetite just enough to not want to order more than I should. (See Walnuts in the glossary.) This idea works for me both before shopping in the grocery store and when going out to eat. With a snack neatly tucked away, that bucket of restaurant bread placed on our table alongside patties of butter doesn't look as appealing. The bread is usually white bread too, and white bread has a high glycemic level. (The GI, or Glycemic index is a measure of the effects of carbohydrates on blood glucose levels.) Restaurant bread is also very high in sodium.

Share Desserts

There was a time I enjoyed the fancy desserts in restaurants. Chocolate mousse or a fancy cheesecake would always win me over. But not now, not with their overabundance of sodium. Now, when we go out, we often order just one dessert. I'll take one bite and Maureen a few more. Then it gets wrapped and taken home for later or for the wee ones who drop by.

Hygienic Tip

Here's a tip from a doctor. The doctor was my father. Whenever he went into a restaurant that he'd not checked out before, he'd visit the men's room. If it was immaculate and had soap and enough towels for everyone, he'd eat there. His theory was that if it was dirty, not well kept that is, and lacked soap and towels, then the cooks, servers, and dishwashers probably weren't exactly "up to snuff." He would take a pass and find another more hygienic place.

Fast-food

Long considered great fun or a necessary adjunct to our hi-speed lives, fast-food is now looked upon as an evil influence to our health. At this writing, many of the eateries known as "fast food" places, have introduced what they refer to as healthier dishes, including salads, lettuce wrapped or grilled burgers, and a few other items that I'll mention soon. Needless to say, fast-food places are still hazardous to the health of the chronically ill and to many healthy people as well.

Still, with some of these places, there is a way to enjoy eating out.

Generally, fast-food means fried food, and often deep-fat-fried food. Fried food is defined as when using a skillet or griddle, and deep-fried or deep-fat-fried is when using a deep pan filled with cooking oil. As mentioned above, many fast-food franchises are offering healthier alternatives including salads, chicken sandwiches, and even grilled burgers. The ubiquitous French fries, however, remain a staple for burger joints even though they now compete with "healthier" choices.

The challenge we face with the healthier choices is that although they have cut down on the trans fats, they have not cut down on the sodium levels or the fat calories. That chicken sandwich is more than likely made with brined chicken that is then salted in-house or marinated with a salty mix Accent (MSG)[1]. To find out, you have to ask the owner or manager of each outlet, or check out the chain's nutritional information online.

The "healthier" salads may or may not be our best choice – it often depends on the dressing. If they have extra virgin olive oil and vinegar available then we're probably in good shape.

Tips for eating fast-food

If you must eat at a fast-food place, try to pick a local establishment. Most chains can't alter their meat or fries and some can't do anything concerning sulfite enhanced foods. Many chain restaurant items are prepared off-site. When ordering, ask them to leave the salt off your burger meat and to please remove any salt on the griddle. Ask them to leave off the cheese and the sauce; in other words, order it "dry." A healthy addition of fresh tomato, onion, and lettuce makes it tasty. If avocado is available and you like it, then enjoy. Always make sure they don't use butter to heat or grill your bun. Commercial sauce is often extremely high with added salt. Some fast-food, or local hamburger places might not be able to comply with your requirements concerning the meat since the meat they use may have been salted at the processing house, a common practice. Additionally, MSG components may have been added to help retain meat "color." Also, best to stay away from those bacon burgers. Way too much sodium, saturated fat, and the calories go through the roof.[2]

Also, fried fish sandwiches are among the worst, especially since they are often deceptively touted as "healthier." They are usually battered before deep-fat frying.[3]

French fries are hazardous to our health. Some locations however, use fresh potatoes and that's okay if you can get them without salt. Chains may use a "potato" that might very well be "stamped" into existence from potato fragments making each fry exactly like the other in color and appearance, and they nearly always arrive at the local facility pre-salted. For fat content, it's the oil they are fried in and how long they stay in that oil that matters to us. Since we have no control over that, we can simply leave them off the order or ask for an exchange like more tomato or lettuce in the sandwich. In some chain restaurants, you can order a baked potato instead of the fries. If so, ask that it not be buttered and if you need a "dressing" for your potato, see if they have low-fat sour cream (not the imitation IMO or similar. Imitation sour cream usually has three to four times more sodium per serving than regular sour cream).

Eating Out While Traveling In America

America has some fairly unique regional foods and meals. Many of these regions are still known for these special dishes, but unfortunately chain restaurants have pretty much altered the terrain into one common gastronomical geography. From Denny's[4] and McDonald's to IHOP, Ruby Tuesdays, Applebee's, Marie Calenders, etc., we can find identical food in any of the fifty states. Like red-top shopping centers with pastel walls, we have been inundated with over-salted commonness.

Locals, however, might retain their area's well-known diet practices like "grits" in the south and "Dungeness crabs" in the northwest, tacos in the southwest to deli sandwiches in New York. Rarely, however, will we find any of these places intentionally serving a no-salt meal. Some are trying to come up with a "low-sodium" meal, but careful, their idea of low-sodium and ours, might not be the same.

One way to be successful when traveling is to be armed with all the information you can obtain before leaving home. A recent development for restaurants is that many now list the nutrient data for their menu items instore and online. However, studies have shown that many are off by an average of about eight-percent. That's okay if you take that into consideration. A few local restaurants scattered around the country also provide similar information on the Web. Their data is derived from an average serving since the cook in one of their restaurants might serve more or less than a cook in another restaurant, therefore the difference.

In 2005, Maureen and I drove from California to upper New York and then down to D.C. and finally back to California through middle America. We spent 21 days on this trip, and I kept detailed notes concerning what we ate and where. In the end, about half our meals came out of a local super-market and were prepared in a motel room where we nearly always had a microwave and a refrigerator.

I also packed along enough no-salt or unsalted items to make sure we always had backup foods.

For the first seven days I was able to have my own bread, but after about seven days in a cooler salt-free bread begins to lose its freshness. Even in zipper lock bags the bread decides it's had it. Reminded me of Felix's question in the Odd Couple movie "What's that green stuff in the refrigerator?" Oscar (Jack Klugman) responded, "It's either very new cheese or very old meat."

The lesson learned on that trip encouraged me to alter recipes a bit. Today, my white bread will last up to 10-days in a cooler. I've added more vinegar and (optionally) potato flour along with soy lecithin, which helps lengthen shelf life and flavor. (If you're using our cookbooks, you can alter the bread recipes to two-tablespoons of vinegar for every 2.5 cups of flour. For each added tablespoon, remove one tablespoon of the primary liquid. You won't taste the vinegar.)

We visited local establishments mostly when we turned to restaurants and learned just how difficult it was to get what we wanted in some places, and how pleasant it was in others. Across the border in Canada, at Niagara Falls, we ate at *The Secret Garden Restaurant*, where I was pleasantly surprised with a low sodium meal. A lettuce wrapped burger cooked without salt. In Buffalo we found *Christina's Restaurant* in a Holiday Inn. They were not only accommodating, the meal was excellent.

From Park City, Utah to D.C. and back we enjoyed meals in a variety of restaurants. In a few places things didn't go as well as we'd like, but when that happens, you can take the lesson with you for your next stop.

Tips for eating in sandwich shops

Shops like Subway, Togo's, Quiznos and some local sandwich shops and even some grocery stores can make acceptable and sometimes tasty vegetarian sandwiches to order. (And always remember the "lettuce wrap" concept if you believe the bread is going to put you over the top for the day.)

The challenge is to get them to make sandwiches without mayonnaise, sauce, and without pickles, olives, marinated anything, peppers, etc. A standard vegetarian sandwich at Subway U.S. locations contains: iceberg lettuce, tomatoes, red onions, green peppers, olives and pickles. Ask them if they will exchange the peppers, olives and pickles for some fresh avocado or more tomatoes and onions. No sauce at all. The extra tomatoes or avocado will make the sandwich juicy enough. And the only sodium you'll really have to count is the bun unless you bring your own, which is highly recommended.[5] Remember too, you can flavor it up with a bit of olive oil and vinegar. (A 6-inch wheat bread at Subway has their lowest sodium level at 360 mg per bun. They promote a "foot long" sandwich with the same bun that has 720 mg of sodium per serving. Your homemade bun might have about 5 mg. It's best to take it along if you know you're going to visit any of the sandwich shops.

A typical sandwich roll in many shops will contain from 350 mg of sodium upwards to about 1500 mg or more. The high-end rolls with garlic or other flavors are also loaded with more salt. If you're stuck out there somewhere and need something to eat, why not order a half a sandwich? You'll be eating half the sodium and half the calories.

Bottom-line tips for eating in restaurants are:

1. Stay clear of menu items using cheese, sour cream or mayonnaise.

2. Consider asking the restaurant to bake, boil or grill unsalted fish or non-brined chicken for you. We stay away from shellfish. Most shrimp have been salted by a processor and sometimes is packaged or presented as "fresh" shrimp. Same with oysters unless fresh, however their natural sodium is high, and of course crab meat is totally out of the question. (3-oz raw Alaskan King crab has 710.6 mg sodium before it's cooked.)

3. Commercial bread is a minefield of problems. I once asked a family style restaurant owner who made his own bread how much salt he used. For my cured palate it tasted excessively salty. He explained that it was in the neighborhood of five-hundred milligrams of sodium

per serving. All that for a one-inch slice. Ever since then, I either avoid restaurant bread altogether or take my own.

4. A good salad made from a cloistered salad bar, or put together in the kitchen is always a very good meal if you can make your own oil and vinegar dressing.[6]

5. Get an extra plate. If you want to order just one meal and split it most waiters will bring you an extra plate. If you estimate the sodium or fat levels are too high, that's a great way to cut them in half and enjoy the evening. Restaurants generally charge an extra plate fee but happily some don't.

6. You might also ask for exchanges and often get them. Fresh veggies for the creamy, or fried foods. Yogurt or sherbet for the heavier desserts.

7. If you order a baked potato, add a tablespoon or two of real sour cream and leave the butter off.

8. Stay away from "all you can eat" restaurants. If you insist in dining at one, take a paramedic along.

Eating out in steak houses.

Steak houses generally serve steaks and lobsters and crab. Most steaks served in these establishments ripple with saturated fats. I suggest you explain to the waiter you would like a lean piece of meat, trimmed of fat before it's cooked and ask to have it grilled or barbecued without use of oil or butter, but definitely not fried or cooked on a griddle.[7] And then eat only about three-ounces of it.

We already know about crab as a no-no. Lobster is iffy. Usually the flavor of a lobster is "enhanced" with melted butter. That raises the stakes much higher. Northern lobster by itself contains 251.6 mg sodium per 3-ounce serving with very little saturated fat[8]. Add butter and the saturated fat level rockets up. (See my lobster recipe in this book.)

Steak houses will also bring you a basket of bread. The cautions listed above for other restaurants are the same here.

Never order the largest steak on the menu, but instead ask for the smallest non-marinated cut. Ask what size it is, and how much it weighs. Ask them to trim the fat off before cooking it. We really don't need more than three-ounces of lean meat (about 49.3 mg of sodium and just 1.807 grams of saturated fat with 123.3 Kcal). Enjoy steak for it's flavor and nutrients as well. Three-ounces of steak contain 17.9 grams of protein and generous amounts of calcium, iron, magnesium, and potassium among other beneficial nutrients. If the largest piece is too large, either plan on taking some of it home or splitting the order.

If you know you're going to a steak house then plan ahead and eat lightly during the day – mostly fruits and veggies. That will help reduce the calorie and saturated fat shock you'll give your body.

Eating out in ethnic-food restaurants

We have a wonderful array of ethnic restaurants in the U.S. that range from Cajun to Chinese, French, Italian, Indian, Japanese, Mexican, Thai, Vietnamese and a plethora of others. Some of these are national or regional chains, while many others are local eateries.

Most ethnic restaurants use salt a bit too generously. The high sodium for most of these foods is not naturally in the food but comes from the added salt (or the processed foods they use as ingredients). Some ethnic recipes use way too much saturated fat for cooking, as well as MSG as a standard ingredient. Again, we must look out for cheeses, creams, too much oil or butter, and even lard.

Maybe this is a good time to tell you about that filming experience. I was the director and camera operator at that shoot. I had a sound man, gaffer (lighting director), and a grip. We lighted the kitchen brightly. They had a line of stovetop burners that looked like it could handle a dozen cooks all at once. Each stovetop burner faced the wall. Behind the cooks who would face the stovetops was a very long stainless steel work area with a higher shelf facing away from the prep chefs who stood behind each of their cooks. The waiters brought the orders to the shelf from the back side, which faced the wall opposite from the stovetops. It was like walking down an alley when moving between the cooks and prep chefs. The flames that came from the burners made the place exceptionally warm. Giant woks were at each station. The restaurant was packed that day, as it usually was.

We filmed during lunch time. The kitchen was humming with activity although efficiently and smoothly, which is what the script called for. So I followed a waiter from the dining table to the kitchen. The order was for a fried-rice dish.

The prep chefs had stacks of fried-rice orders lined up for the cooks when the orders came in. It was their most popular dish. The prep guy would read the order, grab a bucket containing cooked rice, chopped vegetables and meat if it called for it, and then hand the bucket to the cook. The cook would pour a full cup of oil into the wok and heat it quickly. The stovetops are accurately described with the word "flames."

In under a minute the oil would sizzle hot as though boiling and the cook would dump his prepared rice into the wok. He'd stir it while adding some salt mixed with some Accent for under a minute, then adroitly pour the rice onto the plate used by the restaurant. Not a spec of rice would fall out of place. The chef had been doing this forever it seemed. He garnished it with parsley and then it went out to the table with the waiter's proper flair.

One order of rice now contained one cup of coconut oil. I was strong and healthy back then, but I shudder whenever I recall that scene.

Chinese restaurants are not all the same. The last time I ate in one I ordered steamed rice and some fresh steamed vegetables (steamed with unsalted water). They did it, but the wonder in their expressions told me they didn't do that for customers often. My best guess at that restaurant was to not eat their crisp noodles, but alas, I did accept the fortune cookie and later learned one cookie has only 21 mg of sodium and very little fat. I did ask them to not use MSG, soy sauce, or salt, which is a mandatory request that you'll have to make in any Chinese restaurant. MSG comes in a variety of ways and the mixtures or packages don't list the substances as MSG. (See MSG in the glossary.)

Japanese restaurants use teriyaki and soy sauce with most of their recipes. You can ask local Japanese restaurants to leave off the sauces and any added salt. You won't have to worry about fat since the Japanese don't generally serve fat-laden foods. Careful with that sushi though, the rice was probably cooked with salt. Our *No-Salt, Lowest- Sodium International Cookbook* has a very nice sushi recipe in it if you'd like to make your own. There's a URL link listed in it as well where you can visit an excellent chef preparing sushi. His video will clear up any confusion I may have created in writing directions for the recipe.

Indian cuisine uses a lot of curry, which has a health benefit as well as enhancing the flavor of food. Curry powder is largely composed of turmeric, but can also contain cumin seeds, coriander, garlic, cloves, fennel, and more.

Indian restaurants tend to serve lamb or beef for meat but most will have some chicken for you to order. Ask if it's commercial (which probably means brined), or fresh from a supplier who doesn't sell brined chicken. Their soups, as with all restaurants, are too high in sodium.

In most Indian restaurants you can ask for yogurt as well as steamed or fresh vegetables. Ask for steamed rice instead of their standard sauce covered rice. Stay away from fried or stuffed bread, but a Naan might work out for you if you eat just half of it. Naan will have about 170 to 250 mg of sodium. Naan is the Indian version of a flat bread. It is egg-shaped (or teardrop) and might remind you of a pita bread. We have a Naan recipe in *The No-Salt, Lowest-Sodium International Cookbook.*

Tips Concerning Other Food Services

In our fast-paced daily lives we now have access to "complete" meals in grocery stores, delis, gas station mini-marts, and sometimes in places we can't believe. (I expect today's geniuses will arrange for food to arrive via an iSomething futuristic device.)

More than likely very few of those meals has been prepared by a "chef" much less a practicing cook. I have yet to find a meal in any of these places that I could eat, mostly because of the fat and sodium in their food and a few times because of the presentation. I remember while in Los Angeles, CA while working "on the road," being led into an Asian "fast-food" place by a friend. Behind the glass enclosed counter they had at least a dozen tubs of deep fat fried this and thats. When I saw cold grease on some of them I was immediately turned off. My friend bought a buck of sesame fried chicken. The counter helper put it all into a bucket, stuck it into a microwave and heated it for a minute or two. The grease sizzled in the bucket when they handed it over to him. I ate two apples and a banana for dinner that night.

Pizza parlors are also definitely out of the running for heart-health. A single slice of most cheese-only pizzas will have about 400 mg of sodium. Start adding other items and you can get over 1,000 mg of sodium per slice, and that's from a medium size cheese pizza without any of the "deli" meat added.

It's Your Health

As you may have determined, no matter where you are in the world, the best bet is to keep your guard up and make sure the restaurant you visit does it your way not theirs. We've been lucky so far. In some restaurants the waiters have understood what we wanted because guests before us had already put them through the paces. In others we seemed to be the no-salt, low-saturated-fat pioneers.

It's our health so it's up to us to take control. Restaurants want our business, so don't back down.

Another matter concerning eating out. If you are with friends, try to put them at ease before you go out. Let them know that you might not eat a whole lot and if you don't drink alcoholic beverages, let them know that, too.

(Footnotes)

[1]Fat doesn't usually have much sodium in it, but skin does. We cut fat off to decrease

the saturated fat in what we eat.

[1] See MSG in the glossary to learn the many ways it is presented to us.

[2] One-Homemade Bacon, Cheeseburger using a homemade low sodium bun has 1,501 mg sodium. 1-commercial bacon cheeseburger contains 1,949 mg sodium.

[3] One fried fish sandwich, 3-oz fish contains 484.1 mg sodium just for the fish.

[4] At this writing Denny's offers some "low fat" meals, and has been known to offer a "low sodium" breakfast plate. Careful though, the K-calories and sodium levels are still pretty high. To find some nutrient values for Denny's you can visit http://calorielab.com/restaurants/dennys/21

[5] Most buns in sandwich shops are exceptionally high in sodium.

[6] If salad ingredients like the dressing or lettuce feel or taste warm or at room temperature, it's best to not eat them.

[7] Some steak houses and small restaurants in a few parts of the country fry their steaks.

[8] Spiny lobster, raw, 3-ounces, has 151 mg sodium.

[9] Figure based on large flour tortilla shell cooked especially for a salad.

Twenty Top Cooking Tools

If you're already a chef or cook, then you'll have your own idea of what the best tools in the no-salt kitchen might be. Here's our selection and why.

Bread Machine – Since many congestive heart failure patients lose strength and endurance at least during their first year or so, we decided that bread machines were a great item even if only used for kneading the dough. Turns out bread machines help most chronically ill patients including those with Meniere's, Lupus, kidney and liver ailments. Many of our bread recipes are thusly written for the kneading and first rise. We then remove dough, shape it, and bake it in the oven. Our favorite bread maker is posted at megaheart.com on the kitchen page – www.megaheart.com/kit_cabinet.html. These change from time to time since some manufacturers seem to change models more than we change clothes.

Ergonomic jar/lid opener – Same energy challenge as above. For years I was able to simply pop lids off even the most difficult of jars, but after CHF I couldn't do it with the tough ones. Standard bottle lid removers were not easily used either. So we found a product from "OXO," that's triangular in shape with a saw tooth grip. Very little strength required. If a lid is unusually tight I run warm water over the top of the jar for a few moments, then dip the lid only into a bowl of very cold water. Unscrew the lid easily with your hands or use the OXO lid remover again.

Braun Handheld Processor – Lightweight, does the job well, handy for small jobs like chopping nuts, and mixing sauces and salad dressings and pureeing. Particularly easy to use for making fruit Smoothies with fresh fruit and milk or yogurt. It will even crush ice to make a summertime treat. Good mixer that whisks well. Not built for heavy duty jobs. For heavier work we like the Kitchenaid.

Small Rice and Vegetable Steamer – Ease of preparing rice and fresh vegetables. Congestive heart patients generally have little energy or their spouses have more to do than before. So quick tools and comfortable tools have become our choices. The steamer doesn't overcook vegetables if set correctly, which leaves most of the nutrients in them. Great for white, brown and wild rice.

Nonstick Cookware – We encourage nonstick cookware since it requires very little fat to cook meats, vegetables or baked goods. We might add a bit of extra virgin olive oil for flavor but that's about it.

OXO Good Grips Salad Spinner – We found this salad spinner to be the easiest to use and it dries lettuce leaves after washing so thoroughly that you can store lettuce in zip lock bags in your refrigerator for up to one to two weeks without leaf burn.

Zipper Lock Bags – The best for storing fresh vegetables, freshly made bread, leftovers and other items to store in the refrigerator. Can be reused if clean and bag hasn't been storing meat products. Some zipper lock bags are built for freezing as well. These bags are indispensable for saving food and helping to cut down waste.

All-Clad Nonstick Griddle – Recommended when cooking for more than two people. We try to recommend brands because of manufacturer changes, but this griddle is the only nonstick griddle we have found that lasts and lasts and cooks evenly on your stovetop with very little oil. Get the smooth surface version, not the ribbed one. Expensive at first, it will pay for itself in efficient cooking more than a few times. Remember, nonstick requires nonmetal cooking utensils designed to be used with them so as not to scratch surface. Never cut on them, never hit them with cold water after cooking. Store upside down on shelf so other utensils or pots and pans don't damage them. (I must mention that cast iron cookware falls within this category as well. Many of us learned to cook on cast iron and we still enjoy doing so.)

Pizza Pan – We list this because our very low sodium pizza recipe has been the most popular Web site download of any recipe since 1997. Who doesn't love pizza? Make our pizza dough and load it up with your favorite vegetables from mushrooms to thinly sliced zucchini as long as the ingredients are without salt and very low in sodium.

Jelly Roll Pan – Sometimes referred to as a cookie sheet or baking sheet. Use parchment paper to cover pan before baking bread buns, cookies or French fries. Pan stays clean, food doesn't stick with parchment paper and you won't be adding fat. We have many of these since we do so much testing and creating of recipes. Two might work out well in most kitchens.

Frother – This handy gadget is great for making a nonfat milk froth to top hot cereal or a mocha or latte or even your cup of coffee. We also use it to stir up vinegar and oil salad dressings and other light sauces. Comes in battery powered or plug-in versions.

Panini Maker – You can get these for stovetop or electrical plug-ins like our favorite, the Breadman version. Makes a simple sandwich without added butter or oil. Make up your own panini recipes using our no salt bread recipes or your own. Use salt free fresh mozzarella or another low sodium cheese like Heluva Good Low Sodium Cheddar for your best sandwich. Of course, you don't always need cheese to make a panini tasty.

Scone Pan – My personal favorite since I love scones. When I was put on a no-salt diet I thought I'd lost the scones forever. But alas, we have some great no-salt scone recipes and they are easily made in this pan. We use the one from Nordic.

Beater/Mixer – If you don't want a bread machine in your life, you may still want something to knead your dough. A good mixer like the one from Kitchenaid is perfect for this role and of course it's great for mixing batters.

Hand Mixer – Easily operated and necessary for pancakes, waffles, cakes and other light batter.

.

These kitchen items are suggested for use with any recipes, not just ours. We have found these make life in the kitchen a lot simpler. There are of course other kitchen tools that are helpful and necessary, as well as kitchen supplies like parchment paper, aluminum foil, zipper lock bags, freezer containers, etc. Read on for other suggestions.

Additional Suggestions

Large Bread Board
Measuring cups with markers
Plastic utensils for nonstick cookware
Set of good mixing bowls
Elongated measuring spoons to dip into spice jars
Basting Brush
Whisk
4-Cup Measuring (pitcher shaped)
Nylon Turner (some refer to these as spatulas)
Mixing Bowls
Electric Beaters
Elongated Measuring Spoons (handy for standard spice jars)

Twenty No-Salt-Added Products You Want

We've listed scores of no salt added and unsalted products in a previous section. Now, we want to address what we've learned are the most important or possibly the most used products and why you'll want them in your pantry ready for use. If you can't find these locally, please visit megaheart.com/wheretobuy.html. We try to keep supplies and their sources up to date.

No Salt Added Tomato Products – You want to buy these products in bulk when on sale. They include canned tomatoes, tomato sauce, tomato paste. The tomato paste may not state "No Salt Added," but Contadina and other brands make their basic paste without salt. Check the ingredient label to make sure. You'll use these tomato products for soups, stews and sauces. Good brands for tomatoes and sauces are Hunt's, Muir Glen and Del Monte. Other brands also exist including some store branded products.

No Salt Added Eden Organic Beans – The cans will state "No Salt Added." Eden also makes salted beans so make sure you read the labels. Available at *www.healthyheartmarket.com* and possibly at your grocer, or health food store. Use these for salads, soups, stews, chili dishes, etc. Eden has a broad selection of beans. Visit edenfoods.com for the full list of their no salt added products.

Bread Making Ingredients – Our recipes might sound overwhelming at first but after making just one you'll get the hang of it. You don't have to use all these ingredients each time but the items listed below offer extra shelf life, better texture, and more flavor for each loaf or bun you make. See our *No-Salt, Lowest-Sodium Light Meals Book* and *The No-Salt, Lowest-Sodium International Cookbook*, and our Web site for recipes. See our *No-Salt, Lowest-Sodium Baking Book* for standard no-salt bread and muffin recipes.

Ascorbic Acid
Vital Wheat Gluten
Granulated Soy Lecithin
Potato Flour
Bread Machine Yeast or Active Dry Yeast
Onion Powder
Cider Vinegar

Splenda – In my opinion Splenda works well as a sweetener because it is made from sugar but without the calories and without sodium. Bakes, cooks and boils just like sugar.

Ener-g Baking Powder or Featherweight Baking Powder – Ener-g baking powder is double-acting, Featherweight is not. Both work when applied correctly. Basically Featherweight is potassium chloride. Because it is not double-acting, we have to mix it into the batter last and just prior to putting into oven. Ener-g Baking Powder is a mix of calcium carbonate, manganese, delta lactone and citric acid. No sodium.

Ener-G Baking Soda – Ener-G Baking Soda is essentially calcium carbonate. If converting one of your recipes, use three times more Ener-g than baking soda your recipe calls for. That is, 1-teaspoon of standard baking soda would take 3-teaspoons (a tablespoon) of Ener-g. Available from *www.healthyheartmarket.com* or you can locate HHM and this product at *www.megaheart.com/wheretobuy.html*

Spices & Herbs – Needed for flavoring. Many spices also contribute nutrients to our bodies that we might never get elsewhere. You can buy individual spices or rubs. Some spice mixes have salt added, so read the labels carefully. I like to keep a lot of different spices and herbs on hand, but my favorites for general use include thyme, marjoram, sage, curry, cumin, cayenne, paprika, cinnamon, mace, coriander, basil, dried dill, parsley, oregano, and nutmeg. There are others, but if you have the above, you can practically spice any food to taste better. Our favorite commercial rubs are from a company called Nantucket Offshore, however Healthy Heart Market has a few mixes that are also very good. Visit: *www.megaheart.com/wheretobuy.html* to locate Nantucket or Healthy Heart Market. You can find spice mix recipes to make yourself in *The No Salt, Lowest Sodium Light Meals Book*.

Pepper – Specifically cayenne pepper, white pepper, black pepper (coarse and ground), peppercorns and other "hot" spices.

No Salt Chili Powder – Wayzata Bay Chili Powder from Healthy Heart Market, *www.healthyheartmarket.com*. (Williams Original Seasoning (was Grandma's Chili Powder), are recommended in our cookbooks. Wayzata has a hot and a medium version while Williams has four varieties including a very good southwest mix..

Extra Virgin Olive Oil – We prefer extra virgin olive oil to other oils for use in cooking and salad dressings. With its delicate flavor, it's also considered "healthy." If you don't care for olive oil we recommend expeller pressed canola oil.

Unsalted Butter – We choose to use very little butter in our diet, but some recipes work better with it than with oil or applesauce (our favorite oil replacement ingredient). Since you may need butter with a few recipes, make sure it's unsalted.

White Unbleached Flour – Four listed as "best for bread machines" or "bread flour" have a higher level of gluten than standard all-purpose flour. Best for making your bread products.

All-Purpose, Unbleached Flour – All-purpose flour is used for baking cookies, muffins, batter breads and cakes. We store white flour in a dark pantry in an airtight container.

White Whole Wheat Flour – Also produced by some mills as white whole wheat pastry flour. Same nutrients as whole wheat flour. Standard whole wheat flour is heavier in texture and not as easy to work with in no salt bread recipes. Store in air tight container in refrigerator after opening. Bring to room temperature before using.

Unsalted Nuts – Pecans, walnuts, peanuts, almonds. These nutritious nuts will be used in recipes from time to time and can be kept in your freezer in zipper lock bags for a long period. Can be purchased in bulk or large packages at some discount grocery stores.

Dried Fruit – Included are seedless golden or black raisins, cranberry raisins, dates, prunes, apricots, apples, peaches and others that you like.

Unsalted Potato and Tortilla Chips – You don't have to give up chips. A good selection exists for unsalted potato and tortilla chips. Not always found in some markets, you can ask for them and many market managers will happily oblige. The chips come from the same people who make salted chips. Some brand names include Kettle Tim's, Michael's and others. Unsalted tortilla chips include Padrino, El Macero and others. To make a chip dip, mix up some Yo Cheese (See page 225) and stir in some Healthy Heart Market or Nantucket Off-Shore no-salt-added mixes like their Pueblo Mix or HHM's Toasted Onion Dip Mix, which is particularly good. Tortilla chips are always good with your homemade fresh salsa and/or Guacamole.

Breakfast Cereal – Post Spoon Size Shredded Wheat, Erewhon Organic, Crispy Brown Rice (cold and hot) Cereal, Arrowhead Mills Puffed cereals and a few others are our best choices.

Pasta or Noodles – It's always good to have noodles standing by in the pantry for those times when you wonder, "What's for dinner to-night?" and you haven't got an answer. I like the precut lasagna noodles that you don't have to boil before making a lasagna. And don't forget other varieties that work well in pasta salads. Also, rice, white or brown is always good to have on hand. Brown rice is healthier than white, but both are good choices.

Peanut Butter (Unsalted) – The best for a snack or sandwich with your homemade bread. Peanut butter has many healthy attributes, if that is, we don't overdo it. I like to use my own homemade jam when having a P & J for lunch. Once open, remember to store it in your refrigerator.

Additional No-Salt, Low-Sodium Foods We Recommend
Heluva Good Low-Sodium Cheddar Cheese
No Salt Added Ketchup (Enrico's, Hunt's, Del Monte, Others)
Unsalted Corn Tortillas
No Salt Added Ricotta (Whole Foods Markets, others)
Fresh Mozzarella
Rice Vinegar
Cider Vinegar
Balsamic Vinegar
Red & White Wine vinegar
Fresh citrus (lemons, limes, oranges, etc.)
Avocados
No Salt Added canned corn (and frozen)

No Salt Added frozen peas
Sour Cream
No Salt Added honey mustard (We like Mendocino Mustard)
Lindsay Low-Sodium Olives (black)
Canned no salt added green beans
Merino's No Salt Added Pole Caught Albacore tuna
(Other brands available as well)
Ezekiel 4:9 bread

For The Refrigerator – Nonfat or low fat milk, plain yogurt for cook and Yo Cheese, eggs, sour cream, and your choices of meats for a week or more (stored in the freezer unit).

Starter Kit

Check www.healthyheartmarket.com for a great starter kit at discounted price. HHM has filled a basket with all the right foods and ingredients to get you started on a low sodium lifestyle.

Unsalted or No Salt Added Food Products

Many unsalted food products have disappeared from grocery shelves since 1997, including mayonnaise, cheeses, breads and other selections. This list of "processed" foods and ingredients illustrates many of today's available no-salt-added or unsalted, and low sodium products. Others may exist as well. If you have a product you'd like to see added to this list in the future, please send it along via megaheart.com/contact.html. We will revise this book once a year with new additions. If you can't find any of these locally, either visit healthyheartmarket.com, megaheart.com, or search Google, Bing, or Yahoo for suppliers. Consider all brand names registered or trademarked.

Beans, No Salt Added (NSA)

Eden Foods, Organic No Salt Added Beans
Aduki Beans
Black Beans
Black Eyed Peas
Black Soybeans
Butter Beans (Baby Lima)
Cannellini (white kidney)
Garbanzo Beans (Chick Peas)
Kidney Beans
Navy Beans
Pinto Beans

Small Red Beans
Sun-Vista Pinto Beans
Broths / Soups
Better Than Bouillon Lobster Base, Beef Base, Mushroom Base,
Clam Base, Chicken Base
Campbell's Low sodium Cream of Mushroom Soup
Frontier Soups (multiple choices)
Health Valley Beef Flavored Broth
Health Valley Black Bean Soup
Health Valley Chunky Mild Chili
Health Valley Lentil Soup
Health Valley Minestrone Soup
Health Valley Mushroom Barley
Health Valley Organic Vegetable Soup
Health Valley Potato Leek Soup
Health Valley Tomato Soup
Morga Vegetable Bouillon Cubes
Rapunzel Pure Organic Vegetable Bouillon
Rapunzel Vegetable Bouillon Cubes

Bread

ZEVS Flat Greek Pita (Wal-Mart)
Ezekiel 4:9
Mrs. Wright's Very Low Sodium, Safeway Stores
Alvarado Bakery No Salt Sprouted Multi Grain
Trader Joe's Low Sodium

Cereals

Erewhon No Salt Crispy brown Rice Cereal
Erewhon No Salt Brown Rice Cereal
Arrowhead Mills, Whole Grain, Organic, Puffed
Arrowhead Mills, No Salt Added Puffed Corn
Arrowhead Mills, No Salt Added Puffed Millet
Millet Puffs, Nature's Path
Mona's Original Granola All Natural
Post Spoon Size Shredded Wheat
Erewhon Organic Crispy Brown Rice Cereal, No Salt Added
Raw Oats
Quaker Quick Oats

Cheese

Bothwell Unsalted Cheddar Cheese (Manitoba, Canada)
Farmers Cheese (good unsalted, alternative for cream cheese)
Heluva Good Reduced Sodium Cheddar Cheese (contains salt and potassium chloride. No longer has *Low Sodium Cheddar*)
Kutter's Low Sodium (Visit Megaheart.com for link)
Sargento Low Fat Swiss (30 mg slice, contains salt)
Sargento Colby/Cheddar, Muenster (Low-Sodium, contains salt)
Various local and regional brands

Crackers / Cookies

Osem Sunny Wheat Cracker
Devonsheer Plain Melba Toast
Good Health Peanut Butter Pretzels
Ka Me Unsalted Rice Cracker
Koyo Organic Dulsa No Salt Rice Cakes
Liebers, Cracker Snack Unsalted
Lundberg Farms Salt Free Brown Rice Cakes
Lundberg Farms Gluten-Free, Salt Free Brown Organic Rice cakes
Newman's Own Unsalted Popcorn, Organic
Edward & Sons Sesame No Salt, Fat-Free Snaps (gluten free)
Healthy Times Arrowroot Cookies, No Salt
Manischewitz Unsalted Matzos
Streit's: Unsalted Matzos Crackers
Venice Biscotti Chocolate Cookies, No Salt Added

Dried Fruit – Some Packaged as Snacks

Eden Organic No Salt Added Very Low Sodium
Dried Bing Cherries
Dried Cranberries
Dried Apples
Dried Mangos
Dried Pears
Dried Wild Blueberries
Montmorency Dried Tart Cherries
(from Stonehenge, Sensible Foods, Trader Joe's, Others)

Fish, Canned

(High anti-inflammatory food)
Brunswick Sardines in Spring Water
Crown Prince Brisling Sardines
Crown Prince Natural Alaskan Pink Salmon

Crown Prince Natural Solid White Albacore Tuna in Spring Water
Crown Prince Natural Solid White Albacore Tuna in Water
Crown Prince One Layer Brisling Sardines in Oil
Crown Prince Tongol Tuna
Merino's Unsalted Albacore Tuna
Natural Sea Brisling Sardines in Water
Natural Sea Wild Alaskan pink salmon
Natural Value Chuck Tongol Tuna in Water
Natural Value Chunk Tuna in Water
Natural Value Solid Albacore Tuna
Natural Value Traditional Pink Salmon with Skin and Bones
Raincoast Trading Company Pink Salmon
Raincoast Trading Company Sockeye Salmon
Raincoast Tuna Solid White Albacore
Season Blueback Red Salmon
Season Club Skinned & Boneless Sardines in Water
Season Fillets of Mackerel in Water
Season Kipper Snacks
Season Sardines in Tomato Sauce
Season Sardines in Water
Season's No Salt Added Club Sardines in Tomato Sauce
Wild Planet Wild Albacore Tuna

Flour

Eden Organic Hard Red Spring Wheat Flour
Eden Organic Pastry Flour (Soft White Wheat)

Hodgson Mills Organic Flours
Naturally White Unbleached Flour
Oat Bran Flour
Rye Flour
Soy Flour
Whole Wheat Pastry Flour

Bob's Red Mill
10-Grain Flour
Barley Flour
Flaxseed Meal
Gluten Free All Purpose Flour (GF)
Graham Flour
Light Rye Flour

Lowfat Soy Flour
Malted Barley Flour
Organic Hard White Wheat Flour
Organic Unbleached White Flour
Organic Whole Wheat Flour
Potato Flour
Soy Flour
Unbleached White Flour
Unbleached White Pastry Flour
Vital Wheat Gluten
Whole Wheat Flour
Whole Wheat Pastry Flour
Whole Wheat Pastry Flour

Arrowhead Mills
Organic Flax Seed Meal
Rye Flour
Spelt Flour
Stone Ground Whole Wheat Flour

King Arthur
Hi-Gluten Flour
KASL Flour for Pizzas
Organic All-Purpose Flour
Organic White Whole Wheat Flour
Pumpernickel Flour
Rye Flour
Unbleached All-Purpose Flour
Unbleached Bread Flour
Unbleached Pastry Flour
White Whole Wheat Flour
Whole Wheat Flour, traditional

Stone Buhr
Unbleached Cookie Flour (cookies, muffins, pies, cakes, pancakes)
Unbleached White Bread Flour
Whole Wheat Flour

Pillsbury
Bread Flour (contains ascorbic acid)
Unbleached All-Purpose

Pastry Flours
Gold Medal & Others also available

Herbs/Spice mixes/Rubs

Williams Original Chili Seasoning (formerly Grandma's Chili Powder)
Williams Chipotle Chili Seasoning
Williams Tex-Mex Style Chili Seasoning
Williams Chicken Chili Seasoning
Wayzata Bay Chili Powder (healthyheartmarket.com)
Mrs. Dash Unsalted (Most grocery stores)
Frontier (Healthy heart market)
Nantucket Off-Shore (Most have no salt)
Nutrifit Salt and Sugar Free Spice Blends (nutrifitonline.com)
Micky & T's (mickeysrubsandspices.com/) No Salt/No MSG

Meat / Fish, Frozen or Canned

Hormel Breast of Chicken
Salmon, Poached Sockeye (gift www.figis.com) No Salt

Miscellaneous

La Fish Fry, All Natural, No Salt (dry mix for fish, meat, etc.)
Earth's Best Organic Baby Food, No Preservatives, No Salt

Pasta, Noodles

Eden Foods Kamut Spaghetti. Whole Grain
Eden Foods Spinach Ribbons
Most Brands, most varieties are low sodium. Check FDA panels.

Rice/Grains

Brown Rice & Wild Rice
Buckwheat
Eden Organic
Kamut Flakes
Millet
Oat Flakes
Quinoa
Red Quinoa
Rye Flakes
Spelt Flakes

Sauces

Eden Organic No Salt Added Spaghetti Sauce
Enrico's NSA Pasta Sauce
Francesco Rinaldi NSA Pasta Sauce
Diana's Lime Wasabi Grill Crazy
Various local and regional brands

Sandwich Spreads

Arrowhead Mills Organic No Salt Peanut Butter
Laura Scudder's Unsalted Peanut Butter
Lundberg Maranatha Macadamia Butter Roasted, No Salt
MarNatha Unsalted Almond Butter, Crunchy Roasted
MarNatha Unsalted Almond Butter, Raw, Creamy
Nut Butter (Cashews, Almonds, Filberts, Hazelnuts)

Snacks (Each is unsalted)

Azar Nut Company Sunflower Kernels
Barbara's Unsalted Potato Chips
Beritos All Natural Unsalted Tortilla Chips
Blue Diamond Almonds, Oven Roasted, No Salt Added
Brown Rice Snaps
Dan-D-Pak Unsalted Cashews
Dan-D-Pak Whole Premium Cashews
Devonsheer Plain Melba Toast
Garden of Eatin' Blue Chips
Genisoy Soy Nuts
Glenny's Soy Crisps, no salt added
Good Sense Roasted Peanuts
Guiltless Gourmet Unsalted Yellow Corn Tortilla Chips
Health Best Almonds
Health Best Soy Nuts, Dry Roasted
Healthy Heart Market Popcorn
Ka-Ma Rice Crunch
Keenan Farms Pistachio
Kettle Unsalted Potato Chips
Kirkland Unsalted Walnuts, Pecans, Almonds (Cosco)
Klein's Natural Mixed Nuts with Peanuts
Klein's Naturals Almonds, Dry, Roasted
Klein's Naturals Almonds, Roasted
Klein's Naturals Cashews
Klein's Naturals Peanuts, Roasted
Klein's Naturals Pistachios

Klein's Naturals Pumpkin Seeds
Klein's Naturals Sunflower Seeds
Little Bear Yellow Chips
Lundberg Organic Brown Rice Cake
Maisie Jane's Organic Natural Pistachios
Manishewitz Matzo, Thin, Unsalted
Mauna Loa Dry Roasted Unsalted Macadamias
Melissa's Roasted Unsalted Soy Nuts
Michael's Unsalted Potato Chips
Newman's Own Organic Popcorn
Now Foods Corn Off The Cob
Now Foods Roasted Unsalted Sunflower Seeds
Now Foods Soybeans
Old London Unsalted Melba Toast
Padrino's Unsalted Tortilla Chips
Pepita's Pumpkin Seeds
Planters Unsalted Cocktail Nuts
Planters Unsalted Mixed Nuts
Planters Unsalted Peanuts
Royal Oak Gourmet Jumbo Virginia Unsalted Peanuts
Shibolim Whole Spelt K'nockers
Snack Master Turkey Jerky (No Salt Added)
Snak King Unsalted Cashews
Snyder's of Hanover Unsalted Mini Pretzels
Sunflower seeds, Unsalted
Terra No Salt Sweet Potato Chips
Tim's Unsalted Potato Chips
Trader Joe's Organic White Tortilla Chips
Uncle Ray's Unsalted Potato Chips
Virginia Diner Unsalted Gourmet Jumbo Cashews

Soups, No Salt Added

Healthy Valley, No Salt Added (Large Variety of soups)

Spices, Spice blends, Salt-Free

Frontier
Healthy Heart Market
Homemade
McCormick (some)
Mickey T's
Mrs. Dash

Penzeys Spices
Spicehunter
Spiceman
Williams
Wayzata Bay

Tomato Products, No Salt Added

Store Brands like Safeway, Kroger, others.
Academia Barilla, Pitted Cherry Tomatoes
Bella Sun Luci Sun Dried Tomato Halves (Excellent)
Contadina (no salt) tomato paste
Del Monte NSA Diced Tomatoes 14 oz
Del Monte NSA Stewed Tomatoes 14 oz
Del Monte NSA Tomato Sauce 8 oz, 15 oz
Del Monte NSA Basil, Garlic & Oregano Diced Tomatoes
Eden Organic Crushed Tomatoes
Eden Organic Crushed Tomatoes with Basil
Eden Organic Crushed Tomatoes with Onion and Garlic
Eden Organic Diced Tomatoes
Eden Organic Diced Tomatoes with Basil
Eden Organic Diced Tomatoes with Green Chilies
Eden Organic Diced Tomatoes with Roasted Onion
Health Valley Tomato Soup
Heinz NSA Tomato Ketchup
Hunt's No Salt Added Stewed Tomatoes
Hunt's No Salt Added Tomato Paste
Hunt's NSA Tomato Ketchup
Hunt's Whole Tomatoes
Muir Glen canned tomatoes
Muir Glen Organic Tomato Sauce
Muir Glen Organic No Salt Diced Tomatoes
S&W NSA canned tomato sauce
S&W NSA canned tomatoes

Note: Read all ingredient labels. Some imported canned vegetables such as tomatoes might how "0 Sodium" no the FDA food panel, but have added salt, which is listed in the ingredients. An example is a tomato product from Italy called Academia Barilla. They provide the FDA label but the nutrients listed are definitely inaccurate.

Trader Joe's

Most of their dried fruit
Unsalted Peanut Butter
Frozen Fish

Vegetables

Del Monte NSA Corn - Golden Cream Style 14 oz
Del Monte NSA Corn - Golden Summer Crisp 11 oz
Del Monte NSA Corn - Golden Whole Kernel 8 oz, 15 oz
Del Monte NSA Green Beans - Cut 8 oz, 14 oz
Del Monte NSA Green Beans - French Style 14 oz
Del Monte NSA Mixed Vegetables 14 oz
Del Monte NSA Spinach - Cut Leaf 13 oz
Del Monte NSA Sweet Peas 8 oz, 15 oz
Healthy Valley Organic vegetable soup
Libby's Pure Canned Pumpkin

If you have a favorite low sodium product that might be available in large geographic areas, please submit them to us and we'll including them in future printings of this book. Thank you.

To E-mail, just visit megaheart.com and click no the contact page.

RECIPES

NUTRIENT DATA IN THIS BOOK

We use The Nutrition Company's software FoodWorks to analyze all recipes in this book as well as our previous books and at our Web site, Megaheart.com.

FoodWorks is a software that uses USDA data exclusively. For this edition FoodWorks uses the USDA National Nutrient Database for Standard Reference, Release 21: This data forms the basis of nearly all nutrient analysis software systems. It contains information for more than 7000 food items including some name brand foods, primarily in the categories of ready-to-eat breakfast cereals, candies, infant formulas, and fast foods. This database was commonly referred to as Handbook 8 when it was available in printed form.

FoodWorks uses a simple, intuitive food selection process that allows even beginners to quickly master the art of nutrient analysis. Tasks from simple analysis of a recipe to complex multiple-day cycle menus are easily performed. FoodWorks is the offspring of a rich ancestry of analytical software dating back to 1979. More than three decades of effort and experience have resulted in the current edition of FoodWorks.

You may be interested in using FoodWorks at home. It's quite easy. For diets, just select foods eaten and personal data (age, gender, height, weight, etc.). For menus and recipes, simply select the foods or ingredients used. FoodWorks will generate the information you need in seconds! The on-screen help functions and the exclusive *"ShowMe"* tutorials will guide you step-by-step through all the jobs you need to perform.

You can learn more about FoodWorks at *http://www.nutritionco.com.*

The Nutrition Company has been highly supportive of our Web site and our books and for that, we thank them enthusiastically.

Legend

1. The mg numbers after an ingredient reflect the sodium level for that ingredient.
2. (trace) means that an ingredient may have a trace of sodium in it but at any rate the sodium listed by the USDA was too low to affect the recipe.
3. Named products in a recipe mean only that is the product we used to create the recipe. If other no-salt-added or unsalted products are available in your area, then you can use those.
4. Carb Choices for diabetics are listed at the top of each recipe as: Carb Choices. Fiber has been calculated into each listing. When fiber is over 5 grams, it may be subtracted from the carbohydrate value before calculating choice rating. To figure CHO exchange, divide total Carbohydrate by 15.

5 Vegetarian ratings are listed before Carb Choices at the top of each recipe.
Ratings Read: Vegan, Lacto Vegetarian, Lacto-ovo Vegetarian, Flexitarians (See: Glossary for Vegetarians)

6. Splenda has a substitute for most sugars from confectioner's to granulated. When using Splenda Granulated use only half what a recipe calls for.

Note to Vegetarians: Some of our bread recipes use egg white for bread coating prior to cooking. You may use a light coat of oil instead. The purpose is for even browning, and although egg white works better, oil also does the job.

APPETIZERS & DIPS

GUACAMOLE

VEGAN - 0 CARB CHOICES

Makes 1 cup   Sodium Per Recipe: 55 mg   Sodium Per Tablespoon: 3.34 mg

When one of our daughters called and told us her husband had just purchased over 700 acres of avocado and lemon trees we nearly fell off the planet. That's a lot of trees, about 35,000 of them. And that many trees produce a huge number of avocados and lemons. At first I was impressed and then I started laughing and said, "That's a lot of guacamole."

1 ripe medium California avocado (10.9 mg)
1 tablespoon lemon juice (fresh or bottled) (.305 mg)
3 tablespoons Don's nonfat Yo Cheese (34.9 mg)
1 Roma tomato, diced or chopped, seeded (4.55 mg)
1 small onion, chopped (4.4 mg)
¼ teaspoon no salt added chili powder (Wayzata Bay[1]) (trace)

Crush avocado, lemon juice together with fork. When softened add chili powder, sour cream and crush some more. Fold in tomato until evenly distributed. Chill and serve with no salt potato or corn chips.

[1]Wayzata Bay Spice Company available at healthyheartmarket.com.

Guacamole Nutrient Data Per Tablespoon: ***Calories: 19.7, Protein: .496 g, Carbohydrate: 1.845 g, Dietary Fiber: .728 g, Total Sugars: .406 g, Total Fat: 1.335 g, Saturated Fat: .187 g, Monounsaturated Fat: .837 g, Polyunsaturated Fat: .16 g, Cholesterol: .086 mg, Trans Fatty Acids: 0 g, Total Omega-3 FA: .02 g, Total Omega-6 FA: .001 g, Calcium: 8.527 mg, Potassium: 72.6 mg, Sodium: 3.34 mg, Vitamin K: 2.252 mcg***

LOW SODIUM NACHOS

LACTO OVO VEGETARIAN - 1½ CARB CHOICES[1]

Makes 15 Servings

Sodium Per Recipe:138.3 mg   Sodium Per Serving: 9.219 mg

1 bag of unsalted tortilla chips[2] (72 mg)
2 fresh jalapeno peppers or fresh anaheim chilis, seeded, chopped after roasting (6.3 mg)
6 ounces shredded low sodium cheddar[3] or shredded or thinly sliced low-sodium Swiss cheese (60 mg)

Wash peppers, split open, clean out and throw away seeds. Braise over open flame for a few minutes or under preheated broiler, skin side up. Chop finely.

Spread chips on a large lightly oiled or parchment covered jelly roll pan (cookie sheet). Sprinkle chilis over the chips, then grate a light layer of low sodium cheddar or other low sodium cheese, spreading it evenly over chips.

Preheat oven to 350° F. Bake for about 10- minutes or until cheese has melted. Serve hot. Optionals include Yo Cheese, Unsalted Salsa, Cilantro or Guacamole.

[1]Diabetics, nearly all the carbohydrates are in the chips.

[2]Many brands of unsalted tortilla chips are on the market. If you can't find them locally, then check with www.healthyheartmarket.com

[3]We know of only one nationally distributed low sodium cheddar cheese today. Visit: *http://www.megaheart.com/wheretobuy.html* for current availability and merchant.

Low Sodium Nachos Nutrient Data Per Serving: Calories: 207.3, Protein: 5.412 g, Carbohydrate: 21.5 g, Dietary Fiber: 1.786 g, Total Sugars: .626 g, Total Fat: 11.1 g, Saturated Fat: .788 g, Mono-unsaturated Fat: 3.047 g, Polyunsaturated Fat: 3.192 g, Cholesterol: 10 mg, Trans Fatty Acids: 0 g, Total Omega-3 FA: .351 g, Total Omega-6 FA: 0 g, Calcium: 136.8 mg, Potassium: 89.2 mg, Sodium: 9.219 mg, Vitamin K: 1.082 mcg

PARTY SANDWICHES

FLEXITARIAN – 1 CARB CHOICES

Makes 8 4" Luncheon Sandwiches or 32 Party Sandwiches

Sodium Per Recipe: 258.9 mg   Sodium Per Party Sandwich (32): 7.322 mg

This recipe works with chicken, turkey, beef, or pork. We use pesto and either low sodium cheddar cheese or fresh mozzarella[1]. You can cut these to 1" thickness for party appetizers or sandwich length for picnics, or to store in your refrigerator for lunch during the week.

1 Classic French Bread Recipe (17.4 mg)
2 tablespoons extra virgin olive oil
1 recipe Don's Basil Pesto (Page: 270) (.688 mg)
8 ounces thinly sliced cooked meat of choice (153.4 mg[2])
6 ounces low-sodium cheddar (35.7 mg)
½ egg white, whisked with a dash of water[3] 27.4 mg)

Make Classic French Bread dough[4]. When dough is ready, split in half.

Prepare baking pans with parchment paper.

Preheat oven to 400° F.

Roll out first half with rolling pin until thin. Brush dough with one-half the olive oil. Brush or spread half the pesto, then half of the meat and other ingredients on the dough. Cover with cheese. Leave an inch or two of dough on the perimeter uncovered.

Roll tightly length wise to form a log. Baste dough with the egg white.

Set on parchment paper lined baking sheet or in paper lined French bread pan. Roll out second half and do the same. Let dough rise for about fifteen minutes at room temperature.

After dough as risen, place into pre-heated oven, reduce heat to 375° F and bake for 18 to 22 minutes, or until golden brown. Note: Ovens vary. If it takes longer than 22 minutes then write down the time it took on this page.

When done, let cool on rack.

Slice diagonally in 1" to 1 1/2" widths. For picnic or sandwiches to store for future use, slice in 4" to 5" lengths. May refrigerate in zip locked bags.

[1] Some fresh mozzarella is packed in salt water. Wash clean. Sodium level will be about 25 mg per ounce. [2]Approximate. [3] Sodium level figured for half of the egg white since that's about what we use. Whisk all the egg white, however, since splitting it in half is nearly impossible. [4]Recipe is in this book

Party Sandwiches Nutrient Data Per Serving: Calories: 103.2, Protein: 5.045 g, Carbohydrate: 12.8 g, Dietary Fiber: .506 g, Total Sugars: .559 g, Total Fat: 3.403 g, Saturated Fat: 1.341 g, Monounsaturated Fat: 1.269 g, Polyunsaturated Fat: .543 g, Cholesterol: 9.593 mg, Trans Fatty Acids: .002 g, Total Omega-3 FA: .035 g, Total Omega-6 FA: .001 g, Calcium: 41.4 mg, Potassium: 50.1 mg, Sodium: 7.332 mg, Vitamin K: 1.607 mcg

HOT BUFFALO WINGS

FLEXITARIAN – 1 CARB CHOICES

Makes 10 Sodium Per Recipe: 261.3 mg Sodium Wing: 26.1 mg

We had five children around a large round dining table and when we served baked, barbecued, or fried chicken, the arm reach of each child seemed to be like that of the old comic character, "Plastic Man." Except for Maria. She was the youngest and through all those years I hadn't recognized that she always ended up with the chicken wings. After a while she started to say that was because she "liked" them. So, here, just for her and you, are one of my favorite hot chicken wing recipes. Written down and added to his book after receiving a request from a Megaheart.com visitor.

1 dash ground black pepper (.044 mg,)
1 dash unsalted garlic powder (.091 mg,)
1 dash granulated onion powder (.162 mg,)
⅛ teaspoon ground ginger (.072 mg,)
½ cup all-purpose flour (1.25 mg,)
¼ teaspoon paprika (.178 mg,)
¼ teaspoon cayenne pepper (.135 mg,)
10 chicken wings (234.9 mg)[1]

In a small bowl mix together the flour, black pepper, garlic powder, onion powder, ginger, paprika, and cayenne pepper. Place chicken wings in a large non-porous plastic or paper bag along with the flour mix. Shake bag until wings are covered well with the mix. Place on cooking sheet covered with parchment paper. Bake at 325° F for about 20 to 35 minutes (ovens vary), or until golden brown.

Prepare our *Hot Dipping Sauce* (24.4 mg,)[2] (Page 251)

[1] Skin removed. Meat only. If skin on, 38.5 mg sodium per wing.

[2] or *Mr Spice Hot Wing Chicken Sauce* available at healthyheartmarket.com

Hot Buffalo Wings Nutrient Data Per Serving: Calories: 87.6, Protein: 5.982 g, Carbohydrate: 4.872 g, Dietary Fiber: .209 g, Total Sugars: .038 g, Total Fat: 4.709 g, Saturated Fat: 1.312 g, Monounsaturated Fat: 1.849 g, Polyunsaturated Fat: 1.018 g, Cholesterol: 22.3 mg, Trans Fatty Acids: .055 g, Total Omega-3 FA: .06 g, Total Omega-6 FA: 0 g, Calcium: 4.717 mg, Magnesium: 6.851 mg, Potassium: 54.8 mg, Sodium: 21.4 mg, Vitamin K: .114 mcg

TORTILLA CHIPS

VEGAN – 0 CARB CHOICES[3]

Makes 96 Chips   Sodium Per Recipe: 39.5 mg   Sodium Per Chip: .412

We like to make our own chips for parties. It's really very easy and you can give them any flavor you like from plain to onion, garlic, hot pepper and more. We use corn tortillas for this since commercial flour tortillas are usually high in sodium. Most corn tortillas (but not all) are around 5 mg sodium per tortilla. Use our Yo Cheese Spice Dip, Guacamole, or any no-salt-added salsa with these. Also great for tortilla soup.

1 teaspoon cumin, ground (3.528 mg)
½ teaspoon unsalted chili powder[1] (trace)
½ teaspoon granulated onion powder (.648 mg)
12 6" corn tortillas[2] (34.3 mg)
1 tablespoon extra virgin olive oil (trace)
3 tablespoons fresh lime juice (1.012 mg)

You will need parchment paper and a spray bottle or mister.

Preheat oven to 350° F.

Mix together the dry ingredients and set aside.

Cut each tortilla into 8 wedges (across the top like a pizza). This will produce 96 wedges. Place on a parchment paper-covered jelly roll pan (large cookie sheet) in a single layer. If too many for your sheet, then be prepared to bake the remaining chips after the first. Don't try baking two sheets in the same oven.

Mix the olive oil and lime juice together briskly. Spray or sprinkle each wedge until lightly moist. Evenly sprinkle or dust the chips with the spice mix. You can also make up your own flavored mix if you prefer or use one of the spice mixes from any of the popular no salt added commercial mixes.

Bake in preheated oven for 6 to 7 minutes. Rotate pan in oven and bake for another 6 to 7 minutes or until chips are crisp. Don't let them brown.

[1] Adjust for heat. If your chili isn't "hot," then add a tablespoon.

[2] Recipe works with larger tortillas as well. Just add a bit oil/lime juice and spices.

[3]Diabetics: Carbohydrates rated per chip. You can select the number that fit your diet for the day.

Tortilla Chips Nutrient Data Per Chip: Calories: 8.787, Protein: .193 g, Carbohydrate: 1.584 g, Dietary Fiber: .174 g, Total Sugars: .014 g, Total Fat: .234 g, Saturated Fat: .032 g, Monounsaturated Fat: .094 g, Polyunsaturated Fat: .086 g, Cholesterol: 0 mg, Trans Fatty Acids: 0 g, Total Omega-3 FA: .002 g, Total Omega-6 FA: 0 g, Calcium: 6.01 mg, Potassium: 6.13 mg, Sodium: .412 mg, Vitamin K: .035 mcg

YO CHEESE ONION DIP

LACTO OVO VEGETARIAN - 0 CARB CHOICES

Makes One Cup

Sodium Per Recipe: 189.2 mg   Sodium Per Tablespoon: 11.8 mg

Making your own dip allows you to get as creative as you want. This recipe makes it easy to whip together a quick dip. Add some chili powder, garlic, avocados, salsa, or finally chopped scallions. The Yo Cheese recipe is in this book (See: Index)

1 cup nonfat homemade Yo Cheese (186.2 mg)
1 tablespoon Healthy Heart Market Onion Mix (2.459 mg)
1 to 2 teaspoons lime or lemon juice (.581 mg)

Combine all ingredients in small bowl and mix. Eas as that! Add other ingredients if you like.

Works as a dip for unsalted chips or vegetables like celery, carrots, sweet bell peppers.

Onion Dip Nutrient Data Per Tablespoon: Calories: 13.1, Protein: 1.231 g, Carbohydrate: 1.975 g, Dietary Fiber: .023 g, Total Sugars: .132 g, Total Fat: .035 g, Saturated Fat: .015 g, Monounsaturated Fat: .009 g, Polyunsaturated Fat: .003 g, Cholesterol: .459 mg, Trans Fatty Acids: 0 g, Total Omega-3 FA: 0 g, Total Omega-6 FA: 0 g, Calcium: 31.8 mg Potassium: 43.9 mg, Sodium: 11.8 mg, Vitamin K: .023 mcg

GARBANZO BEAN DIP

LACTO OVO VEGETARIAN - 1 CARB CHOICES

Serves 8 to 10 Sodium Per Recipe: 177.7 Sodium Per Serving: 22.2 mg

I remember being somewhere in Florida when I first came across this dip. I was writing a film script for a producer and showed up with some chips and a prepackaged container of "Chickpea" dip. It was okay but not great. So I started playing with it and eventually, using fresh ingredients, I came up with this version. Very tasty and liked by everyone who's tried it. Oh, the script was so good it never made it to the screen.

1 15-ounce can Eden Organic No Salt Added Garbanzo beans (drained & rinsed) (70
3 mg)
¼ tablespoons fresh lemon juice (.587 mg)
¾ teaspoon sesame chili oil (trace)
½ tablespoon extra virgin olive oil (trace)
¼ cup Yo Cheese (Page 233) (93.2 mg)
1 teaspoon no-salt chili powder (trace)
½ cup cucumber, peeled, chopped (2.66 mg)
⅓ cup red onion chopped (3.2 mg)
2 cup red bell pepper, seeded, chopped (1.985 mg)

To make garbanzo dip combine the garbanzo beans, lemon juice, chili oil, olive oil, Yo Cheese, and chili powder in a blender or food processor until smooth. Taste test. If you want more chili powder or lemon add it in. Place into a dipping plate or bowl.

Put cucumbers, onion, bell pepper and tomatoes into a small mixing bowl and gently stir together. Spoon this mixture on top of the Garbanzo dip, leaving an open area near the edge.

Serve with unsalted tortilla or potato chips, carrots, celery, or some homemade crackers.

Garbanzo Bean Dip Nutrient Data Per Serving (8) 1 Carb Choices: Calories: 141.2, Protein: 7.753 g, Carbohydrate: 21.1 g, Dietary Fiber: 5.007 g, Total Sugars: 1.498 g, Total Fat: 2.781 g, Saturated Fat: .221 g, Monounsaturated Fat: .66 g, Polyunsaturated Fat: .469 g, Cholesterol: .459 mg, Trans Fatty Acids: 0 g, Total Omega-3 FA: .009 g, Total Omega-6 FA: 0 g, Calcium: 37.6 mg, Potassium: 135.2 mg, Sodium: 22.2 mg, Vitamin K: 3.046 mcg

Garbanzo Bean Dip Nutrient Data Per Serving (10) (1 Carb Choice): Calories: 112.9, Protein: 6.203 g, Carbohydrate: 16.9 g, Dietary Fiber: 4.006 g, Total Sugars: 1.198 g, Total Fat: 2.225 g, Saturated Fat: .177 g, Monounsaturated Fat: .528 g, Polyunsaturated Fat: .375 g, Cholesterol: .368 mg, Trans Fatty Acids: 0 g, Total Omega-3 FA: .007 g, Total Omega-6 FA: 0 g, Calcium: 30.1 mg, Potassium: 108.1 mg, Sodium: 17.8 mg, Vitamin K: 2.437 mcg

Note: 5.007 g of fiber subtracted from 21.1 g of carbohydrate equals 16.1 g of carbs. Therefore, carb choices computes to 1.

BREAKFAST

Breakfast is often touted as the most important meal of the day and in fact, it is. Breakfast sets us up for the rest of the day. Research has shown that children and adults do much better during the day after a healthy breakfast. Whether you are healthy now or have a chronic illness, breakfast is a must. Please don't skip it. Our bodies need beneficial nutrients spread out over the day. Also, if you're taking medications, you'll want to be as timely with each meal or snack of the day as you are with your medications.

We make sure to include some fiber (like the flaxseed meal in the waffles below) and some protein, (the egg below). Fiber is best found in whole grains, vegetables and fruits.

VERY EASY BELGIAN WAFFLES

LACTO-OVO VEGETARIAN - 1½ CARB CHOICES

Makes 5 Waffles

Sodium Per Recipe: 175.6 mg Sodium Per Waffle: 35.1 mg

Maureen's basic pancake and waffle mix when we first married was, "One, One and One." When I asked what that meant she said, "One flour, one egg, one milk, one baking soda and one melted butter." Sounded simple to me, so I changed a few ingredients but kept the "ones."

1 cup unbleached all-purpose flour (2.5 mg)
1 cup nonfat milk with vitamin A[1] (103 mg)
1 large egg (79 mg)
1 tablespoon grated orange or lemon peel (.18 mg)
1 tablespoon Ener-G Baking Powder (trace)
1 level tablespoon flaxseed meal (trace)

In a small or medium size mixing bowl, beat milk and egg lightly and then stir in the rest of the ingredients..

Bake in a Belgian waffle iron to manufacturer's specifications. Serve hot with favorite topping.

[1] May exchange for 1% low sodium buttermilk. See Buttermilk in Glosssary for available low sodium brands.

Belgian Waffles Nutrient Data Per Serving: Calories: 132.1, Protein: 5.81 g, Carbohydrate: 22.9 g, Dietary Fiber: 1.202 g, Total Sugars: 2.639 g, Total Fat: 1.731 g, Saturated Fat: .374 g, Monounsaturated Fat: .413 g, Polyunsaturated Fat: .242 g, Cholesterol: 43.3 mg, Trans Fatty Acids: 0 g, Total Omega-3 FA: .014 g, Total Omega-6 FA: 0 g, Calcium: 72.2 mg, Potassium: 119.1 mg, Sodium: 35.1 mg, Vitamin K: .105 mcg

CHEESE OMELET

LACTO-OVO VEGETARIAN – 0 CARB CHOICE

Makes One Serving ***Sodium Per Recipe: 82 mg***

Low sodium cheddar, Colby or Muenster cheese make this omelet special. USDA sodium levels for "low sodium" cheese is 5.95 mg sodium. You may have difficulty in finding this. Sargento and Heluva Good have salt in them so their sodium levels range from 25 mg per ounce upwards to 80 mg.

1 large egg (70 mg)
½ teaspoon half & half (1.015 mg)
½ small Roma tomato seeded, sliced and diced (1.55 mg)
1 tablespoon red or green pepper, diced (.07 mg)
1 small button mushroom, diced (.5 mg)
1 tablespoon onion, chopped (.4 mg)
1 ounce low sodium cheddar, sliced or grated (5.954 mg)
spritz of olive oil (trace)

Optional: Garnish with chopped cilantro or parsley, or your own homemade relish or salsa. Healthyheartmarket.com has a nice Sweet Zucchini Relish from Alberto's with very low sodium that works well on top or inside the omelet. (under 5 mg per 2-tablespoons)

Clean vegetables and prepare.

Slice or grate cheese.

Spritz small 6" nonstick pan with olive oil and sauté veggies for about three to four minutes over medium heat. Remove to dish and then lightly spritz with olive oil. Set pan over medium low heat.

Whisk egg with half & half in a small bowl and pour into reheated pan, with a light circular movement spead egg out to edges of pan, set on heat. Cover with lid for about two minutes. Then spread veggies over egg and sprinkle grated cheese over that.

Cover for about two to three minutes or until cheese is melted. Remove and serve hot with homemade unsalted toast spread lightly with your favorite jam.

Cheddar Omelet Nutrient Values Per Serving: Calories: 212.3, Protein: 15 g, Carbohydrate: 6.115 g, Dietary Fiber: 1.522 g, Total Sugars: 3.358 g, Total Fat: 14.8 g, Saturated Fat: 7.661 g, Monounsaturated Fat: 4.61 g, Polyunsaturated Fat: 1.068 g, Cholesterol: 240.8 mg, Trans Fatty Acids: 0 g, Total Omega-3 FA: .152 g, Total Omega-6 FA: 0 g, Calcium: 239.1 mg, Potassium: 371.9 mg, Sodium: 82 mg, Vitamin K: 6.784 mcg

FRENCH TOAST

LACTO-OVO VEGETARIAN – 1½ CARB CHOICES

Serves 2 Sodium Per Recipe: 75.5 mg Sodium Per Serving: 37.7 mg

- **2 French Toast Bread slices (See Page: 209) (7.606 mg)**
- **1 medium egg whisked (61.5 mg)**
- **1 tablespoon nonfat milk with vitamin A (6.297 mg)**
- **cinnamon to taste (trace)**

Preheat large nonstick griddle or nonstick pan over medium flame with a tablespoon of extra virgin olive oil.

In a flat dish large enough to hold one slice of the above bread, whisk together the milk and egg.

Sprinkle cinnamon on both sides of the bread. Dip bread into egg mixture on both sides. and place onto hot griddle or pan.

French Toast Nutrient Data Per Serving: Calories: 183.8, Protein: 7.107 g, Carbohydrate: 24.4 g, Dietary Fiber: 1.022 g, Total Sugars: .875 g, Total Fat: 6.211 g, Saturated Fat: 1.4 g, Monounsaturated Fat: 3.346 g, Polyunsaturated Fat: .783 g, Cholesterol: 94.5 mg, Trans Fatty Acids: 0 g, Total Omega-3 FA: .049 g, Total Omega-6 FA: 0 g, Calcium: 32.5 mg, Potassium: 110.2 mg, Sodium: 37.7 mg, Vitamin K: 2.185 mcg

DON'S BASIC CREPES

LACTO-OVO VEGETARIAN – 0 CARB CHOICES

Makes: 30 6" crepes

Sodium Per Recipe: 391.7 mg Sodium Per Crepe: 13.1 mg

You can make these using standard beaters, a blender, or a food processor. If you thought something as tasty as crepes were off your diet, think again. These are low sodium and just one has only 1.5 grams of total fat. We recommend a good crepe pan.

- **3 large eggs (210 mg)**
- **1⅓ cups 1% cultured low sodium buttermilk (173.3 mg)**
- **¾ cups unbleached, all-purpose flour (1.875 mg)**
- **¼ teaspoon onion powder (.324 mg)**
- **4 tablespoons unsalted butter, melted (6.248 mg)**

Combine the eggs, milk, flour and onion powder in a medium size mixing bowl or blender bowl and beat together on high speed for about a minute or until smooth. It should not be lumpy.

Cover batter and let rest for about a half-hour while you prepare fillings. You may also store this batter in your refrigerator tightly covered for a day. Bring to room temp before using.

When ready to cook, stir in the melted butter.

Heat your crêpe pan or skillet over medium to medium high heat. If using an electric crêpe pan like the Maxim, follow manufacturer's directions. If using a nonstick pan you may proceed without adding oil or butter to the grill, or you may use a little oil or butter for flavoring. For standard pans, brush with a little of the melted butter or use a PAM type olive or canola oil spray.

Pour batter (6" pan will take two-tablespoons, 7" and 8" will take 3 to 4-tablespoons) into your pan[1]. Immediately pick up the crepe pan and tilt and swirl it so that the batter covers most of bottom of the pan.

Loosen the edges of the crêpe with a nonstick or metal pancake turner. Quickly flip the crêpe over. Cook on the other side less than a minute or until lightly golden. Slide it out onto a plate.

Serving suggestions

1. Basic crêpe may be filled with jam and sprinkled with a little powdered or granulated sugar.

2. They may also be filled with ingredients like Ricotta cheese sugar or Splenda®, and a touch of cinnamon. Top with whipped cream, powdered sugar or nothing at all.

3. Serve with freshly cooked or grilled chicken in a light pureed cranberry sauce ladled over the top.

4. Flavor the batter with herbs like a nice Provence mix and fill with leftover or freshly cooked beef such as a tender roast beef or even a nice ground sirloin. Top with a light sauce of sautéed mushrooms mixed with sour cream.

5. Freshly sliced topped with a pureed mix of berries like frozen blackberries and raspberries. Top again with whipped cream and garnish with a strawberry slice. Makes a wonderful dessert.

You may store your cooked crêpes tightly wrapped for up to 3 days in your refrigerator. Freeze with wax paper between each crêpe.

[1]Crêpe pans come in various sizes. We find the 6" crepe to be perfect for our eating plan. For 8" crêpes cut quantity down to 20. You can stretch this recipe with the 6" size up to 40 crêpes after you have gained crêpe making experience. That would cut the sodium down to about 9 mg each and the total fat down to about 1.5 grams with calories per crêpe dropping to 27.

Basic Crêpes Nutrient Values per Crêpe: Calories: 34.2, Protein: 1.37 g, Carbohydrate: 2.885 g, Dietary Fiber: .086 g, Total Sugars: .455 g, Total Fat: 2.286 g, Saturated Fat: 1.266 g, Monounsaturated Fat: .591 g, Polyunsaturated Fat: .139 g, Cholesterol: 26.3 mg, Trans Fatty Acids: 0 g, Total Omega-3 FA: .016 g, Total Omega-6 FA: .041 g, Calcium: 16.4 mg, Potassium: 10.7 mg, Sodium: 13.1 mg, Vitamin K: .158 mcg

OATMEAL PANCAKES

LACTO-OVO VEGETARIAN – 1 CARB CHOICE

Makes: 14 pancakes

Sodium Per Recipe: 281.2 mg ***Sodium Per Pancake: 20.1 mg***

Made Regularly On River Raft Trips by Chef Don's Sister, Dr. "River Guide" Becky, who says, "Perfect for breakfast alongside the river. Hot iron skillet over a fire and you're good for the day."

1¼ cups nonfat milk with vitamin A[1] (128.6 mg)
1 cup rolled oats or Quick Quaker Oats[1] (3.76 mg)
2 large eggs, beaten (140 mg)
1 tablespoon extra virgin olive oil (trace)
½ cup white whole wheat or whole wheat pastry flour (3 mg)
1 tablespoon brown sugar, packed (5.382 mg)
1 teaspoon cinnamon (.598 mg)
1 orange, grated skin only (.18 mg)
2 teaspoons Ener-G Baking Soda (trace)
2 teaspoons Ener-G Baking Powder[2] (trace)

Preheat griddle with light coat of extra virgin olive oil.

Stir together milk with rolled or Quick Quaker Oats in a bowl and let stand for 5 minutes. Add oil and beaten eggs and stir well. Stir in the flour, sugar, orange zest, cinnamon, and Ener-g baking soda and Ener-g baking powder.

Bake on hot greased griddle using 1/4 cup batter for each pancake. Pancakes will not bubble like regular pancakes. Then flip to cook on other side. Serve hot with topping of choice.

[1]Quick Quaker Oats have exactly the same nutrient values as rolled oats.
[2]Ener-g Baking Powder is double-acting.

Oatmeal Pancakes Nutrient Data Per Pancake (without topping) ½-Carb Choices: Calories: 61.8, Protein: 3.399 g, Carbohydrate: 9.92 g, Dietary Fiber: 1.701 g, Total Sugars: 2.244 g, Total Fat: 2.247 g, Saturated Fat: .469 g, Monounsaturated Fat: 1.15 g, Polyunsaturated Fat: .419 g, Cholesterol: 30.7 mg, Trans Fatty Acids: 0 g, Total Omega-3 FA: .023 g, Total Omega-6 FA: 0 g, Calcium: 39.9 mg, Potassium: 102.1 mg, Sodium: 20 mg, Vitamin K: .956 mcg

Nutrient Data using Blackberry Topping as an example 1-Carb Choices: Calories: 77.8, Protein: 3.525 g, Carbohydrate: 13.9 g, Dietary Fiber: 2.178 g, Total Sugars: 5.805 g, Total Fat: 2.291 g, Saturated Fat: .471 g, Monounsaturated Fat: 1.155 g, Polyunsaturated Fat: .444 g, Cholesterol: 30.7 mg, Trans Fatty Acids: 0 g, Total Omega-3 FA: .031 g, Total Omega-6 FA: 0 g, Calcium: 42.5 mg, Potassium: 116.7 mg, Sodium: 20.1 mg, Vitamin K: 2.738 mcg

POOR MAN'S DECAF LATTE

LACTO – 0 CARB CHOICES

Serves 1   Sodium Per Recipe: 15.2 mg

No caffeine, very little sodium and no fat but with lots of flavor. You'll want an inexpensive frother (See: Top 20 Cooking Utensils).

2 tablespoons of nonfat milk with Vitamin A (12.9 mg)
1 packet of Splenda (trace)
1 cup of decaf coffee of choice (2.37 mg)

Brew coffee first. In a clean coffee cup, froth the 2 tablespoons of nonfat milk. Hold the whisk near the top of the milk while frothing. Once it has frothed place into a microwave and heat at high for about 15 to 20 seconds. Keep an eye on it. You will see the milk rise to the top of the cup. At that point remove it from the microwave. Pour one packet Splenda into the cup and then pour in the coffee. The milk will rise with the coffee. Stir a bit and enjoy.

Decaf Latte Nutrient Data Per Cup: Calories: 15.2, Protein: 1.269 g, Carbohydrate: 2.467 g, Dietary Fiber: 0 g, Total Sugars: 1.559 g, Total Fat: .024 g, Saturated Fat: .041 g, Monounsaturated Fat: .014 g, Polyunsaturated Fat: .007 g, Cholesterol: .613 mg, Trans Fatty Acids: 0 g, Total Omega-3 FA: 0 g, Total Omega-6 FA: 0 g, Calcium: 43 mg, Potassium: 211.3 mg, Sodium: 15.2 mg, Vitamin K: 0 mcg

BUTTERMILK WAFFLES

LACTO-OVO VEGETARIAN – ½ -WAFFLE = 2 CARB CHOICES

Makes 2 large round waffles   Sodium Per Waffle: 61 mg

1 cup white unbleached all-purpose (2.5 mg)
½ cup 1% cultured low sodium buttermilk (65 mg)
½ cup orange juice fortified with calcium (1.244 mg)
1 small egg (53.2 mg)
1 tablespoon Ener-G baking Powder (trace)
¼ teaspoon cornstarch (trace)

Preheat waffle iron at a high setting.

Combine all ingredients in medium size bowl and stir vigorously with a wooden spoon. When well mixed, use a measuring cup to pour half of it on the iron for the first waffle. When done, make the second. Serve hot .

[1] Diabetics try using 3/4 cup all-purpose, 1/4 cup Bob's Red Mill soy flour. Waffle carbohydrates will drop to 52.8 g. Half a waffle is 26.4 g.

Buttermilk Waffle Nutrient Data Per Waffle: Calories: 293.9, Protein: 11.5 g, Carbohydrate: 57 g, Dietary Fiber: 1.812 g, Total Sugars: 2.565 g, Total Fat: 3.788 g, Saturated Fat: 1.44 g, Monounsaturated Fat: .784 g, Polyunsaturated Fat: .525 g, Cholesterol: 86.6 mg, Trans Fatty Acids: 0 g, Total Omega-3 FA: .028 g, Total Omega-6 FA: 0 g, Calcium: 166.8 mg, Potassium: 210.5 mg, Sodium: 61 mg, Vitamin K: .244 mcg

OATMEAL

LACTO VEGETARIAN – 4 CARB CHOICES

Serves 2 Sodium Per Recipe: 13.5 mg Sodium Per Recipe: 6.727 mg

Oatmeal can help lower our "bad" cholesterol. For a treat we like to add raisins or dried cranberries and a few other ingredients. When served hot with our special topping it practically becomes as good as any oatmeal breakfast you've ever experienced. For the topping you'll need something like the BonJour Primo Latte froth making device. It really works. (You can find it at megaheart.com/kit_cabinet.html, at amazon.com or at some kitchen stores.)

2 cups filtered low sodium water (trace)
1 medium fresh apple, cubed or diced, skin on (1.82 mg)
⅓ cup seedless raisins or dried cranberries (6.534 mg)
½ teaspoon ground cinnamon[2] (.13 mg)
1 cup Quick Quaker Oats or other unsalted milled oats (2.4 mg)
3 tablespoons nonfat milk with added Vitamin A (20.6 mg)

Put 2-cups of water into pan of choice.

Prepare apple, place into pan along with raisins, cinnamon. Bring to boil.

Put milk into a coffee cup, set aside.

While water is boiling, add the oats, turn heat down a bit and stir for one minute. When done, turn heat off and move the oatmeal to another unused burner.

Using the froth maker, bring milk up to a nice foam. Place milk in the cup into a microwave and heat for about fifteen to twenty seconds or until the foam reaches the top of the cup.

Remove foam from microwave. Serve oatmeal in bowls and lay the foam on top. You may want to make more foam if you divide the oatmeal into three servings.

[1]Diabetics, if you leave out the raisins and apples you'll cut 47 grams of carbohydrates from the recipe total making this a 3 Carb Choices recipe.

[2]Or cinnamon to taste

Oatmeal Nutrient Data Per Serving (with raisins & apple) 4-Carb Choices: Calories: 280.6, Protein: 6.769 g, Carbohydrate: 62.2 g, Dietary Fiber: 7.378 g, Total Sugars: 26.3 g, Total Fat: 3.038 g, Saturated Fat: .514 g, Monounsaturated Fat: .806 g, Polyunsaturated Fat: 1.004 g, Cholesterol: .061 mg, Trans Fatty Acids: 0 g, Total Omega-3 FA: .057 g, Total Omega-6 FA: 0 g, Calcium: 49 mg, Potassium: 451.2 mg, Sodium: 6.727 mg, Vitamin K: 4.438 mcg

[1]Oatmeal Nutrient Data Per Serving (without raisins & apple) 2-Carb Choices: Calories: 151, Protein: 5.609 g, Carbohydrate: 27.9 g, Dietary Fiber: 4.105 g, Total Sugars: .738 g, Total Fat: 2.759 g, Saturated Fat: .448 g, Monounsaturated Fat: .794 g, Polyunsaturated Fat: .921 g, Cholesterol: .061 mg, Trans Fatty Acids: 0 g, Total Omega-3 FA: .04 g, Total Omega-6 FA: 0 g, Calcium: 29.1 mg, Potassium: 150.8 mg, Sodium: 2.55 mg, Vitamin K: 1.483 mcg

SOURDOUGH STARTER

VEGAN – 1½ CARB CHOICES

Makes 4 Cups Sodium Per Recipe: 8.5 mg Sodium Per ½ Cup: 2.125 mg

Make this starter and then use it for bread, pancakes and waffles. See last sentence in instructions for pancake/waffle ideas. Once your starter is ready, remember that consistency varies and for that reason you can't follow sourdough recipes exactly. When making bread or pancakes and waffles, water and flour content always need to be adjusted to the consistency of your sourdough. Use filtered water that does not contain chlorine. Chlorine kills yeast.

- **2 cups white all-purpose flour (5 mg)**
- **2 cups warm water (about 100° F to 105° F) (trace)**
- **2¼ teaspoons active, dry yeast (3.5 mg)**
- **2 teaspoons granulated sugar[1] (trace)**

Combine the ingredients in a medium glass or ceramic bowl, set on a countertop covered with wax or parchment paper in a warm place overnight (about 80° F). Do not use plastic or metal bowls. Cover with a light, dry cloth.

Stir the starter once a day. When it develops a sour smell and it's bubbly, it's ready (about 6 to 7 days). Once it starts to bubble, you'll want to feed it daily with flour and water. When storing, cover the bowl or container with plastic wrap but not tightly. We want it to breathe some.

You will have to use a cup of the starter daily or at least give it away. That's how you'll keep it alive. Each day replace that cup with a cup of warm water (105° to 110° F) and a cup of flour. Cover again.

We store ours in the refrigerator. That way we don't have to feed it every day. But we do have to stir in the liquid that forms or put a cup of water and a cup of flour into it and place it on the countertop at least eight hours before using it. The water should always be about 105° to 110° F. Hot water can kill the yeast. If you store it in the fridge longer than a month, you might need to rebuild it over a three or four day period before using it. Throw it all out if the liquid in the bowl has turned to a pinkish or orangish color. Otherwise stir the liquid back into it and add more flour and water.

For pancakes or waffles, use our existing recipes and exchange one portion of flour for an equal portion of starter. Remember though, you'll have to play with the consistency, since starters vary.

[1] Splenda will not work in this recipe.

Sourdough Starter Nutrient Data Per Half-Cup: Calories: 120.4, Protein: 3.563 g, Carbohydrate: 25.2 g, Dietary Fiber: 1.028 g, Total Sugars: 1.133 g, Total Fat: .347 g, Saturated Fat: .054 g, Monounsaturated Fat: .05 g, Polyunsaturated Fat: .129 g, Cholesterol: 0 mg, Trans Fatty Acids: 0 g, Total Omega-3 FA: .007 g, Total Omega-6 FA: 0 g, Calcium: 5.258 mg, Potassium: 51 mg, Sodium: 1.062 mg, Vitamin K: .094 mcg

LUNCH

Sandwiches for lunch can prove to be filling and full of good nutrients and energy. Adding vegetables to a sandwich and maybe some meat or even a high protein bread are also healthy. High protein bread?

Soy flour has a great deal of protein in it. Our Diabetic bread adaptation not only helps lower carbohydrates, it raises the level of protein. (See Page 187) Good things to add to a sandwich are lettuce, tomato, onion, Yo Cheese Mayo, avocado, raw peeled and sliced cucumbers, extra virgin olive oil and vinegar, and some of your favorite spices or white or black pepper.

Only two of the following recipes are not a sandwich, but don't let that stop you. Leftovers from the night before also can make an excellent lunch. If you're taking a sack lunch to work, then take leftovers like the fried rice on page 186 and it at work if possible.

CHICKEN SALAD or SANDWICH

FLEXITARIAN– 1 CARB CHOICE

Serves 4 Sodium Per Recipe:204 mg Sodium Per Serving: 51 mg

This chicken salad makes a great summer time lunch, or in a sandwich with any of our bread recipes.

1 cup cooked unsalted and non-brined lean chicken breast (76.7 mg)
½ cup red onion, chopped (3.2 mg)
½ cup celery, chopped (40.4 mg)
½ cup light sour cream (80.5 mg)[1]
½ cup unpeeled red or green grapes, halved (1.51 mg)
½ cup apple with skin, chopped (.625 mg)
juice of one fresh lemon (.47 mg)
Options: chopped unsalted nuts (almonds or walnuts) (.567 mg)
dash of pepper to taste (trace)

Mix ingredients together and chill before serving on bed of lettuce or in a sandwich bun.

[1]Data based on ½ cup. You can exchange the sour cream with our Eggless Mayonnaise recipe using homemade Yo Cheese. (See Page: 225)

Chicken Salad Sandwich Nutrient Data Per Serving: Calories: 205.7, Protein: 9.678 g, Carbohydrate: 12.8 g, Dietary Fiber: 2.466 g, Total Sugars: 6.544 g, Total Fat: 14 g, Saturated Fat: 2.887 g, Monounsaturated Fat: 7.207 g, Polyunsaturated Fat: 3.142 g, Cholesterol: 27 mg, Trans Fatty Acids: .007 g, Total Omega-3 FA: .202 g, Total Omega-6 FA: 0 g, Calcium: 66.7 mg, Potassium: 324.8 mg, Sodium: 51 mg, Vitamin K: 7.079 mcg

DEVILED EGG SANDWICH

LACTO OVO VEGETARIAN – 3½ CARB CHOICES

Makes 2 Sodium Per Recipe: 174.8 mg Sodium Per Sandwich: 87.4 mg

2 hard boiled eggs (140 mg)
2 tablespoons yo cheese eggless mayonnaise[2] (23.8 mg)
1 2-inch slice of celery, chopped (6 mg)
white pepper or paprika to taste (trace)
2 homemade sandwich buns (5 mg)

Chop eggs, stir in eggless mayo, celery and paprika and spread on buns. Voila! Deviled egg sandwich lovers will be in seventh heaven.

[1]Diabetics, convert this to a lettuce-wrap sandwich and lower carbs to about 2.6 grams or 0-Carb Choices.[2] See Page: 155

Deviled Egg Sandwich Nutrient Data Per Deviled Egg Sandwich: Calories: 346.3, Protein: 15.6 g, Carbohydrate: 52.7 g, Dietary Fiber: 3.019 g, Total Sugars: 2.934 g, Total Fat: 8.028 g, Saturated Fat: 1.989 g, Monounsaturated Fat: 3.667 g, Polyunsaturated Fat: 1.168 g, Cholesterol: 212 mg, Trans Fatty Acids: 0 g, Total Omega-3 FA: .066 g, Total Omega-6 FA: 0 g, Calcium: 74.4 mg Potassium: 239.6 mg, Sodium: 87.4 mg, Vitamin K: 2.351 mcg

TURKEY AVOCADO SANDWICH

FLEXITARIAN – 3 CARB CHOICES

Makes One Sandwich Sodium Per Sandwich: 90.3 mg

3 ounces thinly sliced (not brined) turkey or chicken (43.5 mg)
1 ounce low sodium Swiss or cheddar cheese (5.954 mg)
1 tablespoon honey mustard (15 mg)
3 slices tomato (3 mg)
1 leaf romaine or iceberg lettuce (2.24 mg)
2 thin slices onion (white or red) (.56 mg)
¼ medium avocado, sliced thinly (3.517 mg)
1 Don's Sandwich Bun (Page: 200) (16.5 mg)

Slice sandwich roll lengthwise, place cheese on top half and toast lightly under broiler until just melted. Toast bottom half lightly at a same time.

Spread mustard on bottom half and lay meat on that.

Pile on the tomato slices, onion slices, lettuce, and avocado. Put sandwich together and Enjoy! Diabetics, cut carbs by making this a lettuce wrap sandwich. Reduces carbs to 15 grams or 1-Carb Choices.

Turkey Avocado Sandwich Nutrient Data Per Sandwich: Calories: 513.1, Protein: 36.3 g, Carbohydrate: 43.8 g, Dietary Fiber: 6.317 g, Total Sugars: 10.5 g, Total Fat: 22.1 g, Saturated Fat: 8.048 g, Monounsaturated Fat: 10.4 g, Polyunsaturated Fat: 2.125 g, Cholesterol: 98.2 mg, Trans Fatty Acids: .012 g, Total Omega-3 FA: .315 g, Total Omega-6 FA: .008 g, Calcium: 260.8 mg, Potassium: 882.2 mg, Sodium: 90.3 mg, Vitamin K: 47 mcg

DON'S CHEESEBURGER

FLEXITARIAN – 4 CARB CHOICES[1]

Makes 4   Sodium Per Recipe: 347.3 mg   Sodium Per Burger: 90.9 mg

I like to serve these to family and friends for a summer time evening barbecue meal. I usually wrap corn on the cob in aluminum foil and set them on the grill to cook. Rotate corn every couple of minutes a quarter a turn at a time. Takes about ten minutes for the corn to cook.

4 Don's Sandwich Buns (Page 200) (22.5 mg)
4 barbecued veggie burger patties (Page 193) (214.2 mg)
½ cup Don's Barbecue Sauce (Page 192) (51.8 mg)
4 ounces low sodium Swiss or cheddar cheese (40 mg)
4 portabella strips cut from cap (about 4-ounces) (20.2 mg)
4 thick slices (1/4" each) large tomato (2.7 mg)
4 large leaves of iceberg lettuce (6 mg)
4 slices of medium size red onion (6.08 mg)

Make slightly larger buns using your favorite unsalted homemade sandwich bun. I usually do this early in the morning or the day before.

Prepare the sauce ahead of time and store in refrigerator.

Slice cheese.

Have mushrooms, tomato, lettuce, and onion ready.

Slice buns in half and cover to retain freshness. We'll toast these over the grill just before using.

Prepare meat.

Set portabellas to back of grill where there's heat but not a direct fire. Keep an eye on them. Don't overcook.

Barbecue the meat until nearly done. Baste with bbq sauce. Set equal portions of cheese on top of each patty. While the cheese is heating and melting, place the bun tops over the meat. Lightly toast the inside of the bottom bun. When done, set lower part of buns on serving trays. Layer mushrooms, onion, tomato and lettuce. Place the top bun and burger on the bottom & enjoy.

Cheeseburger Nutrient Data Per Burger: Calories: 519.1, Protein: 31.6 g, Carbohydrate: 57.6 g, Dietary Fiber: 5.098 g, Total Sugars: 18.3 g, Total Fat: 18.5 g, Saturated Fat: 8.301 g, Monounsaturated Fat: 7.632 g, Polyunsaturated Fat: 1.38 g, Cholesterol: 72.3 mg, Trans Fatty Acids: .242 g, Total Omega-3 FA: .219 g, Total Omega-6 FA: .006 g, Calcium: 263 mg, Potassium: 1116 mg, Sodium: 86.8 mg, Vitamin K: 14.2 mcg

[1]Diabetic Lettuce Wrap Cheeseburger Nutrient Data Per Burger : 1½-Carb Choices: Calories: 330.3, Protein: 26.1 g, Carbohydrate: 25.9 g, Dietary Fiber: 3.893 g, Total Sugars: 16.9 g, Total Fat: 14.4 g, Saturated Fat: 7.721 g, Monounsaturated Fat: 4.983 g, Polyunsaturated Fat: .738 g, Cholesterol: 72.3 mg, Trans Fatty Acids: .242 g, Total Omega-3 FA: .19 g, Total Omega-6 FA: .006 g, Calcium: 256.6 mg, Potassium: 1061 mg, Sodium: 82.7 mg, Vitamin K: 15.6 mcg

DON'S SMOOTHIES

LACTO VEGETARIAN - 1½ CARB CHOICES

Makes 2 8-ounce Servings   Sodium Per Serving: 26.9mg

When it's summertime and the heat rises, a chilled drink with low sodium and lots of nutrients becomes an appealing break. When it gets hot around here I like this drink as a complete lunch. Remember, it's an ice-cold drink so not so quick on the draw when you down it. You can add more ice than we suggest if you like. I also like to replace the half-peach with about three apricots when they are in season. The grams of fiber in this drink are excellent as well. The banana contains half the carbohydrates.

5 fresh strawberries, washed and stems removed (1.35 mg)
1 small ripe banana (1.01 mg)
½ ripe medium peach, sliced (trace)
½ cup nonfat milk with Vitamin A[1] added (51.5 mg)
2 crushed ice cubes from filtered water[2] (trace)

You'll need a handheld or a countertop food processor model.

If you have an ice crusher in your refrigerator then use about a 1/2-inch (in an 8-ounce glass) of crushed ice.

In the processor's puree glass or bowl, add in the peach, banana and washed strawberries. Add milk.

Puree for about thirty seconds or until smooth. Add ice and puree again for a few seconds.

Serve for lunch or a cool break in the day.

[1]The USDA now rates nonfat milk with added Vitmain A as 102.9 mg of sodium per cup. Some cartons may still reflect the old ratings of around 130 mg.

[2]Or about 2-inches of crushed ice from an ice crusher. Have you freshened your refrigerator's water filter lately?

Smoothies Nutrient Data Per Smoothie: Calories: 102, Protein: 3.408 g, Carbohydrate: 23.3 g, Dietary Fiber: 3.226 g, Total Sugars: 15.7 g, Total Fat: .512 g, Saturated Fat: .105 g, Monounsaturated Fat: .083 g, Polyunsaturated Fat: .176 g, Cholesterol: 1.225 mg, Trans Fatty Acids: 0 g, Total Omega-3 FA: .059 g, Total Omega-6 FA: 0 g, Calcium: 92.1 mg, Potassium: 450.9 mg, Sodium: 26.9 mg, Vitamin K: 2.713 mcg

FRIED RICE

LACTO-OVO VEGETARIAN - 2 CARB CHOICES

Serves 2 Sodium Per Recipe: 165.2 mg Sodium Per Serving: 82.6 mg

I first encountered fried rice in Japan while serving with the Marines. It was "hawked" everywhere even through train windows when I traveled from our base camp into Tokyo. I've made variations of their fried rice but I like this one for a quick lunch. I always make it when we have left over rice from another meal. Use either white, brown or even wild rice.

1 tablespoon extra virgin olive oil (trace)
2 medium to large eggs (140 mg)
¼ medium to large sweet red bell pepper, chopped (1.64 mg)
¼ large onion, chopped (1.5 mg)
1 medium zucchini, chopped (19.6 mg)
1 clove garlic, minced (.51 mg)
1 cup cooked white, brown or wild rice (1.3 mg)

In a nonstick pan, over medium heat, scramble the two eggs using 1 teaspoon of the oil, chop and mix well while they cook. When eggs are done, set aside on a dish.

Sauté the red pepper, onion, zucchini and garlic in the same pan in the rest of the oil. When veggies have turned a bright color, put the cooked rice into the pan and stir for a few minutes to heat. Then add the egg, stir for another minute.

Serve in bowls or on a plate immediately. Sprinkle with a little unseasoned rice vinegar if desired. Note: Use your favorite veggies if these don't work for you, like snow or snap peas, asparagus, or grated carrots.

Nutrient Data Per Serving: Calories: 251.1, Protein: 9.762 g, Carbohydrate: 25.2 g, Dietary Fiber: 2.666 g, Total Sugars: 3.751 g, Total Fat: 12.9 g, Saturated Fat: 2.733 g, Monounsaturated Fat: 5.515 g, Polyunsaturated Fat: 3.318 g, Cholesterol: 211.5 mg, Trans Fatty Acids: 0 g, Total Omega-3 FA: .129 g, Total Omega-6 FA: 0 g, Calcium: 57.5 mg, Potassium: 464.1 mg, Sodium: 82.6 mg, Vitamin K: 6.939 mcg

LETTUCE WRAP SANDWICH

Makes 2 Sodium Per Recipe: 98.4 mg Sodium Per Sandwich: 49.2 mg

FLEXITARIAN - ½ CARB CHOICE

Here's a sandwich idea that you can apply to fast food restaurants or even a fancy restaurant – as well as making them at home for a very light summer sandwich. We made a few of these on our coast to coast road trip right after I ran out of no-salt, low-sodium bread. You can use any meat or leave meat out.

2 small slices of lean pork roast, such as pork loin, fat cut off, sliced (about 4-ounces) (51 mg)
1 medium tomato, sliced (6.15 mg)
¼ medium red bell pepper, sliced (1.19 mg)
4 slices from a cucumber, peeled, sliced (.56 mg
⅓ medium red onion, sliced (1.452 mg)
1 tablespoon fresh chopped cilantro (trace)
2 large leafs of iceberg lettuce, chilled (1.5 mg)
1 tablespoon of dressing (See Page: 241) (2.534 mg)

Clean and slice vegetables. Spin-dry lettuce. Place in a small bowl with sliced meat.

Mix the dressing by shaking it together in a small capped container vigorously. Drizzle the dressing on the mix and toss once or twice more.

Clean and spin-dry the lettuce.

Spread the lettuce leaves out, one per serving dish. Evenly lay in the vegetables and slices of meat, then roll. Hold closed with a toothpick.

Lettuce Wrap Sandwich Nutrient Data Per Wrap Sandwich: Calories: 225.7, Protein: 10.4 g, Carbohydrate: 7.647 g, Dietary Fiber: 1.555 g, Total Sugars: 4.81 g, Total Fat: 17 g, Saturated Fat: 5.448 g, Monounsaturated Fat: 8.524 g, Polyunsaturated Fat: 1.537 g, Cholesterol: 45.9 mg, Trans Fatty Acids: 0 g, Total Omega-3 FA: .082 g, Total Omega-6 FA: 0 g, Calcium: 35.1 mg, Potassium: 372.9 mg, Sodium: 49.2 mg, Vitamin K: 10.5 mcg

HUMMUS AVOCADO SANDWICH

VEGAN – NOT EASILY DIABETIC ADAPTABLE

Makes 4 sandwiches (May halve recipe)

Sodium Per Recipe: 101 mg   Sodium Per Sandwich: 25.3 mg

We get our Eden Organic beans from Healthy Heart Market.

8 slices 7-grain bread (See page 208) (40.7 mg)
1 14.5 ounce can Eden No Salt Added Garbanzo beans (35 mg)
4 cloves garlic, minced (2.04 mg)
2 tablespoons fresh lemon juice (.235 mg)
1 medium tomato, thinly sliced (6.15 mg)
1 avocado, pitted, thinly sliced (10.9 mg)
4 leaves Romaine, butterleaf or iceberg lettuce (6 mg)

Drain can of garbanzo beans of all liquid. Using your handheld or other food processor, puree the beans. Add minced garlic and lemon juice while pureeing. Hummus should become smooth.

Lightly toast the bread. Spread the hummus on one piece, and layer the avocado, lettuce and tomato on the other. Join and enjoy.

Save remaining hummus in sealed container in refrigerator for a sandwich during the week. Also works well with our Pita Bread (*The No Salt, Lowest Sodium Baking Book, Page 251*) and other breads in this book.

Hummus Avocado Nutrient Data Per Sandwich: Calories: 573.3, Protein: 19.1 g, Carbohydrate: 104.6 g, Dietary Fiber: 14.3 g, Total Sugars: 15.3 g, Total Fat: 10.1 g, Saturated Fat: 1.261 g, Monounsaturated Fat: 4.866 g, Polyunsaturated Fat: 1.58 g, Cholesterol: 0 mg, Trans Fatty Acids: 0 g, Total Omega-3 FA: .141 g, Total Omega-6 FA: .005 g, Calcium: 107.1 mg, Potassium: 652.4 mg, Sodium: 25.3 mg, Vitamin K: 14.2 mcg

CRANBERRY SANDWICH

FLEXITARIAN - 3½ CARB CHOICES[1]

Makes One Sandwich ***Sodium Per Sandwich: 38 mg***

The Ciabatta bread recipe for this sandwich may be found on page 173 of "The No Salt, Lowest Sodium International Cookbook" You can use homemade French bread or another "crunchy" bread for this recipe as well, but I like the Ciabatta bread best. This is a healthy and tasty sandwich that can be served year 'round.

- **1 Ciabatta bun[2] (1.982 mg)**
- **¼ avocado, thinly sliced (2.72 mg)**
- **1 outer leaf Romaine lettuce (dark leaf) (2.24 mg)**
- **2 tablespoons fresh homemade cranberry sauce[3] (.369 mg)**
- **2 ounces cooked chicken or turkey, sliced (30.5 mg)**
- **2 tablespoons Don's Yo Cheese[4] (23.3 mg)**

Prepare your Yo Cheese at least a day early.

Spread Yo Cheese[3] on lower bun. Spread cranberries on upper bun. Lay chicken or turkey on lower bun, top with avocado and lettuce.

[1] Diabetics, most of the carbs are in the bun. You could adapt this recipe by making a lettuce-wrap sandwich. That would make the sandwich 20.4 grams of carbohydrates or a Carb Choices of 2 otherwise it's a 3.5 Carb Choices sandwich..

[2] Find Ciabatta Bun in *No-Salt, Lowest-Sodium International Cookbook,* or use similar homemade bun like Don's Sandwich Bun.

[3] Or canned such as Ocean Spray®.

[4]See Yo Cheese Page 233.

Cranberry Sandwich Nutrient Data Per Sandwich: Calories: 340.1, Protein: 15.8 g, Carbohydrate: 54.7 g, Dietary Fiber: 5.381 g, Total Sugars: 23.3 g, Total Fat: 7.053 g, Saturated Fat: 1.048 g, Monounsaturated Fat: 4.078 g, Polyunsaturated Fat: 1.01 g, Cholesterol: 27.2 mg, Trans Fatty Acids: .012 g, Total Omega-3 FA: .152 g, Total Omega-6 FA: .005 g, Calcium: 29.2 mg, Potassium: 437.7 mg, Sodium: 38 mg, Vitamin K: 37.2 mcg

PESTO CHICKEN SANDWICH

FLEXITARIAN – 2 CARB CHOICES

Makes 6 Sodium Per Recipe: 357.3 mg Sodium Per Sandwich: 59.5 mg

You'll enjoy our basic pesto, our Sandwich Buns and this sandwich. Grill a juicy skinless chicken breast and use a bit of low sodium Swiss, or low sodium mozzarella with it and wow! Spectacular flavors burst in your mouth.

6 Don's Sandwich Buns (Page 200) (99.2 mg)
1 recipe or 6 servings easy Pesto (Page:252) (4.128 mg)
3 skinless, boneless chicken half-breasts[1] (230.1 mg)
6 medium slices tomato (5.4 mg)
6 thin slices onion (1.62 mg)
3 ounces low sodium Swiss cheese, sliced or grated[2] (11.8 mg)
6 leaves of lettuce (your choice) (1.26 mg)[3]

Lay chicken on work surface, cover with shrinkwrap and pound with mallet lightly until breast is evenly flattened.

Cut breasts in half, filet style. Grill or broil the chicken on a nonstick griddle or in a nonstick pan. If using a standard pan then use a light spritz of olive oil from a spray can.

Lightly toast the opened buns, melt the cheese on the top bun.

Lay each chicken piece on one side of the sandwich bun. Spread the pesto generously across the other bun. Layer with the tomato, onion, lettuce and bring together. Serve hot or warm.

[1]Approximately 4-ounces each or 12-ounces total weight.

[2]Low Sodium Swiss is available in some parts of the country. A half-ounce of standard Swiss usually has 27.5 mg of sodium, which is generally acceptable.

[3]Data figured on inner leaf of Butterhead (Boston/Bibb) lettuce. Iceberg inner leaf would be (11.4 mg) per 6 leaves. Romaine inner leaves would be (.48 mg) sodium.

Nutrient Data Per Sandwich: Calories: 455.6, Protein: 24.9 g, Carbohydrate: 32.5 g, Dietary Fiber: 2.521 g, Total Sugars: 2.988 g, Total Fat: 26.4 g, Saturated Fat: 5.53 g, Monounsaturated Fat: 14.1 g, Polyunsaturated Fat: 4.773 g, Cholesterol: 61.9 mg, Trans Fatty Acids: .015 g, Total Omega-3 FA: .262 g, Total Omega-6 FA: .034 g, Calcium: 193.2 mg, Potassium: 455.5 mg, Sodium: 59.5 mg, Vitamin K: 60 mcg

TACOS FOR TWO

FLEXITARIAN – 1½ CARB CHOICES

Makes 2 Sodium Per Recipe: 133.2 mg Sodium Per Taco: 66.6 mg

May double this recipe. Fresh veggies, a colorful plate, a bit of ground chicken, turkey or beef (or strips of meat if you like), and you've got yourself a healthy dinner.

4 ounces cooked ground lean fowl or beef (107.2 mg)[1]
⅓ teaspoon unsalted chili powder (trace)
⅛ teaspoon garlic powder (.091 mg)
2 tablespoons no-salt-added tomato sauce (8.857 mg)
2 corn tortillas[2] (5.72 mg)
1 teaspoon extra virgin olive oil (.09 mg)
½ cup diced tomato (4.5 mg)
½ cup diced red onion (3.2 mg)
½ cup of iceberg or favorite lettuce, chopped (3.6 mg)
2 ounces low sodium cheddar cheese, shredded or grated (11.8 mg)[3]

Clean vegetables, chop and set aside on your dinner plate.

In a small size fry pan, cook meat with tomato sauce and chili powder and garlic powder. Set aside on a warmer. This taco is also delicious without meat if eaten as a taco salad or "tostada," and served with a dollop of sour cream.

In a medium fry pan, warm the oil over medium high heat coating pan evenly with a paper towel. When pan is hot quickly fry each tortilla on both sides. Remove from pan and cool on paper towel. If more oil is needed for second tortilla, then lightly spritz from a can. Your tortillas shouldn't be oily.

Serve hot.

[1] Based on 4-ounces of ground, lean turkey. Beef and chicken are lower in sodium levels.

[2] USDA figures. Most corn tortillas have no salt and less than 5 mg sodium each. Check your package to make sure they are low sodium before purchasing. Packages generally read 0 sodium or 5 mg sodium.

[3] USDA figures. May not exactly match your supplier's numbers.

***Nutrient Data Per Taco:** Calories: 207.9, Protein: 13 g, Carbohydrate: 22 g, Dietary Fiber: 3.409 g, Total Sugars: 4.984 g, Total Fat: 7.908 g, Saturated Fat: 1.724 g, Monounsaturated Fat: 3.609 g, Polyunsaturated Fat: 1.758 g, Cholesterol: 45 mg, Trans Fatty Acids: .156 g, Total Omega-3 FA: .103 g, Total Omega-6 FA: 0 g, Calcium: 75.6 mg, Potassium: 514.6 mg, Sodium: 66.6 mg, Vitamin K: 11.2 mcg*

EGGPLANT AND BASIL SANDWICHES

LACTO OVO VEGETARIAN – 1 CARB CHOICE

Makes 3 to 4 Sandwiches

Sodium Per Recipe: 40.3 mg Sodium Per Sandwich: 10.1 mg

Even if you think you don't like eggplant, you'll like these. Served with basil, tomato, and fresh mozzarella cheese, these are a light lunch or dinner with plenty of nutrients and flavor. This sandwich does not use bread.

1 small to medium eggplant, peeled (11 mg)
1 level tablespoon dried sweet basil (1.53 mg)
1 medium tomato, thinly sliced (6.15 mg)
4 ounces fresh salt-free or no-salt-added mozzarella[1] (17.9 mg)
spritz of olive oil (trace)
1 tablespoon balsamic vinegar, sprinkled (3.68 mg)

Preheat oven to 450°F.

Wash eggplant. Trim the ends off the eggplant and slice into about 6 to 10 rounds depending on size. Each round will be about 3/8" thick.

Lightly spritz baking sheet by spraying olive oil on it or brushing it on smoothly. Place eggplant rounds on sheet for baking. Spray or brush olive oil on the tops of the eggplant rounds. Bake for twelve minutes.

While baking, slice tomato. Set out sweet dried basil.

When rounds are done, remove from oven. Layer each eggplant slice with a slice of tomato first, sprinkle with dried basil, then salt-free mozzarella. Return to oven for 3 to 6 minutes or until cheese has melted.

Remove from the oven and place three rounds on each of two serving dishes. Drizzle balsamic vinegar on each. We like to use a strawberry flavored balsamic but regular balsamic works well.

Serve warm.

Optional: May substitute mushrooms for eggplant.

[1] Or low sodium Swiss cheese.

Eggplant and Basil Sandwiches Nutrient Data Per Sandwich: Calories: 133.1, Protein: 9.536 g, Carbohydrate: 11.2 g, Dietary Fiber: 5.483 g, Total Sugars: 4.99 g, Total Fat: 6.28 g, Saturated Fat: 3.256 g, Monounsaturated Fat: 2.214 g, Polyunsaturated Fat: .415 g, Cholesterol: 15.1 mg, Trans Fatty Acids: 0 g, Total Omega-3 FA: .086 g, Total Omega-6 FA: 0 g, Calcium: 244.9 mg, Potassium: 457.7 mg, Sodium: 10.1 mg, Vitamin K: 27.7

DINNER

Dinner hour seems to change from country to country. America is made up of so many different cultures that it's a marvel we can even identify a "dinner hour." Even more challenging is trying to figure out what dinner is. It would take an encyclopedia of cultural recipes to fulfill everyone's needs as far as choices go. However, despite the FDA's efforts at building a food pyramid our basic American dinner hour seems to be meat and potatoes.

Prior to and during World War II, our meals were fairly light and consisted of what we could grow or afford. Many of us grew fresh vegetables in victory gardens and pretty much remained lean on the meat. Still, during the war, the federal government needed the meat for our troops. So, to bring about an easing of meat consumption, the government cashed on on the Catholic rule that meat was not to be consumed on Fridays, (fish was), and set Tuesdays as a non-meat day. Back then a huge percentage of Americans were Catholics so the reduction in meat consumption after that mandate became appreciable.

In our house, our mother insisted on a two-o-clock in the afternoon Sunday dinner, whether it was a bowl of tomato soup, (during the war) or years later, a leg of lamb. She loved roast beef and legs of lamb.

After the war we used to have wonderful Sunday dinners with guests, some of them our own friends, others our parent's friends. One of the friends who came over after the war was Greg Boyington, otherwise known as Pappy Boyington of the Baa Baa Black Sheep squadron, a Marine fighter squadron during WW-II. Our father served for his squadron as a flight surgeon. There were others from that era who I remember as well, and all seemed to enjoy our dinners as much as we did.

In college, dinner was something you got when you had time for it. I had a thirty dollar monthly allowance for "three squares" for the month, money provided by the United States Navy for which I would return four years of my life as a Marine (I cheated and gave them six.) I often ended up across the street from the dorm eating at a place that provided those three squares for the whole thirty bucks. Dinner was often a Spencer steak with string beans and a potato. Always the same, which I admit, became a real drag.

Later while serving as a Marine, dinner also meant either a hot plate in your BOQ or pay the Corps your allowance to eat in the O' Club. Since I was an officer the only time I ate in the mess hall was when it was my duty to make sure the mess hall didn't turn into a mess. Part of my time in the Corps, my dinner came out of a small box with the stamp C-Rations imprinted thereon. Although officially known as Type C-ration, we developed other names for it. The soda crackers were so tough we called them John Wayne biscuits.

My best dinner in the Marines was while in the Philippines on a mission.

We'd been in the boondocks for three days without eating anything. Then a typhoon came up. We dug holes and stayed low. The holes were deep and filled with water quickly. It was very dark since no lights, no moon, just clouds, wind, pelting rain and lots of hunger dominated. Suddenly out of nowhere a few troops arrived carrying military green cans the size of an old tomato juice can. Each of us got one can, opened it with the can-opener strung to the dog tag chain around our neck . The content was one whole chicken, in fat, cold. I recall that as the best dinner I've ever had.

After leaving the Corps I spent a lifetime on the road. I discovered that dinners were also suppers or the evening meal, or non-existent. I learned in France that to inform guests it was time to go home was to offer them chocolates, and in Italy, well in Italy nobody wants to break up the party. I ate dinner in a British pub and marveled at the neighborly get-together and the always present bouncer. In Japan, Tahiti, and other locales, the experiences were always just that; an experience to enjoy and to learn.

If there was a common thread that ran through each of the above societies it was that dinner was also a recognized social gathering.

But it's in America that I have been the most surprised. For a long while I traveled coast to coast in small airplanes that I flew, and in large airlines where I sat anxiously wishing I was the one in the cockpit. Always with each trip I ran into gastronomical surprises (airline food excluded). My good fortune was that I traveled before all the red-topped shopping centers appeared with chain restaurants that have attempted to equalize our regional habits as best they could. Why should we even think about enjoying Cajun heat or Kansas City ribs when we can go to Applebee's or McDonald's?

It's not that you can't still find regional delights, but it's not as easy. Touring, traveling, vacationing, and other calls of the road mean we have to search out good spots and then get them to accommodate us. Regional cooking is often worth the effort, but today some regional cooking simply cannot be adapted to our health needs by some restaurants.

Therein lies part of our challenge. Where can we find these wonderful meals or how can we make them without the additional salt, fats, and calories that restaurants add? It is exactly that need that our recipes attempt to respond to when making these meals at home.

Consequently, for dinner we have produced a few recipes here that might sound like regional meals in local restaurants; some of them did come from our travels. Our *No Salt, Lowest Sodium International Cookbook* has recipes that should please you as well and our Light Meals book was drawn from many excursions.

BROILED SWORDFISH

FLEXITARIAN – ½ CARB CHOICE

Serves 2

Sodium Per Recipe: 254 mg   Sodium Per Teaspoon: 127 mg

Quick Mustard Sauce

2 tablespoons white balsamic[1] or white wine vinegar (3.68 mg)
1 tablespoon extra virgin olive oil (.54 mg)
1 teaspoon East Shore, Hain or Mendocino honey mustard (5 mg)
teaspoon dry mustard (trace)
packet of Splenda (trace)

To make the mustard sauce, combine all ingredients and whisk together until well blended. Set aside. Whisk again, just before serving.

2 4.5 to 5 ounce cuts of raw swordfish (244 mg)
½ cup (one small) onion, chopped (1.6 mg)
2 cloves garlic, raw, chopped (1.02 mg)
1 teaspoon extra virgin olive oil (trace)
Optional: Lemon slices for juice.

Set oven rack for broiler Preheat broiler at high setting.

Lightly saute chopped onion and garlic in 1 teaspoon of oil. Spread on broiler pan in area where fish will be placed for broiling. Lay fish on the onions and garlic and set under broiler. Broil on each side for about five-minutes (might take a minute longer). When turning over some onions will stick to the fish. Might sound strange but we want this.

When cooked serve with mustard sauce spread across top of each piece and add lemon wedges to squeeze some juice on top of the mustard sauce. Serve with fresh asparagus and a small baked potato or brown rice.

[1] Of the two, white balsamic is tastier. Sodium data based on balsamic.

Broiled Swordfish Nutrient Data Per Serving: Calories: 274.8, Protein: 27.7 g, Carbohydrate: 6.484 g, Dietary Fiber: .804 g, Total Sugars: 3.2 g, Total Fat: 14.6 g, Saturated Fat: 2.81 g, Monounsaturated Fat: 6.511 g, Polyunsaturated Fat: 4.263 g, Cholesterol: 53 mg, Trans Fatty Acids: 0 g, Total Omega-3 FA: 1.174 g, Total Omega-6 FA: 0 g, Calcium: 24.4 mg, Potassium: 473.9 mg, Sodium: 127 mg, Vitamin K: 2.259 mcg

CRANBERRY CHICKEN

FLEXITARIAN – 1 CARB CHOICES

Serves 4 Sodium Per Recipe: 346.1 mg Sodium Per Serving: 86.5 mg

2 cups of a dry red wine[2] (18.8)
½ cup fresh or not from concentrate orange juice (1.24 mg)
¼ cup balsamic vinegar (14.7 mg)
½ cup Splenda Granulated[3] (trace)
2 cups fresh whole cranberries (4 mg)
4 4 to 5-ounce boneless, skinless chicken half breasts (306.8 mg)
2 tablespoons extra virgin olive oil (.54)
ground black pepper to taste (trace)

In a medium size saucepan, bring first four ingredients to a boil over medium-high heat. Reduce heat to low and simmer for 10 more minutes.

Add fresh uncooked cranberries and simmer until cranberries soften. Add pepper to taste (may use coarsely ground, finely ground or white pepper).

If the sauce is too sweet stir in a bit more vinegar. If it gets too tart, stir in a bit more Splenda Granulated or sugar.

In a larger saucepan or skillet heat the olive oil over medium-high heat. Sear chicken breasts on one side for about 5 to 7 minutes. Turn and brown the other side until breasts are just cooked. Remove breasts from pan and let stand for a few minutes. Slice thinly across the grain of the meat. Spoon a little sauce on each plate and lay breast slices over sauce like shingles on a roof. Then pour a little sauce over the slices, too.

Serve hot.

[1] Diabetics, Splenda cuts carbs down enough for 1 carb choices.

[2] Data based on USDA "Red Wine." May use a nonalcoholic red wine. USDA rates non alcoholic with 32 mg sodium. Alcohol in standard wine will evaporate with the cooking.

[3] Or white granulated sugar. See Nutrients for sugar use below.

[1] Cranberry Duck Nutrient Data Per Serving (with Splenda) : Calories: 350.3, Protein: 27.8 g, Carbohydrate: 17.8 g, Dietary Fiber: 2.362 g, Total Sugars: 10.1 g, Total Fat: 8.34 g, Saturated Fat: 1.334 g, Monounsaturated Fat: 5.299 g, Polyunsaturated Fat: 1.081 g, Cholesterol: 68.4 mg, Trans Fatty Acids: .029 g, Total Omega-3 FA: .113 g, Total Omega-6 FA: 0 g, Calcium: 34.4 mg, Potassium: 572.8 mg, Sodium: 86.5 mg, Vitamin K: 7.351 mcg

Cranberry Duck Nutrient Data Per Serving (with sugar): Calories: 447.1, Protein: 27.8 g, Carbohydrate: 42.8 g, Dietary Fiber: 2.362 g, Total Sugars: 35.1 g, Total Fat: 8.34 g, Saturated Fat: 1.334 g, Monounsaturated Fat: 5.299 g, Polyunsaturated Fat: 1.081 g, Cholesterol: 68.4 mg, Trans Fatty Acids: .029 g, Total Omega-3 FA: .113 g, Total Omega-6 FA: 0 g, Calcium: 34.4 mg, Potassium: 573.3 mg, Sodium: 86.5 mg, Vitamin K: 7.351 mcg

CROCKPOT STEW

FLEXITARIAN – 3½ CARB CHOICES[1]

Serves 4 Sodium Per Recipe: 526.3 mg Sodium Per Serving : 131.8 mg

- **4 small red potatoes, washed, halved, not skinned (40.8 mg)**
- **3 medium size carrots, cleaned, slice in 1-inch pieces (126.3 mg)**
- **1 large onion, skinned, quartered (6 mg)**
- **1 pound lean, top round stew meat, cut into bite size chunks (235.9 mg)**
- **1½ cups Sweet & Sour Zinfandel Sauce[2] (117 mg)**
- **2 tablespoons cornstarch or flour (1.44 mg)**

Prepare the Sweet and Sour Zinfandel Sauce ahead of time, steep it until it's fairly thick. Can be done the day before and refrigerated.

Place ingredients into crockpot in order listed. Set crockpot for slow-cooking at either 6 or 8 hours setting. About one to two hours before the crockpot is finished, remove the vegetables and meat and set them aside in a covered bowl for a return to the pot. Leave the liquid in the crockpot.

Stir 2 to 4 tablespoons of cornstarch or white unbleached all-purpose flour into the liquid in the crockpot until dissolved. Return the vegetables and meat to the crockpot, replace cover and let finish cooking at your original temperature for the balance of time left.

When done, place meat on large platter and place vegetables and potatoes around the meat. Serve hot.

[2] See Page 246. Use all you make. After reducing, it should come out to 1 ½ cups but might reduce to 2-cups at the most. You can make the sauce with Zinfandel wine or the non-alcoholic wine.

[1 & 2]Crockpot Stew Nutrient Data Using Zinfandel Wine only, Per Serving, 2½-Carb Choices: Calories: 363.8, Protein: 29.9 g, Carbohydrate: 40.2 g, Dietary Fiber: 4.845 g, Total Sugars: 5.459 g, Total Fat: 4.129 g, Saturated Fat: 1.372 g, Monounsaturated Fat: 1.48 g, Polyunsaturated Fat: .328 g, Cholesterol: 64.6 mg, Trans Fatty Acids: 0 g, Total Omega-3 FA: .038 g, Total Omega-6 FA: 0 g, Calcium: 44.2 mg, Potassium: 1409 mg, Sodium: 102.6 mg, Vitamin K: 11.1 mcg

Crockpot Stew With Nonalcoholic Zin Sauce Per Serving 3½ Carb Choices: Calories: 512.9, Protein: 32.1 g, Carbohydrate: 59.2 g, Dietary Fiber: 5.862 g, Total Sugars: 21 g, Total Fat: 17.2 g, Saturated Fat: 6.085 g, Monounsaturated Fat: 8.168 g, Polyunsaturated Fat: 1.364 g, Cholesterol: 82.7 mg, Trans Fatty Acids: 0 g, Total Omega-3 FA: .145 g, Total Omega-6 FA: .153 g, Calcium: 85.3 mg, Potassium: 1750 mg, Sodium: 134.8 mg, Vitamin K: 17.6 mcg

Crockpot Stew With Zin Sauce 3½ Carb Choices: Calories: 580.1, Protein: 31.7 g, Carbohydrate: 59.6 g, Dietary Fiber: 5.862 g, Total Sugars: 21 g, Total Fat: 17.2 g, Saturated Fat: 6.085 g, Monounsaturated Fat: 8.17 g, Polyunsaturated Fat: 1.365 g, Cholesterol: 82.7 mg, Trans Fatty Acids: 0 g, Total Omega-3 FA: .145 g, Total Omega-6 FA: .154 g, Calcium: 83.1 mg, Potassium: 1764 mg, Sodium: 131.8 mg, Vitamin K: 17.6 mcg

3-BEAN HOT CHILI 'N PORK

FLEXITARIAN – 1 CARB CHOICES

Makes 10 Cups Sodium Per Recipe: 1024 mg Sodium Per Cup: 93.5 mg

Crockpot Recipe. A terrific slow cooked tenderloin roast. Crockpots are an asset for many of us who just don't have the time or strength or inclination to spend a few hours cooking a great meal. If you work during the day, leaving a crockpot on low is the perfect answer for a hot meal when you arrive home. You can also put a crock-pot meal together for your family when you know you'll be gone during dinner time.

- **1 cup filtered water (trace)**
- **2 14.5-ounce cans no salt added diced tomatoes (105 mg)**
- **1 cup canned no salt added tomato sauce (26.8 mg)**
- **1 6-ounce can no salt tomato paste[1] (166.6 mg)**
- **2 pounds (about 2) small lean pork tenderloins, fat trimmed off (472.7 mg**
- **1 medium onion, chopped (4.4 mg)**
- **4 medium garlic cloves, minced (2.04 mg)**
- **1½ teaspoons no salt added chili powder[2] (Williams, Wayzata Bay or Frontier work well) (trace)**
- **¼ teaspoons white pepper (.03 mg)**
- **1 small jalapeno pepper, seeded and chopped (.14 mg)**
- **1 15-ounce can Eden Organic No Salt Added Black Beans, drained (52.5 mg)**
- **1 15-ounce can Eden Organic No Salt Added Kidney Beans, drained (52.5 mg)**
- **1 15-ounce can Eden Organic No Salt Added Pinto Beans, drained (52.5 mg)**

Prepare onions and jalapeno. You may slice the meat into bite size pieces or cook whole and then pull apart or slice, which is what I like to do. Drain bean cans. Place ingredients into crockpot bowl in order listed. Cover with lid and turn crockpot on for either setting, 6 or 8 hours. Serve hot.

[1] such as Contadina plain tomato paste

[2] may add more chili powder to taste. Wayzata Bay chili powder is hotter than Williams's. Available at www.healthyheartmarket.com

Bean & Chili Pork Nutrient Data Per Serving: Calories: 254.6, Protein: 27.7 g, Carbohydrate: 27.3 g, Dietary Fiber: 7.28 g, Total Sugars: 4.921 g, Total Fat: 3.402 g, Saturated Fat: 1.104 g, Monounsaturated Fat: 1.253 g, Polyunsaturated Fat: .567 g, Cholesterol: 59.1 mg, Trans Fatty Acids: .033 g, Total Omega-3 FA: .032 g, Total Omega-6 FA: .434 g, Calcium: 20 mg, Potassium: 1075 mg, Sodium: 93.5 mg, Vitamin K: 2.992 mcg

ORANGE AND APPLE CHICKEN

FLEXITARIAN – 2 CARB CHOICES

Serves 8 Sodium Per Recipe: 515 mg Sodium Per Serving: 64.4 mg

This crockpot dish may be prepared in the oven as well. Cooking time is different. For the oven you'll bake at 350° F for about 45 to 50 minutes or until chicken is done.

8 large chicken thighs (about 1 ½ pounds), skinless, boneless, pan browned (474.7 mg)
1 tablespoon extra virgin olive oil (trace)
½ cup natural maple syrup (14.5 mg)
3 tablespoons apple cider vinegar (2.235 mg)
1 cup fresh orange juice (2.48 mg)
1 8-ounce can crushed or chunky pineapple in water with juice (2.46 mg)
3 level tablespoons brown sugar, packed (11.6 mg)
2 medium to large Fuji or Gala apples, cut into large bite size pieces (2.5 mg)
¾ cup sliced mushrooms (2.625 mg)
¼ teaspoon cinnamon[1] (.065 mg)
½ teaspoon ground ginger (.288 mg)

After Cooking

level tablespoons cornstarch, set aside for later use (1.26 mg)

Brown the chicken in nonstick skillet or fry pan with 1-tablespoon extra virgin olive oil. While chicken is browning, place all other ingredients into the crockpot except for the cornstarch, and stir. Hold cornstarch aside for later use. When chicken is ready place into crockpot. Cover pot, turn on low setting for 6 hours. Check temperature with thermometer for doneness.

When time is up, mix cornstarch in 1/4 cup of cold water until dissolved, add into the pot and stir. Turn pot on high and cook additional half-hour to forty-five minutes or until chicken is done.

Serve with freshly steamed white or wild rice.

[1] If you like cinnamon a lot, add another ¼ teaspoon. Cinnamon works well as an anti-inflammatory.

Apple Chicken Nutrient Data Per Serving: Calories: 219.1, Protein: 14.2 g, Carbohydrate: 30.7 g, Dietary Fiber: 1.197 g, Total Sugars: 25.3 g, Total Fat: 4.599 g, Saturated Fat: .954 g, Monounsaturated Fat: 2.097 g, Polyunsaturated Fat: .916 g, Cholesterol: 57.3 mg, Trans Fatty Acids: .073 g, Total Omega-3 FA: .092 g, Total Omega-6 FA: 0 g, Calcium: 36.2 mg, Potassium: 368.7 mg, Sodium: 64.4 mg, Vitamin K: 3.854 mcg

MAUREEN'S MUSHROOM CHICKEN STROGANOFF

FLEXITARIAN – 2 CARB CHOICES

Serves 6 Sodium Per Recipe: 572.5 mg Sodium Per Serving 95.4 mg

Quick & Easy. You can cut this recipe in half or you can refrigerate what you don't eat (covered) for up to five days. .

- **1 pound of non-brined chicken tenders[1] (306.8 mg)**
- **1 tablespoon extra virgin olive oil (.27 mg)**
- **¾ cup of chopped onion (4.8 mg)**
- **1 cup sliced mushrooms (3.5 mg)**
- **1 pinch nutmeg (.023 mg)**
- **2 tablespoons unbleached, all-purpose flour (.312 mg)**
- **2 cups nonfat milk with added Vitamin A (205.8 mg)**
- **8 ounces noodles[2] (47.9 mg)**

Prepare noodles or brown rice[2] and set aside where they will keep warm.

In a 12-inch fry pan, heat oil over medium-high flame and sauté chicken tenders until lightly golden and cooked through (about ten to fifteen minutes). Remove from pan and set aside. Reduce heat to medium.

In the same fry pan add onions and sauté until transparent. Add mushrooms and sauté for a few minutes more. Remove from heat and set onion and mushrooms aside. Reduce heat to medium-low.

Combine the flour and one-half cup of the milk in a medium sauce pan thoroughly. Place on burner, raise heat to medium, add balance of milk and mix thoroughly until well blended. Reheat stirring constantly until mixture comes to boil and begins to thicken. Add mushrooms, onions, and nutmeg. Then add chicken and stir until all is well heated.

Serve over noodles or rice with green vegetables like string beans or asparagus. Use sour cream or nonfat Yo Cheese for garnish.

[1] Strips of chicken with no skin, no bone.

[2] Or two cooked cups of brown rice (sodium approx. 12 mg)

Stroganoff Nutrient Data Per Serving (6): Calories: 300.3, Protein: 27.1 g, Carbohydrate: 35.4 g, Dietary Fiber: 1.786 g, Total Sugars: 5.926 g, Total Fat: 5.072 g, Saturated Fat: 1.084 g, Monounsaturated Fat: 2.376 g, Polyunsaturated Fat: .996 g, Cholesterol: 79.2 mg, Trans Fatty Acids: .043 g, Total Omega-3 FA: .095 g, Total Omega-6 FA: .003 g, Calcium: 129.4 mg, Potassium: 489.9 mg, Sodium: 94.9 mg, Vitamin K: 1.79 mcg

PEPPERS STUFFED WITH MEAT

FLEXITARIAN – 2 CARB CHOICE

Serves 6 Sodium Per Recipe: 489.8 mg Sodium Per Serving: 81.6 mg

- **2 cups cooked brown or white rice (3.9 mg)**
- **3 large green bell peppers (19.7 mg)**
- **½ large onion, diced finely (3 mg)**
- **1 cup carrots, chopped (88.3 mg)**
- **½ medium red bell pepper, chopped (1.785 mg)**
- **1 tablespoon extra virgin olive oil (trace)**
- **1 tablespoon garlic clove, minced (1.428 mg)**
- **1 pound lean ground beef (5% fat)[1] (299.4 mg)**
- **1 pinch ground cloves (trace)**
- **½ teaspoon dried oregano (.135 mg)**
- **½ teaspoon dried basil (.238 mg)**
- **4 ounces fresh low sodium mozzarella cheese (17.9 mg)**
- **2 8-ounce cans no salt added tomato sauce (53.7 mg)**
- **cracked black pepper or white pepper to taste (trace)**

Cook rice per package instructions.

Clean bell pepper, cut in half separating top from bottom, remove membrane and seeds. Set aside in 9 x 13 baking dish open side up.

Mix meat, vegetables, and spices with rice.

Mix tomato sauce with a half-cup of filtered water in a bowl.

Fill each bell pepper with the meat mixture. Pour about three-quarters of the tomato sauce over the top of each stuffed pepper. While peppers bake, baste a couple of times with the remaining tomato sauce.

Bake in a 350° F oven for 40 minutes.

At 40-minutes, top with mozzarella cheese, return to oven and cook another 10-15 minutes or until cheese is melted and bubbly. Serve hot.

[1] 1-pound of lean ground turkey is about 450 mg sodium.

Stuffed Peppers Nutrient Data Per Serving: Calories: 326.7, Protein: 25.2 g, Carbohydrate: 32.2 g, Dietary Fiber: 5.233 g, Total Sugars: 9.721 g, Total Fat: 10.3 g, Saturated Fat: 4.217 g, Monounsaturated Fat: 4.4 g, Polyunsaturated Fat: .888 g, Cholesterol: 57 mg, Trans Fatty Acids: .258 g, Total Omega-3 FA: .136 g, Total Omega-6 FA: .006 g, Calcium: 185.2 mg, Potassium: 921.5 mg, Sodium: 81.6 mg, Vitamin K: 15.3 mcg

PORK TENDERLOIN

FLEXITARIAN – 0 CARB CHOICES

Serves 4   Sodium Per Recipe: 265.5 mg   Sodium Per Serving: 66.3 mg

With Special Herb and Spice Rub. This one is easy. Insert garlic cloves, rub with herb and spice mix shown below, bake in oven and serve with stuffed or plain yams and unsalted peas or lightly sautéed string beans. Especially terrific when barbecued using convection heat.

16 ounces, boneless pork roast or tenderloin[1] (261.8 mg)
3 cloves garlic, sliced thinly (1.53 mg)
1 teaspoon dried thyme (.072 mg)
1 teaspoon dried marjoram (.462 mg)
1 teaspoon dried rosemary (.6 mg)
1 teaspoon dried sage (.077 mg)
½ teaspoon ground savory (.168 mg)
½ teaspoon ground white pepper (.06 mg)
1 tablespoon olive oil (.81 mg)

Preheat oven to 325° F. Set rack for middle of oven. (May also be barbecued using convection heat.)

Mix spices together in a small bowl and set aside.

With a sharp knife make stab marks about one-half inch deep throughout the roast. Stuff each hole with a sliver of garlic.

Baste roast with one tablespoon of the olive oil. Rub spice mix on the meat on all sides.

Stick an oven thermometer into the meat. Bake for about 30 minutes per pound or per your supplier's instructions. Make sure the center of the pork reaches at least 170° F on the thermometer.

Serve with yams and green vegetable like green beans or peas.

[1]May cook larger roast or tenderloin, but we recommend that you consume only 4-ounces or less of cooked meat per serving.

Pork Tenderloin Nutrient Data Per Serving: Calories: 171.3, Protein: 26.1 g, Carbohydrate: 1.508 g, Dietary Fiber: .493 g, Total Sugars: .032 g, Total Fat: 6.165 g, Saturated Fat: 1.374 g, Monounsaturated Fat: 3.457 g, Polyunsaturated Fat: .834 g, Cholesterol: 80.3 mg, Trans Fatty Acids: .026 g, Total Omega-3 FA: .057 g, Total Omega-6 FA: .369 g, Calcium: 25.3 mg, Potassium: 512.1 mg, Sodium: 66.3 mg, Vitamin K: 6.003 mcg

SALMON TACOS

FLEXITARIAN – 1 CARB CHOICE

Makes 4 tacos Sodium Per Recipe: 149.4 mg Sodium Per Taco: 37.3 mg

Ever try a fish taco? Don't shrug it off yet if you haven't; this tasty treat will grab your attention and you'll make them again.

The Tomato Salsa

1 large tomato, diced (9.1 mg)
½ medium to large onion diced (3 mg)
3 tablespoons fresh chopped cilantro (trace)
1 teaspoons fresh lemon juice (trace)
½ jalapeno pepper, chopped (.07 mg)
½ teaspoon white pepper (.06 mg)

Chop tomato, cilantro and onion. Mix together a small bowl. Add chopped jalapeno, the lemon juice and white pepper and gently stir together.

The Taco

1 cup shredded iceberg lettuce or Savoy cabbage[1] (7.2 mg)
6 ounces freshly cooked wild salmon (78.2 mg)
2 teaspoons fresh squeezed lemon juice (trace)
4 6-inch corn tortillas (11.4 mg)
¼ cup light sour cream (40.2 mg)

Shred lettuce or cabbage and set aside. Mix ¼ cup of light sour cream and the lemon juice together and set aside.

Heat salmon if already cooked or grilled, if not, cook over medium to high heat until warmed or cooked through. Turn once or twice.

While salmon is heating, spray a fry pan or griddle with light coat of olive oil and cook the tortillas until close to crispy but still foldable.

Place 1.5 ounces of warmed salmon in middle of each tortilla. Spread salsa on the salmon. Lay the shredded lettuce or cabbage on top of the salsa and then drizzle with the sour cream and lemon mix.

Fold and serve hot.

[1]Data figured on Savoy cabbage. Napa or Chinese cabbage would be 49.4 mg sodium per cup. Iceberg lettuce would be about 7.2 mg per cup.

Salmon Tacos Nutrient Data Per Taco: Calories: 160.5, Protein: 12.1 g, Carbohydrate: 17.9 g, Dietary Fiber: 2.566 g, Total Sugars: 2.473 g, Total Fat: 4.824 g, Saturated Fat: 1.584 g, Monounsaturated Fat: 1.536 g, Polyunsaturated Fat: 1.257 g, Cholesterol: 24.1 mg, Trans Fatty Acids: 0 g, Total Omega-3 FA: .67 g, Total Omega-6 FA: 0 g, Calcium: 94 mg, Potassium: 416.3 mg, Sodium: 37.3 mg, Vitamin K: 8.291 mcg

DON'S SPICY BARBECUED CHICKEN THIGHS

FLEXITARIAN – 0 CARB CHOICE

Makes 4 servings Sodium Per Recipe: 283.7 mg Sodium Per Thigh: 35.4

If you like the sweetness of the chicken thigh and you like spices, then this recipe will give you a tasty meal, one that is easy to prepare.

8 small to medium boneless or bone-in, skinless chicken thighs[1] (282.1 mg)
1 teaspoon fresh grated lemon peel (.12 mg)
2 teaspoons Don's Hot Barbecue Spice Mix (1.264 mg)

To Barbecue

Trim all visible fat off thighs.

Rub chicken with spices and the lemon peel.

Barbecue with convection heat. Set over flame last five to ten minutes, turning every few minutes. Serve hot.

For Baking In Oven

Pre heat oven to 350° F.

Trim all visible fat off thighs. Roll chicken thighs in the spices and lemon zest until all thighs are evenly coated.

Bake in 9 / 13 baking dish for 45 to 60 minutes at 350° F.

Serve hot.

[1] Thigh meat only, bone out, skinless, weight approximately 41 grams per thigh for the meat.

BBQ Chicken Thighs Nutrient Date Per Thigh: Calories: 51.1, Protein: 8.115 g, Carbohydrate: .548 g, Dietary Fiber: .135 g, Total Sugars: .286 g, Total Fat: 1.639 g, Saturated Fat: .423 g, Monounsaturated Fat: .5 g, Polyunsaturated Fat: .41 g, Cholesterol: 34 mg, Trans Fatty Acids: .043 g, Total Omega-3 FA: .042 g, Total Omega-6 FA: 0 g, Calcium: 6.141 mg, Potassium: 100.9 mg, Sodium: 35.4 mg, Vitamin K: 1.787 mcg

ST. LOUIS STYLE BBQ RIBS

FLEXITARIAN – 0 CARB CHOICE

Serves 4   Sodium Per Recipe: 370.3 mg   Sodium Per Serving (4): 92.6 mg

I call these St. Louis Ribs because it was in St. Louis I first enjoyed them. Give it a try with my special rib rub below. I also like to knead this rib rub into 96% fat free ground beef when making a burger.

1 rack of small baby back pork ribs, (smallest ribs available)[1] (367.4 mg)
3 teaspoons Don's Rib Rub or to taste (Page 266) (2.873 mg)

Prepare Don's Rib Rub and store in a dry jar for future use.

Sprinkle the spice mix over the meat and rub it in using your hands. It's best to marinate or let this sit covered in a refrigerator for a few hours, but if you're in a hurry, you'll still find it tasty and exciting.

If using an oven, set rack for middle, turn on heat to 325° F either regular or convection.

If using a barbecue, prepare it for convection heat. Set gas barbecue to medium-high heat. If using coals, set pile of coals to one side or one end. Once hot, set ribs on grill where they are away from the flame or coals. Cover with lid and cook for about 60 to 90 minutes. Start with meat side down, then in thirty minutes turn over so meat side is up.

[1]Estimated data. USDA does not provide exact data for baby back pork ribs. Each rib on the small baby back has slightly less than an ounce of meat on them. 6 small ribs will have about 3 to 4-ounces of meat. We weighed them to figure out the meat in ounces and then calculated the USDA figures for the only ribs they list ("Pork, Spare-ribs, Fresh, lean&fat, raw"). The result is about 23 mg of sodium per ounce of meat.

St. Louis Ribs Nutrient Data Per Serving: Calories: 320.3, Protein: 17.7 g, Carbohydrate: 1.398 g, Dietary Fiber: .312 g, Total Sugars: .774 g, Total Fat: 26.7 g, Saturated Fat: 8.557 g, Monounsaturated Fat: 9.742 g, Polyunsaturated Fat: 4.538 g, Cholesterol: 90.7 mg, Trans Fatty Acids: .252 g, Total Omega-3 FA: .189 g, Total Omega-6 FA: 3.657 g, Calcium: 21.9 mg, Potassium: 294.6 mg, Sodium: 92.6 mg, Vitamin K: .714 mcg

BROILED LOBSTER

FLEXITARIAN – 0 CARB CHOICE

Serves 2[1] Sodium Per Recipe: 531.4 Sodium Per Serving: 265.7 mg

This treat is special. Sodium in this recipe is natural and higher than most of our recipes, but lobster lovers will appreciate the fact that we can enjoy a good spiny or rock lobster once in a while. Ask your fish-market rep if the "original" or shipping container lists salt or sodium higher than 150 mg per 3-ounces. Fresh raw lobster is best. We have made the preparation and the cooking of this lobster very easy.

2 5-ounce rock (spiny) lobsters[1] (481.4 mg)
2 tablespoons unsalted butter (3.124 mg)
lemon, sliced into wedges (1.68 mg)

Note: Make sure to time your side-dishes to coincide with the cooking of the lobster.

Fill medium to large pan with enough water to cover the two tails while boiling. Bring water to a boil, lower tails into water and boil at slightly lower heat for exactly 6 minutes. Keep water at a light rolling boil. Pan will not be covered.

While tails are boiling, melt butter over simmer heat in a small pan. When melted squeeze one lemon wedge into butter and stir. Use other wedges as desired. This will be your lobster dipping sauce.

Remove tails to cutting board and let cool for five minutes.

Set rack for oven broiler, turn broiler on.

With sharp food scissors, cut the top shell from the front to the tail. Press the two sides together tightly to help break the meat from the shell (inside). Then slip your finger at the tail (not the front) between the shell and the meat and slip it forward to break meat away from shell. Do this on both sides. Then pull the meat out, close the shell and lay the meat back on the shell and set on broiler pan. Do this with both tails. If shell breaks on you, then lay it on the broiler pan and place the meat on top of it.

Place under broiler for exactly 6 minutes.

Serve immediately.

[1]Meat weight only. Allow about 1-ounce for shell. So, a 6 ounce lobster will have about 5-ounces of meat.

Lobster Nutrient Data Per Full 5-ounce Serving: Calories: 280.6, Protein: 31.2 g, Carbohydrate: 7.538 g, Dietary Fiber: 1.176 g, Total Sugars: 1.059 g, Total Fat: 13.9 g, Saturated Fat: 7.663 g, Monounsaturated Fat: 3.399 g, Polyunsaturated Fat: 1.347 g, Cholesterol: 134.7 mg, Trans Fatty Acids: 0 g, Total Omega-3 FA: .718 g, Total Omega-6 FA: .308 g, Calcium: 87.2 mg, Potassium: 329.1 mg, Sodium: 265.7 mg, Vitamin K: .994 mcg

SESAME CRUSTED FISH

FLEXITARIAN – 1 CARB CHOICE

4 servings   Sodium Per Recipe: 407 mg   Sodium Per Serving: 101.8 mg

Take a hunk of firm fleshed fish, like stripe bass, halibut, cod, yellowtail, tuna or wahoo and give it a crispy sesame crust. Buy your sesame seeds in the Asian or Hispanic section of the market. They're much cheaper than in the spice section. Easily adapted from Scott Leysath's Wild Game cookbook[3]. A great Father's Day gift for the fisherman and hunter. (This recipe also works well with chicken.)

- **4 6-ounce firm fish fillets, skin removed (346.8 mg)**
- **2 tablespoons sesame oil (trace)**
- **3 tablespoons Don's Soy Sauce Replacement[1] (5.325 mg)**
- **1 tablespoon low sodium mustard[2] (15 mg)**
- **½ cup sesame seeds (29.2 mg)**
- **3 tablespoons extra virgin olive oil (trace)**
- **2 tablespoons freshly squeezed lime juice (.605 mg)**
- **2 tablespoons freshly squeezed lemon juice (.305 mg)**
- **1 tablespoon fresh gingerroot, minced (1.728 mg)**
- **3 green onions, chopped (7.2 mg)**

Combine sesame oil, 1-tablespoon of the soy sauce replacement and honey mustard. Rub mixture over both sides of fish fillets. Cover with sesame seeds and lightly press seeds into both sides. Heat oil in a large skillet over medium heat on your good camp stove (or at home). Add fish and cook until sesame seeds are lightly browned on one side. Carefully flip over and cook the other side for 1-minute. Add remaining soy sauce replacement, lemon and lime juice and gingerroot to the pan and cook until fish is lightly cooked. Remove from pan and transfer to plates. Top with chopped green onion.

[1] See page 249

[2] Low Sodium Mustard can be found online at Healthy Heart Market. (http://healthyheartmarket.com/mustards.aspx) or, use 1 teaspoon of Coleman's mustard powder (.165 mg).

[3] For a copy of Scott Leysath's Wild Game cookbook, visit www.arrowhead-classics.com

Crusted Fish Nutrient Data Per Serving: Calories: 514, Protein: 36.1 g, Carbohydrate: 12.4 g, Dietary Fiber: 3.713 g, Total Sugars: 4.388 g, Total Fat: 36 g, Saturated Fat: 5.196 g, Monounsaturated Fat: 16.9 g, Polyunsaturated Fat: 11.5 g, Cholesterol: 102 mg, Trans Fatty Acids: 0 g, Total Omega-3 FA: 2.897 g, Total Omega-6 FA: 0 g, Calcium: 87.9 mg, Magnesium: 135.9 mg, Potassium: 736 mg, Sodium: 101.8 mg, Vitamin D: 0 mcg, Vitamin K: 30.5 mcg

PAN-FRIED CATFISH

FLEXITARIAN – 1 CARB CHOICES

4 servings   Sodium Per Recipe: 419 mg   Sodium Per Serving: 122.8 mg

You'll need to make homemade bread for this one. Adapted from one of Scott Leysath's Sporting Chef[1] *recipes. Excellent flavors. Catfish is a delicious fish. Looks like orange roughy but tastes a whole lot better. The original uses a full cup of half and half for a sauce. For us that's too much fat and too much sodium, so we've converted it to our needs.*

The Sauce

- **½ cup Hot Mustard Sauce (See Page: 254) (73 mg)**

The Fish

- **2 egg whites (109.6 mg)**
- **2 tablespoons nonfat milk (12.9 mg)**
- **4 6 - ounce wild (not farmed) catfish fillets (292.4 mg)**
- **¼ cup unbleached all-purpose flour (.625 mg)**
- **⅛ teaspoon white pepper (add into flour) (.015 mg)**
- **1 cup Don's Garlic Bread crumbs (Page: 195) (2.013 mg)**
- **2 tablespoons extra virgin olive oil (.57 mg)**

Prepare the sauce. Set aside.

Lightly beat eggs with nonfat milk.

Dust the fish first with flour, then dip into egg mixture, then roll in bread crumbs. Heat olive oil in nonstick pan over medium high heat and fry fish until brown on both sides (should take about one to two minutes each side). Drain on paper towels. To serve, place fish on plate and spoon sauce over it. Great with wild rice.

[1] Scott is a professional chef who has a TV show known as "Hunt, Fish, Cook." You can find a special price for his cookbook at *megaheart.com/wheretobuy.html* or you can find it at huntfishcook.com or at any bookstore.

Pan-Fried Catfish Nutrient Data Per Serving: Calories: 337.1, Protein: 33.7 g, Carbohydrate: 19.6 g, Dietary Fiber: .65 g, Total Sugars: 2.188 g, Total Fat: 13.6 g, Saturated Fat: 2.254 g, Monounsaturated Fat: 6.696 g, Polyunsaturated Fat: 2.302 g, Cholesterol: 98.8 mg, Trans Fatty Acids: 0 g, Total Omega-3 FA: .968 g, Total Omega-6 FA: 0 g, Calcium: 44.2 mg, Potassium: 714.3 mg, Sodium: 122.8 mg, Vitamin K: 4.295 mcg

TACO SALAD

FLEXITARIAN - 3 CARB CHOICES[3]

Serves 4 Sodium Per Recipe: 504 mg Sodium Per Serving: 126 mg

8 ounces ground turkey (213.2 mg)
1 8-ounce can no-salt-added tomato sauce (26.8 mg)
2 tablespoons chili powder[1] (trace)
1 tablespoon onion powder (3.726 mg)
2 ears of fresh corn (12.5 mg)
8 cups iceberg lettuce torn into bite-size chunks (57.6 mg)
½ cup thinly sliced or diced carrots (42.1 mg)
½ cup celery, chopped or diced (40.4 mg)
½ cup snow or snap peas, each sliced into three pieces (1.96 mg)
½ cup cucumbers, sliced (1.19 mg)
½ cup red onion, thinly sliced (3.2 mg)
½ cup red pepper[2] (2.98 mg)
1 1 medium to large tomato, chopped (6.15 mg)
½ avocado, chopped (5.44 mg)
4 4-ounces unsalted tortilla chips (16.8 mg)
2 2-ounces Heluva Good® cheddar cheese (20 mg)
Dollop of Sour cream or Don's Yo Cheese (50 mg)

Lightly brown the ground turkey in a medium sized nonstick fry pan. Sprinkle with chili seasoning and onion powder. Add the tomato sauce and simmer while you prepare the salad.

Boil the corn in a small amount of water for about 2 minutes. Remove from pan and trim off kernels. Mix with meat.

Prepare salad with greens and lots of vegetables that you enjoy. Top with the tomato and avocado.

Place 1-ounce tortilla chips on each plate and divide the salad into four servings on top of chips.

Serve the meat/tomato sauce mixture in a small bowl to be heaped on top of the salad. Serve the cheese in a small bowl to be sprinkled on top of the meat mixture. Pass the fresh salsa and sour cream as a garnish and enjoy.

[1] Wayzata Bay, Williams Chili Seasoning or other unsalted chili powder.

[2] Add any other fresh vegetables that you may enjoy in a salad.

[3] Diabetics, the chips contain 73.2 carbohydrates for the recipe.

Taco Salad Nutrient Data Per Serving: Calories: 481.2, Protein: 23.2 g, Carbohydrate: 55.2 g, Dietary Fiber: 9.283 g, Total Sugars: 12.1 g, Total Fat: 20.8 g, Saturated Fat: 3.236 g, Monounsaturated Fat: 6.282 g, Polyunsaturated Fat: 4.703 g, Cholesterol: 74 mg, Trans Fatty Acids: .155 g, Total Omega-3 FA: .502 g, Total Omega-6 FA: .003 g, Calcium: 227.9 mg, Potassium: 1176 mg, Sodium: 126 mg, Vitamin K: 54.3 mcg

MACARONI & CHEESE

LACTO OVO VEGETARIAN – 1½ CARB CHOICES

Serves 4 Sodium Per Recipe: 103.3 mg Sodium Per Serving: 25.8 mg

This recipe was designed for children who must limit their salt/sodium intake. It has been child tested and enjoyed greatly. May double this recipe if you need to.

- **1 cup elbow macaroni (6.3 mg)**
- **1 tablespoons unsalted butter (or canola oil) (1.952 mg)**
- **1 tablespoon all purpose flour (.075 mg)**
- **¾ cup nonfat or 2% milk with vitamin A (77.2 mg)**
- **⅛ tsp teaspoon granulated onion powder (.162 mg)**
- **⅛ teaspoon white pepper (.015 mg)**
- **⅛ teaspoon nutmeg (.044 mg)**
- **3 ounces shredded low-sodium cheddar cheese (17.9 mg)**

Cook macaroni according to package directions and drain.

In a medium-size saucepan over medium heat melt butter and slowly stir in the flour. Cook while stirring until it bubbles or froths (about a minute). Remove pan from heat and add the milk, stirring until well blended, return to heat and cook while continuing to stir until mixture thickens.

When thick, add in the onion powder, pepper, and nutmeg. Stir in cheddar cheese until all the cheese melts. Mixture should be smooth. Pour sauce over cooked macaroni. Option: You can add steamed broccoli to the macaroni and cheese or set it on the side for a complete dish. One-half cup of steamed broccoli adds 14.5 mg sodium and 3 mg of carbohydrates.

Serve hot.

Macaroni & Cheese Nutrient Data Per Serving: Calories: 230.8, Protein: 10.4 g, Carbohydrate: 23.9 g, Dietary Fiber: .929 g, Total Sugars: 3.197 g, Total Fat: 10.3 g, Saturated Fat: 6.357 g, Monounsaturated Fat: 2.759 g, Polyunsaturated Fat: .473 g, Cholesterol: 29.8 mg, Trans Fatty Acids: 0 g, Total Omega-3 FA: .116 g, Total Omega-6 FA: .077 g, Calcium: 214.1 mg, Potassium: 157.9 mg, Sodium: 25.8 mg, Vitamin K: .858 mcg

BARBECUE

Our barbecue recipes will work in gas or charcoal barbecues. My personal preference is charcoal, however, I've also got a large Weber gas BBQ that does just fine. I prefer to cook most solid meat (not ground) using convection heat. Just set the meat to one side and use the heat on the opposite side and then close the lid. Some cooking however is better directly over the heat, like the salmon below, for which I build a "boat."

BASIC BARBECUED SALMON

FLEXITARIAN - ½ CARB CHOICES

Serves 3 Sodium Per Recipe: 165.4 mg Sodium Per Serving (3): 55.1 mg

When you want to barbecue a great piece of salmon, make a boat for it and cook it right over the heat with your barbecue lid closed.

1 12–ounce piece of Alaskan Wild Salmon[1] (159.8 mg)
1 tablespoon (or slightly more) extra virgin olive oil (trace)
2 tablespoons brown sugar (5.04 mg)
1 lemon for juice, cut into wedge (3.4 mg)

Set hot coals across bottom of barbecue (or if using a gas grill, fire it up), cover and let it heat to about 400° F[2].

Build a "boat" out of heavy duty aluminum foil folding it over at least once for a two layer boat. Oil the base with about 1 tablespoon extra virgin olive oil. Spread a little bit of the sugar over the area the fish will cover. Lay fish on that and then drizzle or rub the rest of the oil on the upper layer and layer the rest of the brown sugar over that.

Place boat on grill above hot coals or fire, close lid. Turn salmon over in 4 to 6 minutes depending on heat level. When salmon is turned, cook for another 4 to 6 minutes. Don't overcook it.

Serve hot with homemade unsalted salsa, ear of corn and a nice green salad. Don't forget the lemon wedges for the salmon.

[1]We recommend fresh Alaskan wild salmon, fresh in season. Sockeye is a good choice and usually what is available. "Atlantic salmon," is farm grown and known to have a high level of pesticides.

[2]Salmon will cook well at lower temperatures as well. Just takes a bit longer.

Barbecued Salmon Nutrient Data Per Serving: Calories: 292.8, Protein: 24.1 g, Carbohydrate: 5.885 g, Dietary Fiber: 0 g, Total Sugars: 5.821 g, Total Fat: 18.7 g, Saturated Fat: 2.937 g, Monounsaturated Fat: 11.2 g, Polyunsaturated Fat: 3.077 g, Cholesterol: 70.3 mg, Trans Fatty Acids: 0 g, Total Omega-3 FA: 1.545 g, Total Omega-6 FA: 0 g, Calcium: 11.9 mg, Potassium: 451.2 mg, Sodium: 55.1 mg, Vitamin K: 5.871 mcg

BARBECUED OR CAMPSTOVE-COOKED FRESH TROUT

FLEXITARIAN – 1 CARB CHOICES

2 servings Sodium Per Recipe: 111.5 mg Sodium Per Serving: 55.7 mg

When it's summertime and you really don't feel like heating up the kitchen, the logical place to cook your dinner is outdoors on the barbecue. This preparation works well with most game fish. When cooking whole fish, figure on about 1 pound per person before cleaning and removing the head.

2 whole trout about a pound each, head off and filleted (about ¾ pound meat remaining) (98.6 mg)
1 teaspoon thyme, ground (.77 mg)
1 teaspoon sage (.077 mg)
1 teaspoon marjoram (.462 mg)
½ teaspoon black pepper (.462 mg)
juice of 2 lemons (.94 mg)
½ bunch fresh basil (.2 mg)
2 garlic cloves, minced (1.02 mg)
3 thinly-sliced onion rings (.81 mg)
6 slices tomato (8.1 mg)
2 lengths butcher string, each about 2 feet long.
1 tablespoon extra virgin olive oil (trace)

Mix thyme, sage, marjoram and pepper together. Season fish inside and out with the mix.

Squeeze the juice of 1 lemon into each cavity. Pack equal portion of basil, garlic, onion and tomato into cavity of each fish.

Tie a loop around one end of each fish and make a few more loops around the fish, securing the stuffing.

Brush fish with extra virgin olive oil.

Place on a medium-low heat barbecue grate, or on a camp stove griddle for 5 to 7 minutes, then flip over and cook other side about 7 minutes more or until skin is crisp and fish is just-cooked throughout. To serve, cut string and place fish on plate. Stuffing may be removed or eaten.

Serve hot.

Barbecued Campfire Trout Nutrient Data Per Serving: Calories: 291.2, Protein: 34 g, Carbohydrate: 10.9 g, Dietary Fiber: 2.17 g, Total Sugars: 3.907 g, Total Fat: 12.6 g, Saturated Fat: 2.151 g, Monounsaturated Fat: 6.848 g, Polyunsaturated Fat: 2.811 g, Cholesterol: 93.8 mg, Trans Fatty Acids: 0 g, Total Omega-3 FA: 1.375 g, Total Omega-6 FA: 0 g, Calcium: 158.2 mg, Potassium: 1079 mg, Sodium: 55.7 mg, Vitamin K: 41.7 mcg

BURGER BARBECUE SAUCE

VEGAN – 1 CARB CHOICES

Makes: 2 cups

Sodium Per Recipe: 353.5 mg   Sodium Per 2 tablespoons: 22.1 mg

This sauce is easy to put together and works with with any meat. Optionals of course include adding your own spice mix (or ours).

½ onion, chopped (3.3 mg)
3 cloves garlic, minced (1.53 mg)
¼ cup extra virgin olive oil (trace)
1 6-ounce can no salt tomato paste (166.6 mg)
2 8-ounce cans no-salt-added tomato sauce (146.4 mg)
3 tablespoons red wine vinegar (1.192 mg)
1 cup filtered water (trace)
½ cup light brown sugar or Brown Sugar Twin[1] (30.8 mg)
½ teaspoon sage (.038 mg)
½ teaspoon thyme (.0385 mg)
¼ teaspoon allspice (.366 mg)
2 tablespoons cornstarch (.42 mg)
pinch of cayenne pepper[2] (trace)

Prep all vegetables.

In a medium saucepan, Sauté onions and garlic in one tablespoon of olive oil until translucent.

Add in the rest of the olive oil and the tomato paste, tomato sauce, water, vinegar and brown sugar. Heat over medium heat for about five minutes stirring occasionally.

Add sage, thyme, allspice, cayenne pepper and bring to quick boil. Lower heat to simmer for about fifteen minutes, stirring occasionally.

Stir cornstarch in a small bowl with about ¼ cup of water. When dissolved, add to the sauce and stir until well mixed. Cook while stirring constantly until sauce thickens and develops a gloss.

Cool or use warm. Baste on burger meat while barbecuing. Tastes very good with barbecued chicken and pork ribs, too.

[1]Sugar Twin has approximately 72 mg sodium for the same measurement. Or use Splenda Brown Sugar Blend, or use regular light brown sugar.

[2]Cayenne pepper is hot. Pinch in only what you think you'd like.

Barbecue Sauce Nutrient Data Per Serving: Calories: 79.6, Protein: .986 g, Carbohydrate: 12.3 g, Dietary Fiber: 1.06 g, Total Sugars: 8.264 g, Total Fat: 3.506 g, Saturated Fat: .49 g, Monounsaturated Fat: 2.478 g, Polyunsaturated Fat: .399 g, Cholesterol: 0 mg, Trans Fatty Acids: 0 g, Total Omega-3 FA: .027 g, Total Omega-6 FA: 0 g, Calcium: 17.9 mg, Potassium: 243.8 mg, Sodium: 22.1 mg, Vitamin K: 4.413 mcg

BARBECUED PORK TENDERLOIN

FLEXITARIAN – 1½ CARB CHOICES

Serves 8[1]   Sodium Per Recipe: 501.6 mg   Sodium Per Serving: 62.7 mg

You can barbecue directly over the heat or use convection. Baste the meat about every twenty minutes until done. A very tasty dish for guests.

The Meat

2 pounds of fresh, lean, raw non-brined pork tenderloin (480.8 mg)

The Sweet & Sour Sauce

3 tablespoons cold filtered or bottled water (trace)
2 tablespoons cornstarch (1.44 mg)
½ cup white granulated sugar (trace)
6 tablespoons brown sugar, unpacked (15.1 mg)
½ cup unseasoned rice vinegar[2] (2.38 mg)
½ teaspoon ground ginger (.288 mg)
3 garlic cloves, minced (1.53 mg)

Mix the water and cornstarch and set aside.

Place all other sauce ingredients into a medium saucepan. Stir thoroughly and then add the water and cornstarch mixture. Over medium heat, bring the mixture to a boil, lower the heat and let simmer while stirring frequently until the sauce thickens. Sauce will thicken quickly. Taste test. If you want more sugar, add no more than two tablespoons. When done set aside.

If using a gas barbecue, heat the barbecue with one or two of the jets with the lid closed – leaving a space on the grill that does not take direct heat. We want to cook this tenderloin with convection heat. (Some barbecues have a rack to the rear that is raised above the main grill. If yours does, I suggest using it. Simply place tenderloins on the rack.)

If using a coal barbecue like a Weber, Kingsford, or other, set coals to one side and heat the barbecue with the cover on and the vents open. The base vents should also be open.

After five or ten minutes the barbecue should be about 400° F. Place the two strips of tenderloin[3] over the flameless grill area. We want to cook this meat at about 425° F. Spoon some of the sauce over the meat and close the lid. After fifteen minutes, turn the meat over and spoon more sauce on it. Do this again in fifteen minutes and then again for one last time in fifteen minutes. It will take from 45 minutes to an hour to cook the meat in either the gas or the coal barbecue.

To roast in the oven, set the oven to 350° F, place the pork into a lightly greased baking dish and spread half the sauce over the meat. Bake for a half-hour, turn over and baste with the remaining sauce. Meat may be done in 45 minutes to an hour. Test it since you don't want to overcook it.

Serve with cranberry sauce, steamed unsalted green vegetables like string beans, and potatoes or yams.

[1] Can cut recipe in half to serve 4. We make the above and save the leftovers for sandwiches or a dinner and change the flavor by adding a homemade blackberry sauce as a topping.

[2] Or cider or other vinegar

[3] Most packaged, unbrined tenderloins come with two strips. If you purchase a single strip, then cook according to above. Cooking times will vary.

Barbecued Pork Tenderloin Nutrient Data Per Serving: Calories: 210, Protein: 23.9 g, Carbohydrate: 21.4 g, Dietary Fiber: .056 g, Total Sugars: 19.1 g, Total Fat: 2.474 g, Saturated Fat: .795 g, Monounsaturated Fat: .9 g, Polyunsaturated Fat: .421 g, Cholesterol: 73.7 mg, Trans Fatty Acids: .024 g, Total Omega-3 FA: .019 g, Total Omega-6 FA: .339 g, Calcium: 14.5 mg, Potassium: 468.1 mg, Sodium: 62.7 mg, Vitamin K: .02 mcg

BARBECUE TIPS

Barbecuing is good year 'round. However, in cold climates, it's a bit difficult since the BBQ will be fighting the elements, sometimes losing the battle. Otherwise grilling year around provides us with great cooking.

Here are some key tips that might help you barbecue.

1. Two kinds of heat are used with barbecues. Direct and indirect, which we refer to as convection cooking. Direct means putting your food over the flame or center of heat and indirect or convection means setting the food off to the side of the flame or center of heat.

2. Don't spear meat to turn it. Use long handle tongs.

3. Leave some space between food so that it will cook evenly.

4. Charcoals should be about 75 to 80% gray before cooking with them.

5. Trim fat from meat to avoid flames.

6. If you have sauce left over that has touched raw meat, then we recommend tossing it. Some might say boil it for a few minutes, but bacteria are just too dangerous these days to trust that.

7. Gas grills work better on cold days than do charcoal units.

8. Let meat rest about five minutes or more before slicing. Burgers and hot dogs can be served right away but roasts, steaks, chickens, etc. should rest to allow the juices to resurface.

9. Use barbecue tools instead of kitchen tools.

10. Always clean your barbecue grill after cooking while it's still hot and can be scraped cleanly.

DON'S SPECIAL BBQ SAUCE

VEGAN – ½ CARB CHOICE

Makes 48 tablespoons[1]

Sodium Per Recipe: 310.8 mg   Sodium Per tablespoon: 6.475 mg

This sauce has been used for everything from oysters to steaks and barbecued burgers, chicken and wild game. It was once used in a restaurant in Olympia, Washington with the menu listing, "Oysters Gazzaniga."

2 tablespoons extra virgin olive oil (trace)
1 6 ounce can Contadina tomato paste (166.6 mg)[2]
2 8 ounce cans no-salt-added tomato sauce (53.7 mg)
⅛ teaspoon ground cloves (.639)
1 teaspoon sage (.77 mg)
1 teaspoon marjoram (.462 mg)
1 teaspoon thyme, ground (.77 mg)
1 teaspoon coriander leaf, dried (1.266 mg)
1 teaspoon oregano (.27 mg)
1 teaspoon ground cinnamon (.26 mg)
⅛ to ¼ teaspoon cayenne pepper (.067 mg)
3 tablespoons balsamic vinegar (11 mg)
3 cloves, garlic, minced (1.53 mg)
2 large onions, chopped (12 mg)
1 cup packed brown sugar[3] (61.6 mg)

Mix all ingredients except brown sugar in a medium to large saucepan over medium-high heat. Bring to a slow boil, stirring frequently, then reduce heat to simmer partially covered for up to one hour, stirring occasionally. Stir in brown sugar halfway through the simmering period. Continue to simmer, partially covered until sauce slightly thickens.

Serve hot or brush on meat while barbecuing.

[1]May make fewer or more, depending on thickening you like.
[2]USDA average Data. Contadina brand is lower.
[3]May reduce amount of sugar if you prefer. If you do, taste test for best level.

Barbecue Sauce Nutrient Data Per Tablespoon: Calories: 33.7, Protein: .392 g, Carbohydrate: 6.982 g, Dietary Fiber: .479 g, Total Sugars: 5.731 g, Total Fat: .619 g, Saturated Fat: .09 g, Monounsaturated Fat: .418 g, Polyunsaturated Fat: .078 g, Cholesterol: 0 mg, Trans Fatty Acids: 0 g, Total Omega-3 FA: .008 g, Total Omega-6 FA: 0 g, Calcium: 10.9 mg, Potassium: 92.9 mg, Sodium: 6.475 mg, Vitamin K: 2.386 mcg

SPECIAL VEGGIE BURGER

FLEXITARIAN – 0 CARB CHOICE

Makes 8 patties[1] Sodium Per Recipe: 428.5 mg Sodium Per Patty: 53.6 mg

We often refer to these burger patties as extended, as in stretching the meat to make more patties. But in reality while they also add nutrition they provide a sneaky way to get carrots down your kids (or grandkids). Tasty, healthy and low in fat and cholesterol.

1¼ pounds ground lean (5%) beef[2] (374.2 mg)
½ cup chopped carrots (44.2 mg)
½ cup chopped zucchini (6.2 mg)
½ cup chopped onion (3.2 mg)
½ teaspoon granulated onion powder (.648 mg)
¼ teaspoon white pepper [3](.03 mg)

Clean and prepare vegetables. Work vegetables and spices into meat using your hands or a wooden spoon. Form patties. If you want them for future use, stack together with wax paper between each patty and freeze in zipper lock freezer bag or wrapped in heavy duty aluminum foil.

Barbecue over hot grill with patties placed on a barbecue grill over direct heat. I usually use a grill topper – designed for barbecues – this usually keeps meat from falling through the standard rack type grill[4]. Use a light touch of extra virgim olive oil on the grill since the lean meat will not have enough fat to grill without sticking to the grill.

[1] Plus or minus one.

[2] May also use ground turkey or chicken. Most ground turkey packages come in 20-ounce sizes, which is about 533 mg sodium. If yours are different, adjust recipe accordingly. Check your package for their sodium level. USDA sodium levels will be listed on the FDA label and might vary slightly. We estimate approximately, or a little less than 3-ounces of meat per patty whether beef or turkey burger.

[3] More if you like the pepper flavor.

[4] To see grill topper, visit megaheart.com/kit_cabinet.html

Beef Nutrient Data Per Patty: Calories: 106.4, Protein: 15.5 g, Carbohydrate: 2.132 g, Dietary Fiber: .507 g, Total Sugars: .99 g, Total Fat: 3.59 g, Saturated Fat: 1.605 g, Monounsaturated Fat: 1.529 g, Polyunsaturated Fat: .2 g, Cholesterol: 43.9 mg, Trans Fatty Acids: .242 g, Total Omega-3 FA: .05 g, Total Omega-6 FA: .006 g, Calcium: 13.2 mg, Magnesium: 19.1 mg, Potassium: 307.2 mg, Sodium: 53.6 mg, Vitamin D: 0 mcg, Vitamin K: 1.648 mcg

Turkey Nutrient Data Per Patty: Calories: 114.9, Protein: 12.7 g, Carbohydrate: 2.132 g, Dietary Fiber: .507 g, Total Sugars: .99 g, Total Fat: 5.901 g, Saturated Fat: 1.605 g, Monounsaturated Fat: 2.201 g, Polyunsaturated Fat: 1.436 g, Cholesterol: 56 mg, Trans Fatty Acids: .194 g, Total Omega-3 FA: .082 g, Total Omega-6 FA: 0 g, Calcium: 16.1 mg, Potassium: 227.1 mg, Sodium: 73.4 mg, Vitamin K: 1.861 mcg

GRILLED TOFU

VEGAN – ½ CARB CHOICE

Serves 4 Sodium Per Recipe: 141.4 mg Sodium Per Serving: 35.3 mg

Chimichurri (also spelled Chimmichurri) is not unlike a green or red sauce and is most often used as a marinade for meat. This truly vegan dish combines cumin and our no-salt version of chimichurrie into a barbecued delight.

1 pound extra-firm tofu (64 mg)

Sauce Ingredients

2 cups fresh parsley, loosely packed (67.2 mg)
3 large garlic cloves, chopped (1.53 mg)
½ teaspoon granulated onion powder (.648 mg)
¼ teaspoon white pepper (.03 mg)
⅓ teaspoon red pepper flakes (.18 mg)
2 tablespoons onion, minced (.8 mg)
¼ cup of extra virgin olive oil (trace)
3 tablespoons red wine vinegar (3.576 mg)
3 tablespoons fresh lemon juice (.458 mg)

Spice Rub

½ teaspoon garlic powder (.364 mg)
⅓ teaspoon paprika (.238 mg)
½ teaspoon ground cumin (1.764 mg)
⅓ teaspoon ground fennel seeds (.586 mg)

Oil For Tofu

½ teaspoon extra virgin olive oil (trace)

In your blender pulse-chop sauce ingredients. Don't puree. Set aside.

To prepare the rub, mix ingredients together and set aside.

Slice the tofu lengthwise into two steaks. Brush lightly with the ½ teaspoon extra virgin olive oil. Using your hands press the rub into tofu steaks on two sides. To barbecue, place tofu directly over heat on grill or use a special nonstick grill pan and place directly over heat. (I use a BBQ grill topper.)

Cook for about three or four minutes turn and cook for another three to five minutes. To serve four, cut each of the steaks in half. Serve hot, covered withthe chimichurri sauce.

Grilled Tofu Nutrient Data Per Serving: Calories: 324.3, Protein: 19.4 g, Carbohydrate: 9.912 g, Dietary Fiber: 1.479 g, Total Sugars: .995 g, Total Fat: 25.5 g, Saturated Fat: 3.836 g, Monounsaturated Fat: 7.43 g, Polyunsaturated Fat: 5.092 g, Cholesterol: 0 mg, Trans Fatty Acids: 0 g, Total Omega-3 FA: .072 g, Total Omega-6 FA: 0 g, Calcium: 54.8 mg, Potassium: 222.5 mg, Sodium: 35.3 mg, Vitamin K: 495.5 mcg

BREAD

I remember making bread with my mother. "Don, you knead it." So I did the muscle work while she shaped it afterwards and made whichever bread she had scrolled into her small book of time-worn recipes.

Back then the disruption in that weekly pattern was a single small truck with the words *Helms Bakery* on it. The mobile bakery's logo included the rings familiar with the logo of the Olympics, and rightly so. Helms was the "Official" bread of the Olympics.

And mother tried her darndest to make breads that were much like those on that truck. She also made some terrific Italian and French breads. Now you know the root of my baking skills.

However, the real enjoyment was the scent of fresh bread throughout the house, and we always looked forward to that.

I also remember the high levels of salt used in those breads. Salt is the primary ingredient that keeps commercial bread fresh, although some bakers have always added vinegar, which also helps keep bread fresh.

Today, we need to make our bread without salt, but luckily we have bread machines to do the "muscle" work. Although bread machines can make loaves very easily, they can also serve the purpose of kneading dough for us so that we can make buns, rolls, and smaller loaves as well as longer loaves like baguettes.

Each of our previous books has a selection of bread recipes. Each is a good recipe as written. However, I never seem to make a bread recipe without experimenting with it. I try to push them further along to the point that they stay fresh longer, taste better, and bake without too much trouble.

We have learned that some ingredients enhance salt-free bread to the point of necessity. For instance we know that yeast, ascorbic acid, vinegar, sugar, and gluten are necessary for unsalted bread. Optional ingredients include onion powder (taste), potato flour for bread, pancakes, waffles, and gluten free bread. Also we sometimes add granulated soy lecithin, which retains freshness and offers a nutty flavor, and is important in high grain breads. We have learned too, that extra virgin olive oil or expeller pressed canola oil are best for helping to retain moisture as compared to butter. For ascorbic acid we often use three 500-mg vitamin C tablets crushed in a mortar and pestle.

We recommend using white flour recommended for bread, white whole wheat flour (same nutrients as red whole wheat), and for diabetics, we recommend soy flour for a partial exchange to help lower the carbohydrate level.

The recipe on the next page may be one of the most interesting. It is a no-knead bread. It is one of the world's original bread recipes when yeast was first added to flat bread, so it won't rise very high, but it does have an excellent texture and is a fun conversation starter at dinner parties.

NO KNEAD BREAD

VEGAN – 1 CARB CHOICES
HANDMADE – OVEN BAKED

Makes 1 Loaf[1] Sodium Per Recipe: 14.3 mg Sodium Per Slice: .895 mg

This unique bread is how bread used to be made. This bread has a nice crunch-crust and terrific texture and flavor. Kneading was introduced to bread-making by early commercial bakers.

3 cups white unbleached best for bread flour (7.5 mg)
1 teaspoon Rapid Rise or bread machine yeast (2 mg)
¼ teaspoon ascorbic acid (trace)
1 teaspoon granulated sugar (trace)
1 tablespoon vital wheat gluten (2.79 mg)
2 tablespoons vinegar (.15 mg)
1 tablespoons extra virgin olive oil (.54 mg)
1¼ cups filtered, warmed to 115° F water (trace)

You will use a covered pan in your oven to bake this loaf of bread. You will need two light 100% cotton clothes, floured.

In a medium bowl combine all ingredients in the order listed. Add water and oil and stir until well mixed. Dough will be a bit sticky.

Using stretch plastic, cover the bowl tightly. Allow dough to rest for about 14 to 18 hours in room temperature (around 70° F) or warmer. If making in cooler house turn oven on to 200° F for one minute, then turn off and place in oven with door closed.

Lightly grease and flour-dust a 9" or 10" loaf pan. Either one will work.

When dough is ready small bubbles should appear. Dough does not rise spectacularly but you'll feel that it has risen when you touch it. (We've experienced occasions when bubbles didn't appear and the dough was ready.)

Roll dough out onto a floured work surface. Use additional flour sparingly while working with it since it will be sticky. Fold it over on itself twice. Cover with floured cloth for about fifteen minutes.

When ready, gently but quickly shape the dough into loaf pan shape. Place dough seam side down into your lightly floured pan. Let dough rise in your warmed (about 70° F to 90° F) oven for about two to three hours, possibly a bit more. It does not have to be covered when in the oven. It should double or rise about an inch above the loaf pan.

With loaf still in oven, turn oven on to 475° F. Bake until golden brown. Times will vary from oven to oven. When top is golden brown, turn oven off and let loaf stay in the oven for another 5 to 10 minutes. Test with a finger snap. If it sounds hollow it's done. Remove from oven and roll out of pan to rack for cooling. Slice and serve warm.

[1] You may also make this as a round loaf. Just use a Corningware, iron bowl or other baking pan with a lid to let rise in warm place, then place in oven and bake at 450° F for 30 minutes. After thirty minutes remove lid and bake for another 15 minutes. Bread will be a nice dark golden brown.

No Knead Bread Nutrient Data Per Slice No Knead Bread: Calories: 104.6, Protein: 2.969 g, Carbohydrate: 18.3 g, Dietary Fiber: .689 g, Total Sugars: .333 g, Total Fat: 1.94 g, Saturated Fat: .272 g, Monounsaturated Fat: 1.259 g, Polyunsaturated Fat: .279 g, Cholesterol: 0 mg, Trans Fatty Acids: 0 g, Total Omega-3 FA: .018 g, Total Omega-6 FA: 0 g, Calcium: 4.679 mg, Potassium: 32.1 mg, Sodium: .895 mg, Vitamin K: 1.086 mcg

CLASSIC FRENCH BREAD

LACTO -OVO/VEGAN – 1 CARB CHOICES
BREAD MACHINE KNEAD – HAND SHAPE – OVEN BAKE

Makes 2 loaves[1] Sodium Per Recipe: 46.8 mg Sodium Per Slice: 1.464 mg

If you order a sandwich in a restaurant or sandwich shop with bread similar to this one, you'll probably receive upwards of 1,000 mg of sodium. This very low-sodium recipe is good for curl and regular sandwiches.

2 cups less 2 tablespoons warmed (100° F) filtered water (trace)
4 tablespoons cider vinegar (.30 mg)
1 level unpacked tablespoon grated lemon peel (.36)
5 cups white, unbleached or best for bread flour (12.5 mg)
2 tablespoons potato flour (11 mg)
1 teaspoon malted barley flour (1.114 mg)
¼ teaspoon ascorbic acid (trace)
1 tablespoon white granulated sugar (trace)
1 tablespoon vital wheat gluten (2.25 mg)
1 tablespoon plus 1 teaspoon bread machine yeast (8 mg)

Glaze *(Vegans, use oil instead of egg white)*
½ egg white (whisked with a ¼ teaspoon of water)[2] (27.5 mg)

Place all ingredients in bread pan in order listed. Set bread machine for dough cycle. Dough may rise completely before buzzer sounds. If dough reaches top, or touches lid, remove to a lightly floured bread board. Cut the dough ball into the number of loaves you wish to make. Shape or form either 4 or 6 small round loaves, or two long loaves. Note: You can mix or match. Make one long loaf (about 14 to 16" and two or three rounds, or make all rounds.) For the Party Sandwiches in this book, just split the dough in half and follow the directions in the Party Sandwich recipe (See Page: 138).

For long loaves, roll each half of the dough into a log. Place on a parchment paper covered baking sheet or into a French loaf pan dusted with cornmeal. Baste bread with the egg white/water mix.

Make three diagonal slices about a quarter-inch deep with a sharp knife evenly spaced across the top. Cover with light flour-dusted cloth and let rise for about 45 minutes to an hour or until double in size.[3] Preheat oven to 400° F. When ready, place loaves into oven on rack one third of the way up from the bottom and lower heat to 375° F. Bake 15 to 22 minutes or until golden brown. A finger snap is a good test. If bread sounds hollow it should be cooked through.

Cool on rack at least ten minutes before slicing. Serve warm or reheated or toasted. Excellent bread for panini sandwiches or French toast.

For Small Rounds

Prepare baking sheets with parchment paper and cornmeal sprinkled on paper. When dough is ready, cut into 4 or 6 even pieces. Form into balls, tucking underneath and pinching each one to seal. Place on baking sheets about 3" to 4" apart (These will rise again. Place 4 at the most per sheet). Make two 1/4" deep cross-cuts with a sharp knife across the top. Let rise in warm place for about an hour or until doubled in size. Bake same as loaves above.

[1] Makes 13 to 15" long loaves, data based on 32 slices..

[2] Whisk all the egg white from an egg. You'll end up using only half of it.

[3] In a room temperature of about 70 to 80 degrees F. If you are making two loaves in a French loaf pan, then heat your oven to about 100° F and let rise in there without the cloth cover. When ready to cook, leave in the oven and turn oven on to 375° F and cook for about 25 minutes.

Classic French Bread Nutrient Data Per Serving (with sugar)(Based on 32 slices): Calories: 198.2, Protein: 2.467 g, Carbohydrate: 16.4 g, Dietary Fiber: .712 g, Total Sugars: .486 g, Total Fat: 13.7 g, Saturated Fat: 1.899 g, Monounsaturated Fat: 9.88 g, Polyunsaturated Fat: 1.505 g, Cholesterol: 0 mg, Trans Fatty Acids: 0 g, Total Omega-3 FA: .108 g, Total Omega-6 FA: 0 g, Calcium: 4.294 mg, Potassium: 39.7 mg, Sodium: 1.464 mg, Vitamin K: 8.193 mcg

FIBER WHITE BREAD

LACTO-OVO/VEGAN – 2 CARB CHOICES[2]

BREAD MACHINE KNEAD – HAND SHAPE – OVEN BAKE

Makes 2 loaves Or Makes 16 3'x 4" buns

Sodium Per Recipe: 85.5 mg Sodium Per Slice (32): 1.782 mg

Sodium Per Bun (16): 5.345 mg

This white bread recipe with flaxseed fiber is flexible as well as delicious. You can make cinnamon bread loaves, Parker House rolls, hamburger buns or just plain old sliced bread. It will come out of the oven light and airy and as tasty as any bread you've ever eaten. It's well worth a try. You can use Splenda Granulated as a sugar substitute. If you choose to make rolls or buns, etc. just divide the number of servings into the recipe total to determine sodium level for each serving.

2 cups minus two tablespoons, unsweetened orange juice not from concentrate, with calcium, 105° F to 110° F (17 mg)
6 tablespoons extra virgin olive oil (trace)
4 tablespoons cider vinegar (2.98 mg)
½ teaspoon vanilla extract or flavoring (.189 mg)
5 cups white best for bread flour (12.5 mg)
2 level tablespoons vital wheat gluten (5.365 mg)
2 level tablespoons granular soy lecithin (trace)
4 tablespoons flaxseed meal (4.2 mg)
3 tablespoons potato flour (12.4 mg)
¼ teaspoon ascorbic acid (trace)
2 level tablespoons white granulated sugar (trace)
1 tablespoon plus 1 teaspoon bread machine yeast (7.98 mg)

Glaze *(Vegans, use oil instead of egg white)*

1 large egg white only, whisked with teaspoon of filtered water[1] (27.4 mg)

Place dough ingredients into your bread machine pan in the order listed or in the order your manufacturer suggests. Set for dough and check back in about ten minutes to make sure you have enough liquid or that it doesn't need more flour. If the dough is balling it's okay. Slightly sticky is okay.

Before dough is ready, set the racks in your oven(s) to a place where you can let your dough rise for baking. Heat your oven for 2 minutes at 200° F and then turn it off – leave the door closed. If you have double-ovens, then use both.

Put egg white into a small bowl and whisk with a teaspoon of water. Set aside for use after shaping dough.

When dough is ready, roll out to a lightly floured bread board and slice in half. Work first half into buns or loaves and then work with the second half.

Using a basting brush, baste the top of your dough with the egg white water mix. Place into warmed oven uncovered and door closed or a warm spot in your kitchen covered with a piece of lightly oiled wax paper.

Let rise for forty five minutes in your oven or, if outside your oven, until dough doubles in size.

If using single oven to warm, remove one loaf carefully and set into a warm place. With one loaf still in oven bring heat to 375° F. Bake for about 20 to 35 minutes total or until bread tests hollow with a finger snap. After removing, place second loaf in and bake for 18 to 22 minutes or until done.

Remove after baked and set on wire rack. Let rest for about 10 to fifteen minutes before slicing. May freeze this bread for up to a few months. Freeze slices by placing waxed paper between them first.

For Hamburger Buns

Shape buns by rolling dough out to about ¾" thick, slice into squares with sharp knife, or make rounds with your cutter, set on a jellyroll pan lined with parchment paper, and baste with egg-water mix. Should be able to get 8 buns per jellyroll pan. Bake at 375° F for about 12 to 18 minutes or until golden brown. (Or may bake in oven if you've used the oven for the rise by setting oven temp to 375° F and letting dough bake until golden brown. Should take about 16 to 22 minutes.)

For Parker House Rolls

Roll dough into 1-inch balls and set three balls into each cup of a greased and flour-dusted muffin tin. Baste with the egg-water mix. Let rise for an hour. Bake at 375° F for about 10 to 12 minutes or until golden brown.

[1] One egg mixed with a dash of water whisked. You'll probably only use half the egg white to brush the bread tops. Vegans can leave this step out.

[2]*Diabetics*, most of the carbohydrates are in the flour (476.9 grams for recipe). Exchange 1 cup soy flour for 1 cup of the white flour to lower carb count. Exchange water for orange juice. Replace potato flour with 3 addtional tablespoons of soy flour. (Defatted soy flour lowers carbs and calories even more.)

Fiber White Bread Nutrient Data Per Bun (16) 4-Carb Choices: Calories: 271.4, Protein: 6.52 g, Carbohydrate: 46.9 g, Dietary Fiber: 1.794 g, Total Sugars: 15 g, Total Fat: 6.469 g, Saturated Fat: .887 g, Monounsaturated Fat: 3.889 g, Polyunsaturated Fat: 1.201 g, Cholesterol: 0 mg, Trans Fatty Acids: 0 g, Total Omega-3 FA: .251 g, Total Omega-6 FA: 0 g, Calcium: 22.4, Potassium: 334.9 mg, Sodium: 5.345 mg, Vitamin K: 3.344 mcg

[2] ***Fiber White Bread Nutrient Data Per Slice (32) 1-Carb Choices: Calories: 108.6, Protein: 3.86 g, Carbohydrate: 14.3 g, Dietary Fiber: 1.095 g, Total Sugars: 1.148 g, Total Fat: 4.341 g, Saturated Fat: .58 g, Monounsaturated Fat: 1.934 g, Polyunsaturated Fat: .575 g, Cholesterol: 0 mg, Trans Fatty Acids: 0 g, Total Omega-3 FA: .123 g, Total Omega-6 FA: 0 g, Calcium: 4.741 mg, Potassium: 32.5 mg, Sodium: 1.82 mg, Vitamin K: 1.59 mcg***

DON'S SANDWICH BUNS

LACTO -OVO /VEGAN – 2½ CARB CHOICES[1]

BREAD MACHINE KNEAD – HAND SHAPE – OVEN BAKE

Makes 16 Buns Sodium Per Recipe: 90 mg Sodium Per Bun: 5.628 mg

This recipe has been tested many times. I tried to duplicate the sandwich bun that we used to enjoy in our youth at Bob's Big Boy, in southern California. This was one of the original local chain's that branched out beyond its borders, but for a while it was strictly local. Our father would send my two brothers and me inside while he had the rest of the family outside for car service. He'd give each of us a dollar bill. For that dollar we got two huge burgers, a large order of fries and a giant milkshake and each one of us would get fifteen cents change. Not exactly a homerun on today's health-scale, but it sure was fun back then.

2 cups warmed filtered water (105° F to 110° F) (trace)
¼ cup extra virgin olive oil (1.08 mg)
3 tablespoons cider vinegar (2.235 mg)
5 cups best for bread flour (12.5 mg)
2 tablespoons white granulated sugar (trace)
¼ teaspoon ascorbic acid (trace)
½ teaspoon malted barley flour (trace)
2 tablespoons potato flour (7.75 mg)
¼ teaspoon granulated onion powder (.324 mg)
2 tablespoons vital wheat gluten (5.365 mg)
1 tablespoon granulated soy lecithin (optional) (trace)
1 tablespoon plus 1 teaspoon bread machine yeast (8 mg)

After first rise *(Vegans may use oil baste instead of egg white)*

1 egg white, whisked with ¼ teaspoon water[2] (27.4 mg)
1 tablespoon sesame seeds[3] (3.76 mg)

Place first twelve (12) ingredients into bread machine pan. Set for dough and let the machine knead it.

Prepare two jelly roll pans or the baking sheets you normally use with a layer of parchment paper. Stick into oven or ovens and turn ovens on to 200° F for two minutes. Then turn oven(s) off and let baking sheets stay there. If you have an oven with a proof setting, use that. If you have a large convection oven, you can bake both sheets at the same time. See our economy tip below.

Set an egg on your countertop to let it come close to room temperature. Just before dough is ready, place egg white into a small bowl and whisk lightly with the water. Set aside with pastry brush.

When first rise is completed roll dough onto floured board. Cut in half. Work with each half by itself.

Using your hands press dough down to about three quarters inch (3/4") thick. Cut out buns and place on sheets. We use English muffin rings to cut bun shapes from dough. Baste with egg white and sprinkle with sesame seeds. Place uncovered in your preheated oven and close door. Let rise for 60 minutes.

If you prefer to let dough rise outside the oven, then cover with lightly oiled wax paper or a flour-dusted soft cotton cloth (not Terry towel nor polyester). Let rise outside the oven for about one hour to one and a half hours. When dough doubles in size, it's ready for baking.

Preheat oven to 375° F about fifteen minutes before dough is ready. Bake for about 12 to 18 minutes. (Ovens vary.) When they turn golden brown, they are done. Snap finger lightly on outer crust and if sound is "hollow" then bread is done. Let cool on rack for about twenty minutes before sliced or serving. Let cool for about two hours before storing in zipper lock bags. Freezes well.

Economy tip. When baking any of our bread recipes that are oven baked, you can let rise in the oven. When ready, leave the dough in the oven and turn the oven to the temperature recommended in the recipe. The bread will rise a bit more and bake nicely about the time the oven reaches the set temperature. Typically we find that our bread takes another three to five minutes to brown and be fully baked after chosen temp is reached. Snap a finger on the buns. If you get a hollow sound, turn the oven off, leave buns in for a minute or two more then cool on a rack for twenty minutes. (Let cool another two hours before storing in zipper lock bags. Freezes well.) If baking both sheets in a convection oven, the same rules apply. Upper sheet may finish first.

[1] Diabetics you can exchange one-cup white flour with one-cup Bob's Red Mill Soy Flour. This will lower carbs for the recipe total by 63 grams or 4 grams per bun.

[2] Data is for ½ egg white. That's the most you'd use while brushing the bun tops.

[3] You might need more. Sodium increase would be negligible.

Don's Sandwich Buns Nutrient Data Per Bun: Calories: 190.9, Protein: 5.714 g, Carbohydrate: 32.2 g, Dietary Fiber: 1.384 g, Total Sugars: 1.721 g, Total Fat: 4.147 g, Saturated Fat: .582 g, Monounsaturated Fat: 2.65 g, Polyunsaturated Fat: .654 g, Cholesterol: 0 mg, Trans Fatty Acids: 0 g, Total Omega-3 FA: .036 g, Total Omega-6 FA: 0 g, Calcium: 9.127 mg, Potassium: 75.6 mg, Sodium: 5.628 mg, Vitamin K: 2.15 mcg,

TIPS FOR BREAD BAKERS

1. Set all tools and ingredients you'll need out on your countertop before starting to bake bread, muffins, pies, cakes, etc.

2. Preheat oven about fifteen minutes before you plan to put your baked goods into oven.

3. Warm or proof bread dough in an oven at about 80° F to 100° F, uncovered. If you do this, you can leave the dough in the oven after its rise and just turn the oven on to the desired temperature. (See #4 below).

4. Bread baking does not always require preheating your oven. We let the bread rise in a "proof temp" oven and then when ready just turn it on. (This saves energy and money, by the way.) Timing will change a bit, but results are often excellent. Simply place bread into oven, close door and turn oven to desired temperature. With most ovens, about the time the temperature gets to your selection the bread is nearly fully baked and it will have risen slightly more than it would if placed into a preheated oven. Usual baking time for our recipes using this method, is about 18 to 22 minutes.

DON'S GARLIC BREAD

VEGAN – 2 CARB CHOICES

BREAD MACHINE RECIPE

Makes 1 Loaf Sodium Per Loaf: 88.7 mg Sodium Per Slice : 1.731 mg

This bread is a good breakfast toast or it's exceptional for making bread crumbs for breaded fish or chicken.

1¼ cups orange juice, not from concentrate (3.1 mg)
4 tablespoons olive oil (trace)
2 tablespoons apple cider vinegar (1.49 mg)
3 cloves garlic, minced (1.53 mg)
½ medium onion, diced (1.65 mg
4 cups bread flour (10 mg)
1 tablespoon vital wheat gluten (2.683 mg)
¼ teaspoon ascorbic acid (trace)
3 tablespoons white sugar (trace)
1 teaspoon dried basil or one tablespoon fresh, chopped basil (.238 mg)
1 teaspoon garlic powder (.728 mg)
2 tablespoons chives, chopped (.18 mg)
½ teaspoon coarsely ground black pepper (.924 mg)
2 teaspoons bread machine yeast (4 mg)

Heat orange juice to (100° F to 105° F).

Place balance of ingredients in the bread machine pan in the order suggested or in the order suggested by your bread machine manufacturer.

Select Basic or White Bread cycle for 2 or 2 ½ pound loaf, medium crust, and press Start. Check in ten minutes for moisture. If it needs more liquid, add one or two tablespoons of filtered water. If it seems too sticky or wet, add a few tablespoons of flour.

Cool on rack. If making croutons or bread crumbs, let sit out overnight. Then cut into bite size pieces. Let dry in high room temp or on jelly roll pan in oven set at 200° F for about three hours. Check to make sure bread doesn't brown.

[1]Diabetics, the bulk of carbs are in the flour, orange juice and sugar. You can lower the carbs even more by replacing sugar with Splenda® Sugar Blend for Baking, orange juice with water and exchange 3/4 cup of flour with 3/4 cup soy flour.

Don's Garlic Bread Nutrient Data Per Slice: Calories: 169.1, Protein: 4.423 g, Carbohydrate: 29 g, Dietary Fiber: 1.069 g, Total Sugars: 4.136 g, Total Fat: 3.772 g, Saturated Fat: .526 g, Monounsaturated Fat: 2.511 g, Polyunsaturated Fat: .502 g, Cholesterol: 0 mg, Trans Fatty Acids: 0 g, Total Omega-3 FA: .036 g, Total Omega-6 FA: 0 g, Calcium: 11.1 mg, Potassium: 91.4 mg, Sodium: 1.731 mg, Vitamin K: 3.917 mcg

FOCACCIA

LACTO OVO VEGETARIAN – 2 CARB CHOICES

BREAD MACHINE KNEAD – HAND SHAPE – OVEN BAKE

Serves 12 Sodium Per Recipe: 42.45 mg Sodium Per Slice: 3.533 mg

Change topping to one of your choice, but this one works very well. Cut as wedges for serving. Makes up to 16 servings. Freeze the bread you don't use right away[1].

1 cup plus 1-tablespoon warmed filtered or low sodium water (trace)
2 tablespoons plus 1 teaspoon extra virgin olive oil (trace)
2 tablespoons cider vinegar (1.49 mg)
3 cups white unbleached (best for bread) flour[2] (6.25 mg)
2 level tablespoons sugar (trace)
1 tablespoon vital wheat gluten (4.5 mg)
¼ teaspoon ascorbic acid (trace)
¼ teaspoon granulated onion powder (.648 mg)
2¼ teaspoons bread machine yeast (4.5 mg)

The Topping

2 tablespoons extra virgin olive oil (trace)
1 medium onion, diced (4.4 mg)
2 garlic cloves (1.02 mg)
1/3 cup low sodium cheddar cheese (30 mg)
1 tablespoon rosemary or basil, dried (1.65 mg)

Place first nine ingredients into bread machine in order listed or in your manufacturer's suggested order. Set machine for dough and start.

Prepare one baking sheet by covering it with parchment paper.

A few minutes before dough is ready set your oven to about 200 degrees for two minutes and then turn it off. Leave door closed. (If you live in a warm area and your house is warm, you can let the shaped bread rise there.) Set racks for lower middle of oven.

While dough is working in the bread machine, cook onions in nonstick pan, coated with olive oil, over medium or low heat until they are carmelized. Set aside.

Remove dough and shape into a ball. Roll dough in a small bowl with enough olive oil to completely coat it. Set ball down on breadboard and press until it's about 1/2 inch thick. Form a circle or an oblong focaccia by stretching the dough as you would pizza dough. It will pretty much take up most of a jellyroll pan's space. True Italian focaccia is oblong.

Press thumb and fingers into dough to make imprints on top, (small pockets).

Sprinkle the chopped garlic across the top, sprinkle with rosemary or if you prefer dried basil (basil provides an excellent flavor). Then lay the onions on and press them in, then sprinkle the cheese over the entire area staying at least an inch away from the outer edges.

Let rise for fifteen minutes in a warm area covered with a flour-dusted light cloth, or under wax paper, or uncovered in a warmed oven (Oven should be about 80° F to 90° F).

If letting it rise outside the oven, then preheat the oven to 400° F. After rise, bake for about 15 to 20 minutes or until rich golden brown.

If you let the focaccia rise in the oven, leave it there and turn the oven on to 400° F. Bake for about 15 to 20 minutes or until finger snap-test sounds hollow. A rich golden brown color will pretty much mean your focaccia is done. If it rises higher than expected it may need more time to bake.

[1] Generally no-salt bread should be kept in the freezer if not used within three days of baking. Since no-salt bread lacks preservatives (salt being one of them), they can spoil even though they retain that "fresh" feel and appearance.

[2] Not all flour companies declare their product is best for bread or breadmaking. We use Arrowhead Mills, King Arthur and Bob's Red Mill white unbleached flour, and Stone Buhr's "Great for Bread Making" white unbleached flour in our tests.

[3] Diabetics, most of the carbs are in the flour. If you exchange 1 cup of defatted soy flour you can subtract 72 grams of carbs from the recipe total.

Focaccia Nutrient Data Based on 12 Servings: Calories: 200.1, Protein: 5.901 g, Carbohydrate: 27.7 g, Dietary Fiber: 1.29 g, Total Sugars: 2.622 g, Total Fat: 7.156 g, Saturated Fat: .699 g, Monounsaturated Fat: 3.339 g, Polyunsaturated Fat: .612 g, Cholesterol: 6.25 mg, Trans Fatty Acids: 0 g, Total Omega-3 FA: .045 g, Total Omega-6 FA: 0 g, Calcium: 62.3 mg, Potassium: 69.3 mg, Sodium: 4.545 mg, Vitamin K: 2.852 mcg

Diabetic (Soy Flour & Splenda® Blend for Baking Exchange) Focaccia Nutrient Data Based on 12 Servings: Calories: 183.6, Protein: 8.914 g, Carbohydrate: 21.1 g, Dietary Fiber: 2.54 g, Total Sugars: 2.182 g, Total Fat: 7.222 g, Saturated Fat: 2.167 g, Monounsaturated Fat: 4 g, Polyunsaturated Fat: .685 g, Cholesterol: 7.087 mg, Trans Fatty Acids: 0 g, Total Omega-3 FA: .074 g, Total Omega-6 FA: 0 g, Calcium: 81.6 mg, Potassium: 274.6 mg, Sodium: 5.075 mg, Vitamin K: 3.371 mcg

ROSEMARY BAGUETTES

VEGAN – ½ CARB CHOICES

BREAD MACHINE KNEAD – HAND SHAPE – OVEN BAKE

Makes 32 1" Slices

Sodium Per Recipe: 25.8 mg Sodium Per Slice: .805 mg

Why not grow your own rosemary as well as other herbs like thyme, and sage? Dry out your rosemary and then use in this recipe. Delicious.

1 cup distilled water, warmed to about 105°F (trace)
1 tablespoon cider vinegar (.745 mg)
1½ tablespoons extra virgin olive oil (.405 mg)
½ teaspoon vanilla extract (.189 mg)
3 cups less two-tablespoons white unbleached bread flour (7.185 mg)
2 tablespoons potato flour (7.75 mg)
1 level tablespoon vital wheat gluten (2.25 mg)
¼ teaspoon ascorbic acid (1.664)
2 level teaspoons sugar (trace)
½ teaspoon onion powder (.648 mg)
1 tablespoon dried rosemary[1] (1.65 mg)
2½ teaspoons bread machine yeast (5 mg)

Place ingredients into bread machine in order listed. Set machine for dough.

Prepare baguette pans by lightly coating with extra virgin olive oil and dusting with cornmeal.

Set pan on large jelly roll pan or baking sheet.

Set rack to lower third. Turn oven on 200° F° for two minutes, then turn off. Leave door closed.

After dough has risen in machine roll out to lightly floured breadboard and slice in half. Roll into two logs that stretch to about 14" to 16" but about 2" in diameter. Place into the warmed oven. Let rise for 45 minutes to an hour.

Leave dough in oven. Turn oven on to 400° F and bake for 16 to 20 minutes or until deep golden brown. Remove and cool on rack for at least ten minutes. Slice 1" thick to serve with soup, stew, chili or salads. (Can also be used for sandwich buns or burgers.)

[1] Another teaspoon or two is acceptable if you want more rosemary flavor.

Rosemary Baguettes Nutrient Data Per Slice: Calories: 52.2, Protein: 1.515 g, Carbohydrate: 9.595 g, Dietary Fiber: .412 g, Total Sugars: .316 g, Total Fat: .782 g, Saturated Fat: .116 g, Monounsaturated Fat: .483 g, Polyunsaturated Fat: .118 g, Cholesterol: 0 mg, Trans Fatty Acids: 0 g, Total Omega-3 FA: .008 g, Total Omega-6 FA: 0 g, Calcium: 3.609 mg, Potassium: 31.1 mg, Sodium: .805 mg, Vitamin K: .416 mcg

BUTTERMILK SANDWICH BUNS

LACTO-OVO VEGETARIAN – 2½ CARB CHOICES

BREAD MACHINE KNEAD – HAND SHAPE – OVEN BAKE

Makes 12 buns Sodium Per Recipe: 264.6 mg Sodium Per Bun: 33 mg

Perfect for hamburgers and lunch sandwiches.

1	**cup 1%, slightly warmed cultured low-sodium warmed buttermilk[1] (130 mg)**
⅓	**cup warmed filtered or no sodium water (trace)**
2	**tablespoons apple cider vinegar (1.49 mg)**
1	**large egg (70 mg)**
3¾	**cups white unbleached bread flour (9.375 mg)**
¼	**cup potato flour (15.5 mg)**
1	**teaspoon granulated lecithin (trace)**
4	**tablespoons extra virgin olive oil (1.08 mg)**
1	**tablespoon white granulated sugar (trace)**
1	**tablespoon vital wheat gluten (2.25 mg)**
¼	**teaspoon ascorbic acid[2] (trace)**
½	**cup quick oats (milled oats) (1.88 mg)**
1	**tablespoon bread machine yeast (6 mg)**

Glaze

½	**large egg white, whisked with water (27.4 mg)**

Warm the buttermilk in microwave to about 80° F.

Add ingredients to your bread machine in order listed. Set on dough cycle and when dough has risen, bring out onto lightly floured bread board.

Set egg out on countertop after you start bread machine to bring it to room temperature. About ten minutes before dough is ready, separate egg white , throw out the yolk, and whisk it with a quarter to half teaspoon of filtered water. You'll use this to glaze the bun shaped dough with a brush.

When dough is ready, press down on dough with palms until dough is about a 3/4" thick. With a sharp knife or pizza cutter, cut or shape buns into rectangle of about 2" x 4". Cut out 12 buns. With the last few you may have to roll together the dough scraps and shape to bun. Tip: We use a muffin cutter to cut out round burger buns.

Place these on jelly roll pan baking sheets covered with parchment paper (6 to a sheet).

Glaze all buns with the egg white mix using a basting brush.

Cover with flour-dusted light-weight cloth. Place in warm spot and let rise for one hour. If placing into a warmed or a proofing oven, let rise uncovered about 45 minutes or until double in size.

Four dough that rose outside the oven, preheat oven to 375° F. and bake for 14 to 20 minutes or until golden brown. For dough that rose inside the oven, just turn the oven on to 375° F and back for about 15 to 18 minutes.

Cool on rack.

When cooled store in zipper lock bags for about 3 days or freeze or refrigerate for longer storage (in the bags).

[1] You may use dry buttermilk mix instead. Works just as well. Sodium is lower at (85 mg). Prepare powder buttermilk mix according to package.

[2] You can obtain ascorbic acid at healthyheartmarket.com or locate it at megaheart.com/wheretobuy.html

Buttermilk Sandwich Buns Nutrient Data Per serving: Calories: 234.5, Protein: 8.054 g, Carbohydrate: 39.5 g, Dietary Fiber: 1.871 g, Total Sugars: 3.524 g, Total Fat: 6.714 g, Saturated Fat: 1.41 g, Monounsaturated Fat: 3.619 g, Polyunsaturated Fat: .913 g, Cholesterol: 21.8 mg, Trans Fatty Acids: 0 g, Total Omega-3 FA: .051 g, Total Omega-6 FA: 0 g, Calcium: 60.8 mg, Potassium: 154.2 mg, Sodium: 33 mg, Vitamin K: 2.966 mcg

WHITE WHOLE WHEAT BREAD

VEGAN – 1 CARB CHOICES

BREAD MACHINE RECIPE

Makes 1 2-cup loaf

Sodium Per Recipe: 23.8 mg ***Sodium Per Slice (15): 1.589 mg***

- **⅔ cup plus 1 teaspoon filtered water (trace)**
- **1 lemon, grated peel only (.36 mg)**
- **1 tablespoon extra virgin olive oil (trace)**
- **2 tablespoons cider vinegar (1.49 mg)**
- **2 teaspoons sugar (trace)**
- **1 cup unbleached white flour (2.5 mg)**
- **1 cup unbleached white whole wheat flour[1] (6 mg)**
- **2 tablespoons vital wheat gluten (4.5 mg)**
- **1 tablespoon of potato flour[2] (5.72 mg)**
- **⅛ teaspoon ascorbic acid (trace)**
- **1½ teaspoons bread machine yeast[3] (3 mg)**

Place ingredients into your bread machine pan in the order your manufacturer suggests or in the order listed above. Make sure to keep sugar away from the yeast until the machine is started.

Set machine on either basic bread, medium crust or Whole Wheat Rapid Rise, Medium Crust.

[1] Same nutrients as red whole wheat

[2] If no potato flour on hand, then add 1 level tablespoon of unbleached white or white whole wheat flour. Potato flour adds moisteness to most baked goods.

[3] May use rapid rise yeast.

White Whole Wheat Nutrient Data Per Slice: Calories: 73.6, Protein: 2.547 g, Carbohydrate: 13.6 g, Dietary Fiber: 1.368 g, Total Sugars: .66 g, Total Fat: 1.162 g, Saturated Fat: .166 g, Monounsaturated Fat: .693 g, Polyunsaturated Fat: .193 g, Cholesterol: 0 mg, Trans Fatty Acids: 0 g, Total Omega-3 FA: .012 g, Total Omega-6 FA: 0 g, Calcium: 5.297 mg, Potassium: 57.6 mg, Sodium: 1.39 mg, Vitamin K: .719 mcg

FRENCH TOAST BREAD

LACTO OVO - 1½ CARB CHOICES

BREAD MACHINE RECIPE

Makes 1 Loaf (12 Slices)

Sodium Per Bread Recipe: 45.6 mg Sodium Per Bread Slice: 3.803 mg

One slice of this French toast[1], topped with natural maple syrup or our wild blackberry sauce is enough for a whole breakfast. Serve with fresh orange juice and a light dusting of powdered confectioner's sugar.

- **⅞ cup of warmed filtered water (trace)**
- **3 tablespoons olive oil (trace)**
- **2 tablespoons cider vinegar (.30 mg)**
- **⅛ teaspoon vanilla (.047 mg)**
- **2 level tablespoons light or reduced fat sour cream (18.3 mg)**
- **2¾[1] cups white unbleached best for bread flour (6.875 mg)**
- **2 tablespoons potato flour (11 mg)**
- **½ teaspoon malted barley flour (trace)**
- **1 tablespoon granulated soy lecithin (trace)**
- **¼ teaspoon ascorbic acid (trace)**
- **1 tablespoons vital wheat gluten (2.958 mg)**
- **2 tablespoons sugar (trace)**
- **⅛ teaspoon granulated onion powder (.162 mg)**
- **2 teaspoons bread machine yeast (4 mg)**

Place all ingredients into bread machine pan in order listed or in the order your manufacturer lists. Remember to not put sugar in contact with yeast.

Set for white bread, medium crust. When done, cool for about a half hour before slicing ¾ inch to one-inch pieces for French toast

[1]For French Toast See Page: 145

French Toast Bread Nutrient Data French Toast Bread Alone Per Slice: Calories: 149.8, Protein: 4.087 g, Carbohydrate: 23.8 g, Dietary Fiber: 1.021 g, Total Sugars: .326 g, Total Fat: 4.018 g, Saturated Fat: .715 g, Monounsaturated Fat: 2.506 g, Polyunsaturated Fat: .483 g, Cholesterol: 1.292 mg, Trans Fatty Acids: 0 g, Total Omega-3 FA: .033 g, Total Omega-6 FA: 0 g, Calcium: 11.5 mg, Potassium: 69.1 mg, Sodium: 3.803 mg, Vitamin K: 2.119 mcg

NO YEAST PIZZA CRUST

VEGAN - 1 CARB CHOICES

Makes 1 16" pizza Serves: 12

Sodium Per Recipe: 114.2 Sodium Per Slice: 9.53 mg

Ever want a quick pizza without having to wait a few hours to make yeast dough? Try this recipe. Ener-G Baking Powder makes the crust possible and it's quite good and cracker thin. See the yeast pizza crust on the next page for a standard pizza crust.

2 cups all purpose flour (5 mg)
½ teaspoon dried basil (.238 mg)
¼ teaspoon onion powder (.324 mg)
¼ teaspoon ground or dried oregano (.067 mg)
⅛ teaspoon dried thyme (.096 mg)
⅛ teaspoon savory (.042 mg)
4 teaspoons Ener-G baking powder (trace)
⅔ cup nonfat milk with Vitamin A (68.5 mg)
¼ cup extra virgin olive oil (trace)
Spritz oil for pizza pan (trace)

Preheat oven to 425°F.

Combine first 9 ingredients in a medium size mixing bowl, stirring with spoon or hands until bowl is clean and ball is formed. Knead about eight to ten times or until ball is without lumps.

On a lightly floured board, roll dough out to shape of your pizza pan, which should be about 16" in diameter or 10" x 15" jelly roll pan. Roll as think as you can get it. This is a tough dough to roll so it will take some body weight.

Spritz pizza pan with light coat of oil and place rolled dough on it. Roll in pan to get dough to edges if necessary. Pinch edges. (You can brush oil on the edge if you like, but it's not necessary.)

For crispy crust, bake for 10-minutes, then remove and place topping on crust, then back into oven and cook for another 15 to 20 minutes.

Calories: 179.4, Protein: 6.177 g, Carbohydrate: 17.5 g, Dietary Fiber: .649 g, Total Sugars: .853 g, Total Fat: 9.355 g, Saturated Fat: 3.608 g, Monounsaturated Fat: 4.608 g, Polyunsaturated Fat: .705 g, Cholesterol: 14.4 mg, Trans Fatty Acids: 0 g, Total Omega-3 FA: .095 g, Total Omega-6 FA: 0 g, Calcium: 125.1 mg, Potassium: 68.8 mg, Sodium: 9.513 mg, Vitamin K: 4.665 mcg

YEAST PIZZA CRUST

VEGAN – 1½ CARB CHOICES

Makes 1 thick 15-inch crust. *Serves 12*

Sodium Per Recipe: 15.8 mg *Sodium Per Serving: 1.316 mg*

2½ cups unbleached bread flour (6.25 mg)
2¼ teaspoons rapid rise yeast (1-package) (3.5 mg)
¼ teaspoon ascorbic acid (trace)
½ teaspoon dried basil (.238 mg)
½ teaspoon dried oregano (1.35 mg)
1 garlic clove, minced (.51 mg)
1 teaspoon granulated sugar (trace)
1 tablespoons cider vinegar (.745 mg)
1 cup filtered water (115° to 130° F)
2 tablespoons extra virgin olive oil (trace)
1 tablespoon cornmeal (.377 mg)

Stir together 2 1/2 cups flour, rapid rise yeast, ascorbic acid, basil, oregano, clove, and sugar in medium size bowl. Stir warmed water and olive oil into flour mixture. If dough needs more flour to ball up into a smooth and elastic dough, add flour one-tablespoon at a time. Knead on lightly floured surface until smooth and elastic, about 5 to 6 minutes. Cover with floured cloth and let rest for about 15 minutes.

Lightly oil a 15-inch round pan[1] for a thick crust. Sprinkle cornmeal across the pan. Shape dough for pan on flour dusted board by pressing down with palms, then stretching dough either by tossing (if you know how) or you might try lightly using a rolling pin. Shape dough into smooth ball. Divide and roll dough to fit desired pan(s). Top pizza as desired. (see Pizza Toppings tip below)

For crisp crust bake at 400° F for ten minutes, then remove from oven (leaving oven on) spread topping and then bake for another 15 to 20 minutes.

If you want a soft crust, bake pizza for 25 to 30 minutes at 400° F.

Pan pizza fans, let the dough rise for about 30 minutes.

[1] For a thin crust use about 2/3 of the dough for the same pan. Or you can make two 12" rounds.

Pizza with Yeast Nutrient Data Per Slice:alories: 123.5, Protein: 3.247 g, Carbohydrate: 21.4 g, Dietary Fiber: 1.083 g, Total Sugars: .444 g, Total Fat: 2.616 g, Saturated Fat: .369 g, Monounsaturated Fat: 1.712 g, Polyunsaturated Fat: .369 g, Cholesterol: 0 mg, Trans Fatty Acids: 0 g, Total Omega-3 FA: .028 g, Total Omega-6 FA: 0 g, Calcium: 7.68 mg, Potassium: 58.9 mg, Sodium: 1.316 mg, Vitamin K: 2.905 mcg

CINNAMON SWIRL BREAD

VEGAN – 2 CARB CHOICES

BREAD MACHINE KNEAD – HAND SHAPE – OVEN BAKE

Makes 2 loaves (32 slices)

Sodium Per Recipe: 84.7 mg   Sodium Per Slice: 2.646 mg

With raisins and unsalted walnuts. For breakfast toast or a party, this bread is great right out of the oven. Easy to make using your bread machine dough cycle. Will freeze in a tightly sealed zipper lock bag.

2 cups of filtered water, warmed to about 105° F (trace)
3 tablespoons extra virgin olive oil (trace)
2 tablespoons cider vinegar (1.49 mg)
½ teaspoon vanilla extract (.189 mg)
5 cups white unbleached bread flour (12.5 mg)
2 tablespoons vital wheat gluten (4.5 mg)
¼ teaspoon ascorbic acid (trace)
2 teaspoons ground cinnamon (1.196 mg)
2 tablespoons white granulated sugar (.252 mg)
1 tablespoon bread machine yeast (6 mg)
1 cup seedless black raisins, not packed, at buzzer[1] (17.4 mg)

Filling

1 cup black or golden seedless raisins, packed (17.4 mg)
½ cup chopped unsalted almonds[2] (.69 mg)
3 tablespoons white granulated sugar (.378 mg)
3 tablespoons brown sugar, packed (16.1 mg)
2 tablespoons ground cinnamon (3.536 mg)

After shaping loaves in pan

tablespoon cinnamon (1.768 mg)
tablespoon sugar (.126 mg)

Warm water to about 110° F to 115° F. Place water, oil, vinegar into bread machine basket. Cover with flour, gluten, ascorbic acid, 2-teaspoons of cinnamon, the sugar and the yeast on a dry spot on top. When raisin buzzer sounds, add ½ cup raisins[1].

Set machine for dough cycle.

While machine is working, mix together the last five ingredients: 1-cup raisins, ½-cup chopped almonds, 3-tablespoons white granulated sugar, 3-tablespoons brown sugar, 2-tablespoons ground cinnamon. You can add two tablespoons of melted unsalted butter to this mix to make it richer and stick to the dough better, but it's not necessary, especially if you want to keep the total fats low.

When dough is ready, roll out onto a lightly floured breadboard and cut in half. Flatten each half one at a time to about 3/8 to ½" thick in an oblong shape. You can use a rolling pin. Sprinkle half of the cinnamon nut mix over the surface, spreading it evenly with your hands if you like. Roll very tightly lengthwise into a log. You want to stretch the dough a bit when you do this. Pinch the bottom edge together to close tightly. Push the ends in to make it fit into a 7" lightly greased loaf pan with the pinched bottom on the bottom of the pan.

Do the second one the same way.

Sprinkle the tops with the cinnamon sugar mix. (I like to baste the top of the dough with a bit of egg white whisked with a few drops of water and then sprinkle the cinnamon-sugar mix. Added sodium would be about 1 mg per serving.)

Place in a warm spot, lightly covered with a very light cloth or wax paper and let rise for about an hour.

Bake at 375° F for 20 to 30 minutes. They will turn golden brown on top. Test for doneness before removing.

Serve warm or reheated. To reheat use a microwave for only 20 seconds. Toasts beautifully.

[1] Some bread machines do not have "raisin buzzers." Some machines knead for only 20 minutes. Best to know your machine and add the raisins 5 minutes before the kneading process is completed.

[2] Optional

Cinnamon Swirl Nutrient Data Per Slice: Nutrient Values Per Slice: Calories: 309.7, Protein: 3.312 g, Carbohydrate: 27.1 g, Dietary Fiber: 1.67 g, Total Sugars: 9.169 g, Total Fat: 21.7 g, Saturated Fat: 2.924 g, Monounsaturated Fat: 15.5 g, Polyunsaturated Fat: 2.488 g, Cholesterol: 0 mg, Trans Fatty Acids: 0 g, Total Omega-3 FA: .159 g, Total Omega-6 FA: 0 g, Calcium: 23.8 mg, Potassium: 119 mg, Sodium: 2.646 mg, Vitamin K: 12.8 mcg

HAWAIIAN SWEET BREAD

LACTO-OVO VEGETARIAN – 2½ CARB CHOICES[1]

BREAD MACHINE KNEAD – HAND SHAPE – OVEN BAKE

Makes 18 Buns, Or 2 loaves (32 slices)   Sodium Per Recipe: 148.5 mg

Sodium Per Bun (18): 8.249 mg   Sodium Per Slice (32): 4.64 mg

This dough can be used to make buns, loaves or dinner rolls.

2 cups warmed filtered water (trace)
2 tablespoons white wine vinegar (1.49 mg)
1 teaspoon vanilla (.378 mg)
2 tablespoons honey (not wild) (1.68 mg)
1 large egg (70 mg)
3 tablespoons extra virgin olive oil (.81 mg)
¼ cup granulated sugar[1] (trace)
4¾ cups white best for bread flour (11.9 mg)
1 cup whole wheat pastry or white whole wheat flour (6 mg)
¼ cup potato flour (15.5 mg)
1 tablespoon granular or soy lecithin (trace)
2 tablespoons vital wheat gluten (5.365 mg)
¼ teaspoon ascorbic acid (trace)
1 tablespoon plus 1-teaspoon bread machine yeast [2](8 mg)

Glaze

½ large egg white & water beaten just before dough

Place all ingredients except the single egg into bread machine pan and set machine for dough. (Read directions below before starting.)

This is a large recipe. You can knead this in any machine that will make a two or two and a half pound loaf. If you use the smaller of the two, allow the first rise to take place in a large lightly greased bowl, covered tightly and set into a warm location (about 80° F to 90° F).

If letting rise in a two and half pound machine, lightly grease the machine lid. When dough rises to lid, take out and shape into buns, rolls or two loaf pans and let rise in warm area for another 45 minutes to an hour.

Baking suggestion: *If baking two loaves,* allow rise to take place in an oven with a proof setting or an oven that is warmed to about 80° F.

When dough has risen leave in place and turn oven on to 375° F and bake bread until oven reaches that temperature. Then bake until top is golden brown.

For buns you will have about 6 to 9 on a baking sheet. I use parchment covered pans. If you make large buns you'll get 6 per pan and only 12 buns. To shape buns, roll in individual balls of equal size after first rise. Place on baking sheet and press down gently to flatten a bit. Baste with the beaten egg white. Let rise in warm oven uncovered. Set racks apart before doing so. When baking, bake only one sheet at a time. (If you have a double oven you may use one for the rise or both for the rise of separate sheets and then bake at same time.)

The first batch can be baked by leaving in the oven if you use that for the rise by turning on oven to 375° F. Let oven heat to that temperature. If the buns aren't done, let cook until tops are lightly browned. Remove first batch and bake next batch for about 12 to 18 minutes or until lightly browned.

[1] May exchange one cup of flour with Bob's Red Mill Soy Flour. Buns are 2½ Carb Choices.

[2] We prefer Fleischmann's Bread machine yeast since it contains a bit of ascorbic acid.

[3] You will probably use up to a half of the egg white. Data is for half. Sodium level for using all the egg white would be 54.8 mg sodium.

***Hawaiian Bread Nutrient Data Per Bun (18) 2½-carb Choices**: Calories: 204.4, Protein: 6.09 g, Carbohydrate: 37.3 g, Dietary Fiber: 1.901 g, Total Sugars: 4.822 g, Total Fat: 3.5 g, Saturated Fat: .55 g, Monounsaturated Fat: 1.865 g, Polyunsaturated Fat: .681 g, Cholesterol: 11.8 mg, Trans Fatty Acids: 0 g, Total Omega-3 FA: .029 g, Total Omega-6 FA: 0 g, Calcium: 11.9 mg, Potassium: 128.9 mg, Sodium: 8.249 mg, Vitamin K: 1.588 mcg*

***Hawaiian Bread Nutrient Data Per Slice (32) 1½ Carb Choices**: Calories: 115, Protein: 3.426 g, Carbohydrate: 21 g, Dietary Fiber: 1.07 g, Total Sugars: 2.713 g, Total Fat: 1.968 g, Saturated Fat: .309 g, Monounsaturated Fat: 1.049 g, Polyunsaturated Fat: .383 g, Cholesterol: 6.609 mg, Trans Fatty Acids: 0 g, Total Omega-3 FA: .017 g, Total Omega-6 FA: 0 g, Calcium: 6.719 mg, Potassium: 72.5 mg, Sodium: 4.64 mg, Vitamin K: .894 mcg*

SEVEN GRAIN BREAD

VEGAN – 2 ½ CARB CHOICES[1]
BREAD MACHINE RECIPE

Makes 1 Loaf Sodium Per Recipe: 58.2 mg Sodium Per Slice: 3.367 mg

This updated version of our popular 7-grain bread is as healthy as they get. Great for sandwiches including our Hummus Sandwich.

1½ cups plus 1 tablespoons warmed orange juice with calcium (about 100° F) (3.746 mg)
3 tablespoons homemade applesauce, warmed to 80° F to 100° F (.097 mg)
1 tablespoon olive oil (room temperature) (trace)
1 tablespoon apple cider vinegar (.745 mg)
2 cups unbleached white flour (5 mg)
2 cups whole wheat flour[1] (12 mg)
¾ cup 7-grain mix[2] (7.5 mg)
½ cup light brown sugar packed, or ¼ cup Splenda Brown Sugar Blend (42.9 mg)
2½ teaspoons bread machine yeast[3] (5 mg)
2 oranges, grated rind zest only (.36 mg)

Place warmed orange juice in your bread machine. Put ingredients into machine in order listed.

Set machine for white bread, medium crust.

If your machine chooses bake time by loaf size or weight, choose 2 pound size or a 3 hr 30 minute cycle.

Serve with dinner, for sandwiches or as a crispy toast in the morning, topped with your favorite jam.

[1] Diabetics bulk of carbs are in flour and sugar. Use Splenda Brown Sugar Blend and exchange 1/2 cup whole wheat flour with soy flour to lower carbs. Lowers carb choices to 2. (Defatted soy flour lowers carbs even more.)

[2] Or use White Whole Wheat or Whole Wheat Pastry flour.

[3] We use Bob's Red Mill 7-Grain Cereal

[4] If using Splenda Brown Sugar Blend, add ¼ teaspoon yeast.

7-Grain Nutrient Data Per Slice (16) 2½-Carb Choices : Calories: 189.9, Protein: 5.209 g, Carbohydrate: 38.2 g, Dietary Fiber: 3.634 g, Total Sugars: 6.965 g, Total Fat: 2.446 g, Saturated Fat: .311 g, Monounsaturated Fat: 1.298 g, Polyunsaturated Fat: .362 g, Cholesterol: 0 mg, Trans Fatty Acids: 0 g, Total Omega-3 FA: .022 g, Total Omega-6 FA: 0 g, Calcium: 43.2 mg, Potassium: 145 mg, Sodium: 3.637 mg, Vitamin K: 1.348 mcg

Diabetic Version 7-Grain Nutrient Data Per Slice (16) 2-Carb Choices: Calories: 172.1, Protein: 5.937 g, Carbohydrate: 31.3 g, Dietary Fiber: 3.551 g, Total Sugars: 2.103 g, Total Fat: 3.376 g, Saturated Fat: .424 g, Monounsaturated Fat: 1.29 g, Polyunsaturated Fat: .333 g, Cholesterol: 0 mg, Trans Fatty Acids: 0 g, Total Omega-3 FA: .021 g, Total Omega-6 FA: 0 g, Calcium: 36.2 mg, Potassium: 120.7 mg, Sodium: 1.524 mg, Vitamin K: 1.277 mcg

MUFFINS / CAKES

Ovens use heat averaging. Whether electric or gas it will rise above and drop below the temperature you set it at. For instance, if you set your oven for 350° F, then it could rise as high as 450° F and drop as low as 250° F. That's one reason we preheat for some baked items and also a reason why we don't want to keep popping the door open. A demonstration by a professional ovenmaker or repairman would illustrate that when we open the oven door we immediately lose about 100° F or more of heat. If we keep popping the door open to "check" our baking, then it will take longer to bake and might cause our cake, muffins or bread to collapse. Along those same lines, our freezer/refrigerator units do much the same. In their case however, the compressor is driving the freezer and the freezer puts the cold air into the refrigerator. Open the refrigerator too long, and the cold escapes forcing the compressor on again to chill down the freezer so that it can pump cold air back into the refrigerator.

What's this got to do with muffins, which are also known as "little cakes?"

Well, muffins and cakes need their cooking temperature constant. Open the oven door at the wrong time and poof, your cake or muffins may drop on you (same with bread, by the way).

When we make cakes like our applesauce cake, or muffins such as our cranberry muffins, we preheat for about ten to fifteen minutes, then put the muffins/cakes into the oven, close the door and set the timer. We check with an oven light if we need to take a look. At the given time, we check through the oven window and if the cake or muffins aren't quite done we allow a few more minutes. Only then do we open the door and use a long wooden skewer to test the muffins/cakes. If the stick is dry when we pull it out we remove the baked item.

Timing is everything. When we test the cakes we do it quickly. If they have to cook more, we want the door closed as soon as possible. We usually give them another three to five minutes and that generally suffices.

By the way, to help keep your muffins or cakes moist, exchange one or two teaspoons of your flour with equal parts of potato flour. As it does with our bread recipes, potato flour will add "freshness" and an extra day or two of life to the cakes.

Our cakes freeze well, but should be thawed by letting them sit out to reach room temperature.

APPLESAUCE CAKE

LACTO-OVO VEGETARIAN – 2½ CARB CHOICES

Makes 12 Servings   Sodium Per Recipe: 95.1 mg

Sodium Per Serving with walnuts: 7.925 mg

Sodium Per Serving without walnuts: 7.73 mg

This cake can be made with or without unsalted walnuts. The walnuts raise the total fats from .6 grams per serving to 7.2 grams. Walnuts offer a huge bonus with nutrients we need. See Walnuts in our glossary.

- **2 cups raw apples, diced (2.5 mg)**
- **1 large egg (70 mg)**
- **1 cup sugar (trace)**
- **½ cup expeller pressed canola oil (trace)**
- **¼ teaspoon vanilla (.095 mg)**
- **1 teaspoon cinnamon (.26 mg)**
- **1 cup white unbleached All Purpose flour(2.5 mg)**
- **1 cup not packed seedless golden raisins (17.4 mg)**
- **1 cup unsalted walnuts, chopped Optional:[1] (2.34 mg)**
- **1 tablespoon Ener-G Baking Soda (trace)**
- **2 teaspoons Ener-G Baking Powder (trace)**

Preheat oven to 350° F about fifteen minutes before baking. Lightly grease and flour an 8 x 8 inch baking pan.

With a large spoon, stir all ingredients together until smooth.

Bake 50 minutes. Test with toothpick before removing. Stick pick into center and pull out. If sticky, cook for 5 minutes more or until done..

[1]1 cup chopped unsalted walnuts have 76.3 grams of total fat. You may reduce amount you use or leave them out altogether to help cut calories.

Applesauce Cake Nutrient Data Per Serving With Walnuts: Calories: 225.4, Protein: 3.558 g, Carbohydrate: 38.7 g, Dietary Fiber: 2.033 g, Total Sugars: 26.3 g, Total Fat: 7.551 g, Saturated Fat: .81 g, Monounsaturated Fat: 1.412 g, Polyunsaturated Fat: 4.891 g, Cholesterol: 17.6 mg, Trans Fatty Acids: .002 g, Total Omega-3 FA: 1.003 g, Total Omega-6 FA: .109 g, Calcium: 50.8 mg, Potassium: 173.6 mg, Sodium: 7.925 mg, Vitamin K: 1.672 mcg

Applesauce Cake Nutrient Data Per Serving Without Walnuts: Calories: 161.6, Protein: 2.073 g, Carbohydrate: 37.3 g, Dietary Fiber: 1.38 g, Total Sugars: 26 g, Total Fat: 1.193 g, Saturated Fat: .213 g, Monounsaturated Fat: .541 g, Polyunsaturated Fat: .291 g, Cholesterol: 17.6 mg, Trans Fatty Acids: .002 g, Total Omega-3 FA: .118 g, Total Omega-6 FA: .109 g, Calcium: 41.3 mg, Potassium: 130.6 mg, Sodium: 7.73 mg, Vitamin K: 1.409 mcg

Diabetic Version Without Walnuts, using Splenda® Blend for Baking, 2-Carb Choices: Calories: 129.4, Protein: 2.073 g, Carbohydrate: 29 g, Dietary Fiber: 1.38 g, Total Sugars: 17.7 g, Total Fat: 1.193 g, Saturated Fat: .213 g, Monounsaturated Fat: .541 g, Polyunsaturated Fat: .291 g, Cholesterol: 17.6 mg, Trans Fatty Acids: .002 g, Total Omega-3 FA: .118 g, Total Omega-6 FA: .109 g, Calcium: 41.2 mg, Potassium: 130.4 mg, Sodium: 7.73 mg, Vitamin K: 1.409 mcg

CRANBERRY MUFFINS

LACTO OVOVEGETARIAN – 2½ CARB CHOICES

Makes 20 Muffins

Sodium Per Recipe: 514.4 mg Sodium Per Muffin: 25.7 mg

3 cups fresh/frozen cranberries[1] (35.1 mg)
¾ cup low fat (2%) buttermilk (97.5 mg)
¾ cup homemade applesauce, pureed[2] (trace)
1¼ cups white granulated sugar (trace)
5 large egg whites (350 mg)
1½ teaspoons vanilla extract or flavoring (.567 mg)
1¼ cups white unbleached flour (3.125 mg)
1 cup whole wheat pastry flour (3.125 mg)
1 teaspoon ground cinnamon (.598 mg)
¾ teaspoon ground cloves (3.827 mg)
1 cup golden raisins. not packed (17.4 mg)
¼ cup chopped unsalted walnuts (.585 mg)
1 tablespoon Ener-G Baking Powder (trace)
4 teaspoons Ener-G Baking Soda (trace)

Prepare muffin cups. If using a muffin pan (recommended) place paper cups into pans. If cups are not nonstick, Spritz with canned oil such as canola or olive oil (Pam type). Set aside.

Preheat oven to 350° F.

Mix dry ingredients in a separate bowl.

Combine sugar, homemade salt-free and sugar-free applesauce, and buttermilk until well mixed. Add in egg whites and vanilla, stir.

Beat together the wet and dry until batter is smooth.

Spoon in the cranberries and then spoon batter into muffin cups, up to top edge and place into oven. You may bake on two different shelves at the same time.

Bake at 350° F for 23 to 30 minutes. When done, a toothpick should come out dry.

[1] May use other fruit or a combination of fruit. Suggestions include pitted dates, frozen blueberries, frozen strawberries.

[2] May exchange for same measurement expeller pressed canola oil or extra virgin olive oil. If you do, add 1432 calories to the recipe total and 162 grams total fat.

Nutrient Data Next Page

Cranberry Muffins Nutrient Data Per Muffin Using Sugar: Calories: 250, Protein: 10.8 g, Carbohydrate: 47.6 g, Dietary Fiber: 8.732 g, Total Sugars: 17.5 g, Total Fat: 2.993 g, Saturated Fat: .731 g, Monounsaturated Fat: .662 g, Polyunsaturated Fat: 1.112 g, Cholesterol: 53.8 mg, Trans Fatty Acids: 0 g, Total Omega-3 FA: .222 g, Total Omega-6 FA: 0 g, Calcium: 87.3 mg, Potassium: 505 mg, Sodium: 25.7 mg, Vitamin K: .62 mcg

Diabetic Version Cranberry Muffins Using Splenda® Blend for Baking - 2 Carb Choices – Nutrient Data Per Muffin; Calories: 225.8, Protein: 10.8 g, Carbohydrate: 41.4 g, Dietary Fiber: 8.732 g, Total Sugars: 11.3 g, Total Fat: 2.993 g, Saturated Fat: .731 g, Monounsaturated Fat: .662 g, Polyunsaturated Fat: 1.112 g, Cholesterol: 53.8 mg, Trans Fatty Acids: 0 g, Total Omega-3 FA: .222 g, Total Omega-6 FA: 0 g, Calcium: 87.3 mg, Potassium: 504.9 mg, Sodium: 25.7 mg, Vitamin K: .62 mcg

Remember when figuring Carb Choices, that when Dietary Fiber is more than 5 grams, we can subtract the total fiber grams from the total carbohydrate and come up with a number for the Carb Choices calculation. In the above example Dietary Fiber: 8.732 g is subtracted from Carbohydrate: 41.4 g for a total of: 32.688 grams. That fits well within the 2-Carb Choices chart.

EASY CHOCOLATE CAKE

VEGAN – 2 CARB CHOICES

Serves 12 Sodium Per Recipe: 23.4 mg Sodium Per Serving: 1.95 mg

1½ cups white unbleached all-purpose flour (3.75 mg)
1 cup sugar (trace)
3 tablespoons unsweetened cocoa (3.40235 mg)
6 tablespoons olive oil (1.62 mg)
1 teaspoon vanilla (.378 mg)
1 tablespoon apple cider or white vinegar (.745 mg)
1 cup warm water (trace)
1 tablespoon Ener-G baking powder (trace)

Preheat oven to 350° F about ten minutes before you put pan in. Make sure oven is at 350° F when you finish mixing batter.

Mix first three dry ingredients together in 9" square pan*.

Make 3 indentations with tablespoon. Pour oil in one, Vinegar in second and vanilla into third. Pour water over all and stir in the baking powder with fork until mix is just blended. Place in preheated oven immediately.

Bake in preheated oven at 350° F for 35 - 40 minutes. Lightly oil pan, then dust with white flour before placing batter in. Bake on middle rack. When done, cool on rack for about a half-hour before frosting. (For Frosting for this cake see next page.) *Will also work in a single 8 x 8 or round 9 x 9 x 2" pan.

Nutrient Data Per Serving: Calories: 186.6, Protein: 1.88 g, Carbohydrate: 30 g, Dietary Fiber: .898 g, Total Sugars: 16.8 g, Total Fat: 7.093 g, Saturated Fat: 1.066 g, Monounsaturated Fat: 5 g, Polyunsaturated Fat: .782 g, Cholesterol: 0 mg, Trans Fatty Acids: 0 g, Total Omega-3 FA: .055 g, Total Omega-6 FA: 0 g, Calcium: 58.6 mg, Potassium: 165.4 mg, Sodium: 1.95 mg, Vitamin K: 4.144 mcg

EASY CHOCOLATE CAKE ICING

VEGAN – 1 CARB CHOICES

Serves 12   Sodium Per Recipe: 24.4 mg   Sodium Per Serving: 2.037 mg

Use with Easy Chocolate cake or any other cake or muffins that you might want to frost. Diabetics add this to cake totals.

- **2 squares semi sweet cooking chocolate (10 mg)**
- **2 to 3 tablespoons nonfat milk with vitamin A[1] (12.9 mg)**
- **1 cup confectioner's sugar (1.2 mg)**
- **1 teaspoon vanilla extract/flavoring (.378 mg)**

Melt chocolate over low heat in double boiler or saucepan.

Stir melted chocolate and vanilla into sugar.

Add in milk slowly, making sure you are reaching proper consistency for icing/frosting. You may end up using only 1 tablespoon of milk. Work up to no more than 3 tablespoons.

Beat with wooden spoon until thick. If you put in too much milk, add more confectioner's sugar to thicken. If icing is left over, may freeze for later use.

[1] According to the USDA nonfat milk with added vitamin A has lower sodium than milk without vitamin A. The data shown here is for two tablespoons.

Nutrient Data Per Serving: Calories: 65.3, Protein: .286 g, Carbohydrate: 13 g, Dietary Fiber: .083 g, Total Sugars: 12.4 g, Total Fat: 1.546 g, Saturated Fat: .953 g, Monounsaturated Fat: .004 g, Polyunsaturated Fat: .005 g, Cholesterol: .051 mg, Trans Fatty Acids: 0 g, Total Omega-3 FA: 0 g, Total Omega-6 FA: 0 g, Calcium: 4.829 mg, Potassium: 20 mg, Sodium: 2.037 mg, Vitamin K: 0 mcg

RICH CHOCOLATE CAKE OR CUPCAKES

LACTO-OVO VEGETARIAN – 4 CARB CHOICES[1]

Makes One Single (18 pieces)
or Double-Layer Cake (12 servings) or, Makes 24 cupcakes
Sodium Per Recipe: 385.5 mg Sodium Per Piece (18): 21.4 mg
Sodium Per Slice Double-Layer (12):32.2 mg
Per Cupcake (24) : 16.1 mg Per Cupcake Splenda Blend (24): 16.1 mg

Perfect for that birthday where you don't want all 70 of those candles lit up. A bit high in fat and sugars, this lowered sodium chocolate cake should be reserved for special occasions. This recipe also makes a two layer cake using 9" cake pans, 24 cupcakes or one 9" x 13" baking dish. Diabetics see nutrient section for data when using Splenda. Cupcakes drop to 1 Carb Choice.

2 cups sugar or 1-cup Splenda Granulated (trace)
¾ cup cocoa (no salt added or included) (12.3 mg)
2 cups all-purpose flour[1] (5 mg)
1 tablespoon Ener-G baking powder (trace)
1 teaspoon vanilla extract (.378 p mg)
3 large egg whites (164.3 mg)
2 large egg yolks (16.3 mg)
1 teaspoon cream of tartar (.515 mg)
½ cup expeller pressed canola oil (trace)
1 cup light sour cream[2] (161 mg)
⅞ cup filtered no sodium water, room temperature (trace)
1 cup semi-sweet chocolate chips (25.7 mg)

Preheat oven to 350° F.

Prepare cake pans or muffin tins, whichever you are making. For baking dishes or pans, lightly oil and flour dust them. Nonstick muffin cups (paper) work well without dusting.

Sift together into a large bowl the first 4 ingredients. Set aside.

Separate eggs, setting aside the yolks. In a medium bowl, beat the egg whites with the cream of tartar until stiff. Set aside.

In another medium or small bowl beat the oil, two of the egg yolks, vanilla, and sour cream until blended. Beat in the water. Stir in the chocolate chips.

Pour the wet ingredients (but not the egg whites) into the dry ingredients and stir together with a large spoon, mixing batter quickly until it's smooth. Using a large plastic spatula, bring the egg whites into the batter and stir until evenly distributed.

Pour the batter into a prepared 9" x 13" baking dish or into two prepared round 9" cake pans depending on a single-layer or a double-layer cake. If making cup cakes, use 24 standard size muffin cups.

Bake at 350° F for 45 minutes or until a toothpick comes out of center dry. (Cup Cakes take about 35 to 40 minutes.)

[1] If you use Softassilk or other cake flour, use 2¼ cups instead of the 2-cups listed here.

[2] Check the FDA label for sodium to make sure it's close to the USDA figures we show. Adjust if necessary. FDA labels aren't exact USDA figures.

Rich Chocolate Cake Nutrient Data Per Slice Double-Layer (12): Calories: 342.2, Protein: 5.67 g, Carbohydrate: 63.7 g, Dietary Fiber: 2.699 g, Total Sugars: 41.6 g, Total Fat: 8.487 g, Saturated Fat: 4.685 g, Monounsaturated Fat: 2.718 g, Polyunsaturated Fat: .842 g, Cholesterol: 41.6 mg, Trans Fatty Acids: .002 g, Total Omega-3 FA: .148 g, Total Omega-6 FA: .109 g, Calcium: 45.7 mg, Potassium: 281.5 mg, Sodium: 32.1 mg, Vitamin K: .722 mcg

Nutrient Data Continued Next Page

Rich Chocolate Cake Nutrient Data Per Cake Slice (18 Slices Cake): Calories: 228.1, Protein: 3.78 g, Carbohydrate: 42.5 g, Dietary Fiber: 1.8 g, Total Sugars: 27.7 g, Total Fat: 5.658 g, Saturated Fat: 3.123 g, Monounsaturated Fat: 1.812 g, Polyunsaturated Fat: .561 g, Cholesterol: 27.7 mg, Trans Fatty Acids: .002 g, Total Omega-3 FA: .099 g, Total Omega-6 FA: .072 g, Calcium: 30.5 mg, Potassium: 187.7 mg, Sodium: 21.4 mg, Vitamin K: .481 mcg

Note: Use Splenda Sugar Blend for Baking for below results. One half cup = 96 gm carbohydrate = 384 calories

Rich Chocolate Cake Nutrient Data Per Cupcake (24): Calories: 171.1, Protein: 2.835 g, Carbohydrate: 31.9 g, Dietary Fiber: 1.35 g, Total Sugars: 20.8 g, Total Fat: 4.243 g, Saturated Fat: 2.342 g, Monounsaturated Fat: 1.359 g, Polyunsaturated Fat: .421 g, Cholesterol: 20.8 mg, Trans Fatty Acids: .001 g, Total Omega-3 FA: .074 g, Total Omega-6 FA: .054 g, Calcium: 22.8 mg, Potassium: 140.8 mg, Sodium: 16.1 mg, Vitamin K: .361 mcg

[1]Diabetic Version - Carb Choices 1½ - Rich Chocolate Cake Nutrient Data Per Serving (24 Cupcakes using Splenda Blend for Baking: Calories: 138.8, Protein: 2.835 g, Carbohydrate: 23.5 g, Dietary Fiber: 1.35 g, Total Sugars: 12.5 g, Total Fat: 4.243 g, Saturated Fat: 2.342 g, Monounsaturated Fat: 1.359 g, Polyunsaturated Fat: .421 g, Cholesterol: 20.8 mg, Trans Fatty Acids: .001 g, Total Omega-3 FA: .074 g, Total Omega-6 FA: .054 g, Calcium: 22.8 mg, Potassium: 140.6 mg, Sodium: 16.1 mg, Vitamin K: .361 mcg

PUMPKIN CAKE

LACTO-OVO VEGETARIAN – 2½ CARB CHOICES

Serves: 16   Sodium Per Recipe: 148.7 mg   Sodium Per Slice: 9.295 mg

Here's a terrific cake for Thanksgiving or when you just feel like having pumpkin flavor. Years ago in Los Angeles, California, while growing up, we used to visit a restaurant downtown that had a great pumpkin cake. I'm not sure of it's recipe, but like a lot of others I've tried to replicate it for no salt and lower sodium. I'm sure theirs had lots of saturated fat in it, but fat in this recipe is very low. Ener-G Baking Powder is available from Healthy Heart Market.

1½ cups sugar (trace)
1½ cups unbleached all-purpose (4.11 mg)
2 teaspoons Ener-G Baking Powder (trace)
1 tablespoon Ener-G Baking Soda (trace)
1½ teaspoons ground cinnamon (.39 mg)
¾ cup expeller pressed canola oil (trace)
1⅔ cups canned pumpkin, no salt (2.353 mg)
2 large eggs, beaten slightly (140 mg)

Preheat oven to 325° F.

Prepare a 7" x 11" baking dish (glass or ceramic) by lightly greasing it. Dust it with whole wheat pastry or whole wheat flour.

In a small bowl, beat eggs slightly.

In a larger bowl, using a wood spoon, blend together the sugar, flour, baking powder, baking soda, and cinnamon until well mixed. Using your spoon, blend in the oil until well mixed. Fold in the pumpkin until evenly blended. Fold in the beaten eggs and mix until evenly distributed. About a minute. Like all cakes, try not to over-mix or over-beat. Place in oven immediately.

Bake at 325° F for 35 to 40 minutes, or until a toothpick stuck in the middle comes out dry. Cool on rack, turn out and frost with your choice of frosting or the one below.

The Frosting

1 cup confectioner's sugar (1.2 mg)
2 tablespoons orange juice[1] (.31)
1 orange, grated peel (zest) only (.36 mg)

Stir orange juice into sugar until it begins to turn to a frosting texture. If you need more juice, add it one teaspoon at a time. Fold in the zest when nearly done. Spread on cake evenly.

[1] May need more. If so add 1/4 teaspoon at a time.

Nutrient Data Per Serving: Calories: 251.6, Protein: 1.906 g, Carbohydrate: 37.3 g, Dietary Fiber: .516 g, Total Sugars: 26.4 g, Total Fat: 11 g, Saturated Fat: .97 g, Monounsaturated Fat: 6.719 g, Polyunsaturated Fat: 3.015 g, Cholesterol: 26.4 mg, Trans Fatty Acids: .04 g, Total Omega-3 FA: 1.875 g, Total Omega-6 FA: 1.905 g, Calcium: 30.6 mg, Potassium: 35 mg, Sodium: 9.295 mg, Vitamin K: 7.892 mcg

Splenda Baker's Tips

When using Splenda instead of sugar, you'll get texture changes. A few recipes can deal with an all granulated Splenda, but some breads, cakes and muffins need some sugar. Bread especially needs a little sugar to work with the yeast. Muffins and cakes will change texture but more to the light side than the heavy. Try a muffin recipe with Splenda Blend for Baking to help cut calories and carbohydrates. To convert and figure total carbs for your recipe use the below. Also find more about Splenda in the glossary.

Splenda Sugar Blend for Baking (use ½ as much as sugar)
one half cup = 96 gm carbohydrate = 384 calories
one half teaspoon = 2 gm carbohydrate = 16 calories

Splenda also has a confectioner's sugar replacement that works with frosting.

GINGER CAKE

LACTO-OVO VEGETARIAN – 4 CARB CHOICES

Makes 9 Squares

Sodium Per Recipe: 203.4 mg   Sodium Per Serving: 22.6 mg

Easy to make, not too sweet, just like the ginger cake mom made, except sodium is much lower.

2¼ cups unbleached all-purpose flour (5.625 mg)
⅓ cup Splenda or granulated sugar (trace)
1 cup Grandma's or B'rer Rabbit dark or Robust molasses or similar molasses with no salt (124.7 mg)
3 tablespoons warm filtered water (trace)
1 tablespoon cider vinegar (.745 mg)
½ cup expeller pressed canola oil (trace)
1 large egg (70 mg)
1¼ teaspoons ground ginger (.72 mg)
1¼ teaspoons ground cinnamon (.325 mg)
⅛ teaspoon ground cloves (1.276 mg)
1 tablespoon Ener-G® Baking Powder (trace)

Preheat oven to 325° F with rack in the middle.

Lightly grease and flour dust a 9 x 9 x 2 Pyrex or other baking pan[1].

In a large bowl, using a beater (mixer) at slow speed blend the first twelve ingredients – for about a half minute. Increase beaters to medium and blend for another two minutes. Then add the baking powder and blend for another minute. (Make sure to scrape bowl occasionally to include all ingredients.)

Pour/scrape into pan and place in oven. Batter will be thick.

Bake for 45 to 50 minutes or until a wood toothpick inserted into middle of cake comes out clean.

Serve warm with a dollop of whipped cream.

[1] We have tested this in other size pans with best results pointing to the 9 x 9 x 2 pan/dish.

Nutrient Data Per Serving: Calories: 269.5, Protein: 3.968 g, Carbohydrate: 60.1 g, Dietary Fiber: 1.087 g, Total Sugars: 28.3 g, Total Fat: 1.705 g, Saturated Fat: .294 g, Monounsaturated Fat: .747 g, Polyunsaturated Fat: .45 g, Cholesterol: 23.5 mg, Trans Fatty Acids: .003 g, Total Omega-3 FA: .156 g, Total Omega-6 FA: .145 g, Calcium: 88.9 mg, Potassium: 596 mg, Sodium: 22.6 mg, Vitamin K: .862 mcg

CHOCOLATE SCONES

LACTO-OVO VEGETARIAN – 3 CARB CHOICES

Makes 8 Sodium Per Recipe: 250.5 mg Sodium Per Scone: 31.3 mg

This recipe has been child tested and passed with flying colors.

2 cups unbleached all-purpose flour (5 mg)
½ cup granulated sugar (trace)
¼ cup firmly packed dark brown sugar (15.4 mg)
2 tablespoons Ener-G Baking Powder (trace)
¼ granulated onion powder(.324 mg)
⅓ cup unsalted butter (8.315 mg)
⅓ cup low sodium buttermilk[1] or 2% milk (43.3 mg)
3 ounces unsweetened chocolate (20.9 mg)
1 large egg (70 mg)
1½ teaspoons vanilla extract (.567 mg)
½ cup chopped unsalted walnuts (optional) (1.17 mg)

Preheat oven to 350°F

We use a Nordic nonstick scone pan with eight sections, but you can also bake this on a cookie sheet or jelly roll pan. Use parchment paper for a liner.

Melt the chocolate per package instructions.

In a medium size bowl sift together the flour, granulated sugar or Splenda Granulated, brown sugar, baking powder, and onion powder.

Slice the butter into thin chunks and then work them into the flour with either a pastry blender or your hands. When the mix is coarse you're ready for the next step.

In a same size or larger bowl, using a spoon, combine the milk, melted chocolate, egg, vanilla, and unsalted walnut pieces. Add the milk mixture to the flour mixture, scraping it all in. Knead together with your hands to combine. Batter will be thick and nearly solid when done.

Pat the dough into the Nordic pan wedges. If using a baking sheet make an 8-inch-diameter circle with the batter in the center of the baking sheet. Cut into 8 wedges with a sharp or serrated knife. Bake for 18 to 20 minutes. Test with a toothpick; when it comes out dry scones are done.

Move to rack, slide off sheet by pulling on paper. If using Scone pan, let cool for five minutes then remove to rack.

[1] See Buttermilk in Glossary for low-sodium buttermilk brands

Chocolate Scone Nutrient Data Per Scone: Calories: 379.5, Protein: 7.34 g, Carbohydrate: 49.2 g, Dietary Fiber: 3.143 g, Total Sugars: 20.6 g, Total Fat: 19.3 g, Saturated Fat: 9.243 g, Monounsaturated Fat: 4.682 g, Polyunsaturated Fat: 4.124 g, Cholesterol: 48.2 mg, Trans Fatty Acids: 0 g, Total Omega-3 FA: .762 g, Total Omega-6 FA: .205 g, Calcium: 58.4 mg, Potassium: 193.3 mg, Sodium: 31.3 mg, Vitamin K: 2.04 mcg

SIDE DISHES

Side dishes, also known as "sides," are an important part of many meals. They offer the opportunity to add nutrients as well as colorful or tasty food to a full entree. Sides allow us to create and present different ideas. For instance, on page 233 you'll find our Yo Cheese recipe. It's not exactly a "side dish," but it works well with salads and dips. Your search for low sodium cheeses, low sodium mayonnaise, and a low sodium salad dressing base ends right here. Plain yogurt converted to the consistency of cream cheese and all in your refrigerator. It's a recipe you can easily make and refrigerate for use with many meals, snacks and even party dips.

BOSTON BAKED BEANS

VEGAN – 2 CARB CHOICES

Serves 6 *Sodium Per Recipe: 104.9 mg* *Sodium Per Serving: 23.1 mg*

1 can Eden Organic No Salt Added Small Red Beans or white beans, with liquid (52.5 mg)
2 tablespoons filtered water[1] (trace)
¾ teaspoon granulated onion powder (.972 mg)
1 bay leaf, whole (.138 mg)
¼ cup dark brown sugar[2] (15.4 mg)
2 teaspoons dry mustard (.33 mg)
1 medium onion, diced (4.4 mg)
¼ cup tablespoons Grandma's molasses[3] (31.2 mg)

Place beans with juice and water with the bay leaf and onion powder into a medium size pot and place over medium-high heat on stovetop, uncovered. Bring to a boil. Lower to simmer and add the rest of the ingredients. Simmer, stirring occasionally for about 45 minutes. Remove bay leaf. Serve hot.

[1] You might need to add another one-quarter cup of water during or right after the boil. We don't want it wet, but the consistency of liquid in cans often changes from one can to the next.

[2] See Splenda in glossary for brown sugar substitute.

[3] Baker's Tip: Spray measuring cup with light coat of oil before pouring molasses in. Then pour into the beans. Cup will be clear.

Boston Baked Beans Nutrient Data Per Serving: Calories: 147.7, Protein: 5.192 g, Carbohydrate: 32.4 g, Dietary Fiber: 6.35 g, Total Sugars: 17.6 g, Total Fat: .36 g, Saturated Fat: .029 g, Monounsaturated Fat: .227 g, Polyunsaturated Fat: .073 g, Cholesterol: 0 mg, Trans Fatty Acids: 0 g, Total Omega-3 FA: .031 g, Total Omega-6 FA: 0 g, Calcium: 48.3 mg, Potassium: 512.1 mg, Sodium: 17.5 mg, Vitamin K: .145 mcg

MOCK SAUSAGE

FLEXITARIAN – 0 CARB CHOICES

Makes 8 2-ounce Servings

Sodium Per Recipe: 371.2 mg ***Sodium Per Sausage: 46.4 mg***

I enjoyed sausages before my initial heart failure diagnosis. Back then I thought the dear old sausage was gone forever. But alas, I finally came up with a recipe that works well. Since then others have tweaked it, including more than one national magazine.

12 ounces lean ground turkey or chicken (319.8 mg)
3 ounces lean ground pork (47.6 mg)
1 teaspoon dried sage (.0777 mg)
½ teaspoon cumin seed, lightly toasted (1.764 mg)
½ teaspoon no salt added garlic powder (.364 mg) tea-
½ spoon granulated onion powder (.648 mg)
½ teaspoon freshly ground black pepper (.462 mg)
¼ teaspoon crushed red pepper flakes (.135 mg)
¼ teaspoon dried oregano (.067 mg)
¼ teaspoon dried tarragon (.248 mg)

Combine all of the ingredients in a medium size bowl. Form the mixture into eight 2 to 3-inch-diameter patties. Heat a nonstick pan or skillet over medium heat. Brown the patties on both sides about 4 minutes per side or until cooked through. Serve hot.

Mock Sausage Nutrient Data Per Serving: Calories: 94, Protein: 9.335 g, Carbohydrate: .538 g, Dietary Fiber: .153 g, Total Sugars: .109 g, Total Fat: 5.832 g, Saturated Fat: 1.808 g, Monounsaturated Fat: 2.346 g, Polyunsaturated Fat: 1.072 g, Cholesterol: 41.2 mg, Trans Fatty Acids: .117 g, Total Omega-3 FA: .06 g, Total Omega-6 FA: 0 g, Calcium: 12.5 mg, Potassium: 141.5 mg, Sodium: 46.4 mg, Vitamin K: 2.378 mcg

MASHED POTATOES WITH FLAIR

LACTO OVO-VEGETARIAN – 1 CARB CHOICES

Makes 8 Servings

Sodium Per Recipe: 345 mg   Sodium Per Serving: 43.1 mg

Succulent, sweet and full of nutrients, but be careful to not overeat. Rutabagas and turnips are high in sodium levels.

2 medium rutabagas, washed, peeled quartered (154.4 mg)
2 medium white potatoes, washed, peeled, quartered (25.6 mg)
4 tablespoons shallots, diced (4.8 mg)
1 tablespoon unsalted butter (1.562 mg)
⅛ teaspoon white pepper[1] (.044 mg)
2 tablespoons half & half (12.3 mg)

After preparing rutabagas and potatoes, place into medium pot, cover with water and bring to a boil. Lower heat to a simmering boil and continue to cook for about 25 minutes or until done.

Drain water, mash together with shallots, unsalted butter, white pepper, and shallots using hand masher. Stir with large wooden spoon, mash more until smooth.

Serve hot.

[1] Add more pepper to taste but no more than 1/4 teaspoon total.

Mashed Potatoes Nutrient Data Per Serving: Calories: 97.3, Protein: 2.535 g, Carbohydrate: 19.2 g, Dietary Fiber: 4.162 g, Total Sugars: 6.979 g, Total Fat: 1.713 g, Saturated Fat: .956 g, Monounsaturated Fat: .401 g, Polyunsaturated Fat: .179 g, Cholesterol: 3.816 mg, Trans Fatty Acids: 0 g, Total Omega-3 FA: .08 g, Total Omega-6 FA: .038 g, Calcium: 61.6 mg, Potassium: 608.1 mg, Sodium: 43.1 mg, Vitamin K: 1.456 mcg

MUSHROOM MIX

VEGAN – 0 CARB CHOICES

Makes: 12*[1] *Sodium Per Tablespoon: .58 mg

This easy to make and healthy mix can be used as a delicious topping or ingredient for any meat dish from burgers to steaks and can even be added to omelets.

1 tablespoon extra virgin olive oil (trace)
4 cloves garlic, minced (2.04 mg)
1 cup (2.5 ounces) mushrooms, chopped (2.8 mg)
2 tablespoons fresh parsley, chopped (2.128 mg)

In a saucepan, heat olive oil over medium high heat. Add garlic first. Sauté for two minutes stirring frequently. Add mushrooms and do the same for another two minutes. Add parsley and continue sautéing for one minute

Use as a topping for meat.

[1] 12-tablespoons depending on moisture in the mushrooms.

Mushroom Mix Nutrient Data Per Tablespoon: Calories: 12.8, Protein: .254 g, Carbohydrate: .54 g, Dietary Fiber: .101 g, Total Sugars: .121 g, Total Fat: 1.152 g, Saturated Fat: .155 g, Monounsaturated Fat: .833 g, Polyunsaturated Fat: .124 g, Cholesterol: 0 mg, Trans Fatty Acids: 0 g, Total Omega-3 FA: .009 g, Total Omega-6 FA: 0 g, Potassium: 24.1 mg, Sodium: .581 mg, Vitamin K: 5.89 mcg,

GREEN BEANS With MUSHROOMS

VEGAN – 0 CARB CHOICES

Makes 8 Sodium Per Recipe: 24.3 mg Sodium Per Serving: 3.04 mg

This is a terrific side for many dishes. It especially works well with our chicken recipes.

1 tablespoon extra virgin olive oil (.27 mg)
4 tablespoons diced shallots[1] (1.6 mg)
8 large mushrooms, sliced (9 mg)
green beans (approx ½ to ¾ pound) (13.2 mg)

Wash and blanch beans in boiling water for 2 minutes. Drain and rinse in cold water.

Sauté shallots and mushrooms in oil Add beans and reheat. Serve hot.

[1] May replace shallots with garlic.

Green Beans with Mushrooms Nutrient Data Per Serving (8): Calories: 30.5, Protein: 1.266 g, Carbohydrate: 3.185 g, Dietary Fiber: .81 g, Total Sugars: .591 g, Total Fat: 1.804 g, Saturated Fat: .252 g, Monounsaturated Fat: 1.233 g, Polyunsaturated Fat: .227 g, Cholesterol: 0 mg, Trans Fatty Acids: 0 g, Total Omega-3 FA: .013 g, Total Omega-6 FA: 0 g, Calcium: 12 mg, Potassium: 137.9 mg, Sodium: 3.04 mg, Vitamin K: 1.036 mcg

ROASTED VEGETABLES

VEGAN – 1 CARB CHOICES

Serves 4

Sodium Per Recipe: 100 mg Sodium Per Serving: 25 mg

This is a good recipe for presenting vegetables in a "new light." No-salt, minimum potassium, lower carbohydrate, and lots of flavor.

2 medium carrots (120 g) or 12 to 16 mini-carrots (84.2 mg)
1 medium red bell pepper, julienned (4.76 mg)
1 medium onion, cut into 1/2-inch wedges (4.4 mg)
1 tablespoon plus 1-teaspoon sesame seeds (1.317 mg)
2 level teaspoons Splenda Granulated (trace)
3 tablespoons Soy Sauce Replacement[1] (5.325 mg)
1 teaspoon extra virgin olive oil (trace)

Preheat the oven to 425°F.

Place carrots, red pepper, and onion into a medium bowl with the olive oil. Stir until veggies are coated with the oil. (Might need a bit more oil, depending on size of vegetables.)

Place the oil covered veggies in a single layer on a parchment paper covered baking sheet or one that is nonstick.

Sprinkle sesame seeds evenly over veggies.

Bake on middle rack for about 8 minutes. Turn the veggies. Bake for 6 to 8 more minutes, or until the vegetables begin to brown around the edges and are tender.

The Sauce

While veggies are baking, stir together the Splenda, Don's Soy Sauce and cider vinegar in the same bowl.

When veggies are done, place them in a serving dish or on a platter. Drizzle the sauce over all veggies but don't stir them.

[1] Either in *The No Salt, Lowest Sodium Cookbook*, or *The No Salt, Lowest Sodium International Cookbook* or Page 257.

Roasted Vegetables Nutrient Data Per Serving: Calories: 60.6, Protein: 1.454 g, Carbohydrate: 10.9 g, Dietary Fiber: 2.322 g, Total Sugars: 6.05 g, Total Fat: 1.683 g, Saturated Fat: .24 g, Monounsaturated Fat: .572 g, Polyunsaturated Fat: .716 g, Cholesterol: 0 mg, Trans Fatty Acids: 0 g, Total Omega-3 FA: .021 g, Total Omega-6 FA: 0 g, Potassium: 267.9 mg, Sodium: 25 mg, Vitamin K: 5.61 mcg

NUTTY TOPPED YAMS

VEGAN – 2 CARB CHOICES

Serves 4 Sodium Per Recipe: 57.9 mg   Sodium Per Serving: 14.5 mg

While researching for our "No Salt, Lowest Sodium International Cookbook" we came developed a variety of tasty and healthy recipes. Not all could be put into the new book. Here's one we wish we had included. The concept is African where sweet potatoes are a big part of their diet. Another huge part of their diet includes legumes or peanuts. While baking the yam you'll put together the stuffing. Remember to not over-bake the yam.

large yams (approximately 3 cups cooked) (40.5 mg)

The Topping

2 teaspoons extra virgin olive oil (.18 mg)
⅔ cup chopped onion (about one small onion) (4.224 mg)
1 tablespoon of minced garlic cloves (about 2 large) (1.428 mg)
1 tablespoon grated fresh ginger (.78 mg)
¼ teaspoon ground cumin (.882 mg)
dash or pinch of red pepper flakes (cayenne) (trace)
dash or pinch of white pepper (trace)
⅓ cup chopped unsalted peanuts (2.831 mg)
⅔ cups chopped fresh tomato (5.994 mg)
¼ teaspoon (1-packet) Splenda (trace)
1 tablespoon fresh lemon juice (.154 mg)
2 level teaspoons unsalted peanut butter (.908 mg)

Bake yams in jackets at 400° F for about 40 to 50 minutes or until just done. Don't over bake them and don't peel them after cooking.

In a medium saucepan, sauté onion, garlic, and ginger in oil. Add spice and peppers. Cook another minute. Add peanuts, tomatoes, Splenda or 1/4 teaspoon of sugar, and lemon juice. Reheat while stirring gently for another minute. Add peanut butter and stir gently until combined.

Slice yams (or sweet potatoes) lengthwise to serve. Top each half with hot peanut mixture (topping). Serve warm.

Nutrient Data Per Serving: Calories: 251.2, Protein: 5.861 g, Carbohydrate: 39.2 g, Dietary Fiber: 6.654 g, Total Sugars: 2.936 g, Total Fat: 8.988 g, Saturated Fat: 1.265 g, Monounsaturated Fat: 4.974 g, Polyunsaturated Fat: 2.279 g, Cholesterol: 0 mg, Trans Fatty Acids: 0 g, Total Omega-3 FA: .037 g, Total Omega-6 FA: 0 g, Calcium: 44.5 mg, Potassium: 1135 mg, Sodium: 14.5 mg, Vitamin K: 6.468 mcg

YO CHEESE

LACTO OVO VEGETARIAN – 0 CARB CHOICES

Makes 32 Level Tablespoons (2 cups)

Sodium Per Recipe: 372.4 mg[1] Sodium Per Tablespoon: 11.6 mg

You can use this as a cream cheese and even for dips for your guests who will never guess it's just plain yogurt. And better yet, lots of calcium, very low in calories and carbohydrates.

2 pounds or 4-cup container plain nonfat Yogurt[2](372.4 mg)

Use a tightly woven sieve or if your sieve is loosely woven, line it with food rated cheesecloth. Spread cheesecloth open, then double it. You want enough to cover the bottom of the sieve and up the sides for about four inches. A tightly woven sieve works well without the cheesecloth.

Place sieve so that it is suspended in a larger bowl that will fit into your refrigerator (bowl should have low sides and hold sieve up).

Pour or spoon all the yogurt into the sieve. (Clean and save the container to store the results in.)

Place into refrigerator. After about three hours take out and drain the water from the bowl and return to fridge. Do the same in another three hours. After that you can drain the final amount at the 24 hour mark. What you end up with is a dense, creamy cheese like texture known as Yo-cheese.

Store in the original container or a smaller plastic container you can place an airtight lid on.

Use Yo Cheese as a cream cheese, sandwich spread, mayonnaise replacement, salad dressing base, dip for vegetables, or unsalted chips. You can mix granulated onion powder, unsalted chili powder, or chives and minced or finely diced green onions or any other flavor you want for dips or salads in this.

Works great for topping raspberries, blueberries or strawberries. Excellent spread when mixed with just a bit of Splenda or sugar for our homemade salt-free toasted bagels.

[1] Best estimate for final measurement is based on 1/2 of container's lost liquid. Recipe may have fewer calories than listed or 372.4 mg

[2] We have found, after testing many brands of Plain nonfat Yogurt, that either Nancy's or Dannon's Plain nonfat Yogurt works the best when attempting to obtain the texture of cream cheese. Other regional brands probably work as well.

Diabetics: 3 tablespoons will put you at .5 carb choices.

Yo Cheese Nutrient Data Per Tablespoon (32 tablespoons): Calories: 11.6, Protein: 1.194 g, Carbohydrate: 1.592 g, Dietary Fiber: 0 g, Total Sugars: 0 g, Total Fat: .031 g, Saturated Fat: .015 g, Monounsaturated Fat: .009 g, Polyunsaturated Fat: .001 g, Cholesterol: .459 mg, Trans Fatty Acids: 0 g, Total Omega-3 FA: 0 g, Total Omega-6 FA: 0 g, Calcium: 30.5 mg, Potassium: 39 mg, Sodium: 11.6 mg, Vitamin K: 0 mcg

BROWN RICE

LACTO OVO-VEGETARIAN – 1½ CARB CHOICES

Serves 4 Sodium Per Recipe: 57 mg Sodium Per Serving: 14.2 mg

Mushrooms & Asparagus give this side dish a wonderful flavor. Top with some parsley and it's just the right filler for many meals.

½ cup brown rice (6.475 mg)
1½ teaspoons extra virgin olive oil (trace)
½ pound fresh mushrooms[1] (11.5 mg)
½ medium onion, diced (2.2 mg)
2 cloves garlic, chopped or minced (1.02 mg)
2 tablespoons light or low fat sour cream (25 mg)
¼ pound asparagus spears (2.4 mg)
¼ cup chopped parsley (8.4 mg)

Cook rice according to package instructions either with filtered water or with a homemade unsalted chicken broth. (See page: 231)

Steam asparagus spears until they turn bright green and set aside.

When rice is about ten to fifteen minutes from being cooked, prepare the mushroom mix.

Place oil in a saute pan and heat over medium flame. Add mushrooms and chopped onion. Saute, stirring gently until lightly browned and softened, about 8 minutes. Add the garlic halfway between the 8 minutes.

Stir the mushroom mixture and sour cream into the hot cooked rice. It will fluff or should fluff before you add other ingredients.

Garnish with the asparagus spears and parsley and serve.

[1] Your choice

Brown Rice Nutrient Data Per Serving: Calories: 137.5, Protein: 5.464 g, Carbohydrate: 23.4 g, Dietary Fiber: 2.403 g, Total Sugars: 2.839 g, Total Fat: 3.208 g, Saturated Fat: .81 g, Monounsaturated Fat: 1.098 g, Polyunsaturated Fat: .925 g, Cholesterol: 8.333 mg, Trans Fatty Acids: 0 g, Total Omega-3 FA: .022 g, Total Omega-6 FA: 0 g, Calcium: 25.3 mg, Potassium: 341.9 mg, Sodium: 14.2 mg, Vitamin K: 74.9 mcg

SOUPS & SALADS

Soups

If making soup seems a mystery to you, then you're in luck. Soup making is really easy, especially with the right recipes in hand.

Soup is the world's healer. It warms us, soothes our aches when we are ill, and it's always full of great nutrients.

Another secret about soup making is that most soups are made pretty much like each other; even though ingredients are different, the method of getting to the final soup is often the same.

Broth or stock based soups require your homemade broth be made at least a day ahead of time. Maureen has developed a chicken broth that is so inexpensive and easy to make, and gives you chicken leftovers for salads, sandwiches or other chicken dishes, that you might find yourself making broth more than ever before (Page 239). We store extra broth in the freezer or if it's to be used soon, in the fridge. Use either plastic containers or Mason jars. Leave room for expansion if freezing. We freeze in jars with lid off. After frozen we secure with lid.

Most soups begin by heating extra virgin olive oil in a stock pot, followed by sautéing fresh vegetables called for in the recipe. We often add garlic and other herbs, which helps enrich the soup's flavor. Once vegetables are softened, we add in the spices and meat if meat is called for. At this point we add our broth or other liquid, bring all to a boil, and then reduce heat to a simmer. The final step sometimes requires puréeing. After that we either refrigerate it for overnight flavor enhancement or we serve it hot.

Salads

Our basic vinaigrette recipe for use at home and at restaurants consists of extra virgin olive oil, balsamic vinegar or lemon juice with a pinch of sugar. Essentially, the mix is three parts of oil to one part of vinegar or lemon juice and sugar or Splenda from a packet. See Glossary for Splenda data.

We also like to make avocado dressing. Just mash a little avocado into the basic vinaigrette until smooth and you've got a terrific dressing.

We have a Yo Cheese recipe in this book that's also good for salad dressings. The Yo Cheese is naturally acidic and works well in dressings.

Pasta is a nice addition to salads, but cook al dente. We want the pasta to absorb some of the salad dressing without becoming mushy.

After cleaning "greens" and drying, store in zipper lock bags in the refrigerator.

CHILI CHICKEN & BLACK BEAN SOUP

VEGAN – 1½ CARB CHOICES

Serves 8 Sodium Per Recipe: 532.4 mg Sodium Per Serving: 66.6 mg

Soups are a wonderful way to use up ingredients and leftovers from other recipes. They are also an excellent entrée.

- **2 teaspoons extra virgin olive oil (.18 mg)**
- **1 fresh green jalapeño chili, seeded and chopped (.14 mg)**
- **1 medium onion, chopped (4.4 mg)**
- **3 cloves, garlic, chopped (1.53 mg)**
- **½ teaspoon cumin (1.764 mg)**
- **½ teaspoon Don's Italian Seasoning[1] (.247 mg)**
- **¼ teaspoon ground thyme (.138 mg)**
- **1 teaspoon granulated onion powder (1.296 mg)**
- **⅛ teaspoon white pepper (.15 mg)**
- **4 cups Maureen's Chicken Broth[2] (86.7 mg)**
- **1 14.5 ounce can no salt added tomatoes[3] (42.8 mg)**
- **6 no salt corn tortillas cut into strips (1.6 mg)**
- **1 pound boneless, skinless chicken breast (288 mg)**
- **2 14.5 ounce cans Eden Organic Black beans (105 mg)**

Sauté pepper with garlic & onion in olive oil in stockpot until onion is translucent. Add spices, stir and cook for another minute. Add chicken broth and tomatoes with juice and bring to boil. Add the tortillas and simmer for another 15 minutes or until tortillas dissolve.

Cut chicken into bite size pieces. Add chicken, simmer until cooked through-about ten minutes. Add the black beans and heat about 5 more minutes or until soup is heated through.

Garnish with a dollop of sour cream and fresh chopped tomatoes. Cilantro or lemon juice is nice, too.

[1] Use Don's Italian Seasoning, See Page: 239)

[2] See pages 48-49, *No Salt, Lowest Sodium Light Meals Book.* (Reprinted in this book with permission. See Page: 231) Or use Swanson or other brand unsalted Chicken Broth. Swanson is 45 mg sodium per cup. Add 12 mg sodium per serving.

[3] This is a USDA figure, so we use it. However, most cans of no-salt-added tomatoes that we have found contain at least 72 mg of sodium some as high as 175.

Chili Chicken Black Bean Soup Nutrient Data Per Serving: Calories: 204.7, Protein: 21.3 g, Carbohydrate: 22.4 g, Dietary Fiber: 1.415 g, Total Sugars: 2.741 g, Total Fat: 3.373 g, Saturated Fat: .69 g, Monounsaturated Fat: 1.377 g, Polyunsaturated Fat: .522 g, Cholesterol: 37.6 mg, Trans Fatty Acids: 0 g, Total Omega-3 FA: .041 g, Total Omega-6 FA: 0 g, Calcium: 34.5 mg, Potassium: 433.7 mg, Sodium: 66.6 mg, Vitamin K: 4.524 mcg

EASY COLD WINTER NIGHT CHILI

FLEXITARIAN – 1 CARB CHOICES

Makes 8 Servings

Sodium Per Recipe: 468.3 mg ***Sodium Per Serving: 58.5 mg***

With or without meat this is an excellent chili. The Canon's Sweet Hots are available from Healthy Heart Market if you can't find them locally.

2 teaspoons extra virgin olive oil (trace)
1 large onion, diced (6 mg)
½ pound lean ground beef (149.7 mg)
1 tablespoon Grandma's chili powder (trace)
1 can Eden Organic Kidney beans[1] (52.5 mg)
1 can no salt added pinto beans (52.5 mg)
1 14.5-ounce can no salt added tomatoes[2] (105 mg)
1 can no salt added tomato sauce (26.8 mg)
1 tablespoon Canon's Sweet Hots[3] (trace)

In the same medium to large size saucepan you'll use for the whole recipe, sauté onions in olive oil until translucent. Add meat and cook until done. Drain the fat and add chili powder to the meat.

Add all ingredients and bring to a low boil. Turn heat down and simmer for a half hour.

Serve hot.

May be refrigerated and reheated in a microwave. If chili gets too thick, add some filtered water and reheat.

[1] A variety of no salt added pinto beans can be found today. Some include Sun Vista, Health Valley and Eden No Salt Added Organic. There may be other NSA brands of kidney beans available as well.

[2] Official USDA numbers state that a can of no salt added tomatoes has only 19 mg of sodium. We believe this is an error, especially since that would mean the can contained only one and a half tomatoes. All cans we have found on the market come to about 105 to 175 mg of sodium per can. We list 105 here for S&W canned NSA tomatoes.

[3] Available at healthyheartmarket.com or www.sweethots.com

Cold Winter Night Chili Nutrient Data Per Serving: Calories: 161.2, Protein: 14.2 g, Carbohydrate: 22.4 g, Dietary Fiber: 10.3 g, Total Sugars: 3.468 g, Total Fat: 1.654 g, Saturated Fat: .682 g, Monounsaturated Fat: .655 g, Polyunsaturated Fat: .17 g, Cholesterol: 17.6 mg, Trans Fatty Acids: .097 g, Total Omega-3 FA: .027 g, Total Omega-6 FA: .002 g, Calcium: 13.7 mg, Potassium: 711.6 mg, Sodium: 58.5 mg, Vitamin K: 2.218 mcg,

CHILLED MANGO SOUP

VEGAN – 1½ CARB CHOICES

Serves 2 Sodium Per Recipe: 7.501 mg Sodium Per Serving: 3.75 mg

If you like mangoes, you'll love this cold soup. Recently, Maureen visited Maui, Hawaii with some of her friends, and when served this dish she knew she had a winner.

½ cup cold mango juice[1] (3.286 mg)
½ cup cold filtered water (trace)
¼ jalapeno chili pepper, seeds removed, diced (.035 mg)
1 cup fresh or frozen mango (3.3 mg)
1 lime, juice from (.88 mg)

Wash jalapeno, clean insides, remove all seeds and then dice. If using fresh mango, peel, seed and measure. For a little more "kick," add a ¼ teaspoon ground ginger or ¼ onion chopped. Place all ingredients into a processer and puree until mix is smooth. Add a bit more water if you like. Chill in refrigerator for a few hours before serving. Serve chilled.

[1]Mango juice is often a combination with other ingredients such as apple juice, mango puree, orange juice, banana puree and lemon juice. For this recipe we used Trader Joe's Mango Juice.

Mango Soup Nutrient Data Per Serving: Calories: 85.3, Protein: .602 g, Carbohydrate: 22.6 g, Dietary Fiber: 1.643 g, Total Sugars: 19.2 g, Total Fat: .266 g, Saturated Fat: .061 g, Monounsaturated Fat: .09 g, Polyunsaturated Fat: .057 g, Cholesterol: 0 mg, Trans Fatty Acids: 0 g, Total Omega-3 FA: .033 g, Total Omega-6 FA: 0 g, Calcium: 13.4 mg, Potassium: 176.7 mg, Sodium: 3.75 mg, Vitamin K: 3.767 mcg

SOUP MAKER TIPS

1. Start with Maureen's unsalted, very low sodium chicken broth/stock. See next page.

2. Use fresh ingredients, such as produce from the farmers market or your local specialized produce stand. If using canned beans like Eden Organic, drain and rinse them first.

3. Sauté veggies in extra virgin olive oil first.

4. Use fresh herbs and spices to enliven soups and to help with color.

5. We like to puree part of the soup and add it back into the rest of the soup.

6. Many soups can be "punched up" in flavor with a sqeeze of lime or lemon juice (per serving) or a few tablespoons of balsamic vinegar in the soup near the end of cooking.

7. Top with dollops of sour cream, or grated no salt added cheese or other toppings like fresh basil and parsely.

MAUREEN'S CHICKEN BROTH

FLEXITARIAN – 0 CARB CHOICES

Makes 10 cups Sodium Per Recipe: 216.8 mg Sodium Per Cup: 21.6 mg

1 2 ½ to 4-pound nonbrined fryer, whole (87.9 mg)
4 quarts filtered water (see instructions) (trace)
2 stalks celery with some leaves, 1 inch pieces (27.2 mg)
1 large onion, quartered (6 mg)
2 cloves garlic, minced (1.02 mg)
2 med. carrots, peeled and cut into 1 inch pieces (84.2 mg)
8 black peppercorns (8 mg)

Remove parts from chicken cavity. Put it into a large stockpot and cover with the water. Add rest of ingredients and bring all to a boil over moderate heat. Lower the heat to a constant simmer. Skim any scum that rises to the top. Cook for about 2 to 3 hours. Remove the chicken to a platter. Strain the liquid through a sieve with a fine mesh. Discard the vegetables. Cool both broth and chicken. Remove the chicken meat from the bones. The meat can be used in soups, casserole dishes, fried rice, salads, sandwiches, etc. Chill both the broth and the meat in the refrigerator – this can be overnight if you choose to make soup the following day. Remove the fat that rises to the surface of the broth. You can save broth in canning jars in your refrigerator for future use; it will keep for up to a week. Or you can freeze the broth in quart jars; fill only three-fourths full to allow for expansion.

Maureen's Chicken Broth Nutrient Values Per Cup: Calories: 40.6, Protein: 2.703 g, Carbohydrate: 3.158 g, Dietary Fiber: .705 g, Total Sugars: 1.282 g, Total Fat: 1.944 g, Saturated Fat: .55 g, Monounsaturated Fat: .78 g, Polyunsaturated Fat: .432 g, Cholesterol: 11.3 mg, Trans Fatty Acids: 0 g, Total Omega-3 FA: .024 g, Total Omega-6 FA: 0 g, Calcium: 12.9 mg, Potassium: 100.3 mg, Sodium: 21.6 mg, Vitamin K: 2.677 mcg

MAUREEN'S PLAN FOR A SINGLE CHICKEN

After separating meat from bones and while broth is chilling in the fridge, dice one-third of the meat for use in soup. Make variations of chicken soup including chicken noodle, or a southwest version by adding a can of diced chopped tomatoes and no-salt corn and 6 low-sodium corn tortillas cut into strips. Finish it off with some chili powder, onion powder, and oregano.

Dice another third to make into a chicken salad using chopped celery, green onion, onion powder, plain yogurt or sour cream, chopped apples, grapes, or dried cranberries. Use as a salad or in sandwiches.

I usually reserve the last third for a chicken casserole. Depending on seasonings you can make it into enchiladas, a chicken/noodle casserole, or any of your specialties. I usually add a can of tomato sauce and southwest seasonings for a taco filling.

POPPY SEED SALAD DRESSING

VEGAN – 0 CARB CHOICES
Makes Approximately 4 tablespoons
Sodium Per Recipe: 4.434 mg   Sodium Per Tablespoon: 1.0759 mg

This is a terrific salad dressing. You may exchange the 1 teaspoon of sugar with ½-packet Splenda. Works with most green salads. Spinach and Romaine are best. Add in cucumbers, sliced tomatoes, diced low sodium cheddar and some avocado. You can double this recipe.

3 tablespoons raspberry vinegar (3.576 mg)
2 tablespoons extra virgin olive oil (.27 mg)
1 teaspoon sugar or ½ packet of Splenda (trace)
¼ teaspoon poppy seeds (.588 mg)

Whisk together vigorously with fork or mini-whisk.

Delicious over fresh spinach, with fresh berries and a few walnuts or served with sliced fresh tomatoes and sliced cucumbers.

Poppy seed Salad Dressing Nutrient Data Per Serving: Calories: 66.8, Protein: .036 g, Carbohydrate: 1.129 g, Dietary Fiber: .034 g, Total Sugars: 1.054 g, Total Fat: 6.823 g, Saturated Fat: .94 g, Monounsaturated Fat: 4.935 g, Polyunsaturated Fat: .76 g, Cholesterol: 0 mg, Trans Fatty Acids: 0 g, Total Omega-3 FA: .052 g, Total Omega-6 FA: 0 g, Calcium: 3.265 mg, Potassium: 5.705 mg, Sodium: 1.075 mg, Vitamin K: 4.064 mcg

SALAD DRESSING EXTRAORDINAIRE

VEGAN – 0 CARB CHOICES
Makes 4 tablespoons
Sodium Per Recipe: 7.63 mg   Sodium Per Tablespoon: 1.84 mg

While traveling from coast to coast in our pickup truck, my wife created this easy to make salad dressing. We used it on freshly cut vegetables, salads and even sandwiches. It proved to be our "on the road" crutch for kicking up otherwise familiar foods. We made enough for 10 days before leaving home and stored the small bottle in our ice chest. It's also low in sodium, cholesterol and carbohydrates. Give it a try, I think you'll really like it. You may double it or go for a bottle full. Just keep the proportions the same.

2 tablespoons white balsamic vinegar (7.36 mg)
2 tablespoon extra virgin olive oil (.27 mg)
2 teaspoons sugar or 1 packet of Splenda[1] (trace)
¼ teaspoon dry mustard powder (trace)

Place in small container and shake well before each use. Refrigerate for future use.

[1] One packet of Splenda equals ¼ teaspoon measurement, and the sweetness of two-teaspoons sugar.

Salad Dressing Extraordinaire Nutrient Data Per Tablespoon: Calories: 76.1, Protein: .07 g, Carbohydrate: 3.181 g, Dietary Fiber: 0 g, Total Sugars: 2.803 g, Total Fat: 7.037 g, Saturated Fat: 1.012 g, Monounsaturated Fat: 3.381 g, Polyunsaturated Fat: 2.325 g, Cholesterol: 0 mg, Trans Fatty Acids: 0 g, Total Omega-3 FA: .03 g, Total Omega-6 FA: 0 g, Calcium: 2.472 mg, Potassium: 9.727 mg, Sodium: 1.84 mg, Vitamin K: 1.47 mcg

RASPBERRY VINAIGRETTE SALAD

VEGAN – 1 CARB CHOICES

Serves 4 Sodium Per Recipe: 188.6 mg Sodium Per Serving: 47.1 mg

Here's an easy to make, delicious salad treat. It's perfect for summer patio dinners or served with your favorite barbecue meal. It's also a great salad for winter evenings while curled up by the fireplace. Always a favorite.

The Vinaigrette

tablespoons raspberry vinegar (.45 mg)
tablespoons extra virgin olive oil (trace)
tablespoon sugar or ½ packet of Splenda (.126 mg)
teaspoon dry mustard (trace)

The Salad

1 package (6-ounce or equivalent) Mixed Salad Greens (55.9 mg)
1 cup red, seedless grapes (3.2 mg)
½ cup unsalted walnuts, toasted until oily (1 mg)
4 ounces grated low-sodium Swiss[1] (127.9 mg)

Whisk together the first four ingredients.

In a medium salad bowl, mix the last four ingredients and top with the dressing. Toss and serve. Delicious!

[1] There are various low sodium Swiss cheese products with sodium levels as low as 25 mg per ounce. To grate slices, roll them up like a cigar and then grate.

Raspberry Salad Nutrient Data Per Serving: Calories: 277.4, Protein: 10.4 g, Carbohydrate: 15.2 g, Dietary Fiber: 2.013 g, Total Sugars: 3.445 g, Total Fat: 20.9 g, Saturated Fat: 5.449 g, Monounsaturated Fat: 7.443 g, Polyunsaturated Fat: 6.885 g, Cholesterol: 18.2 mg, Calcium: 277.4 mg, Iron: 1.456 mg, Potassium: 372.2 mg, Sodium: 47.1 mg, Vitamin K: 3.308 mcg

POTATO SALAD

LACTO OVO VEGETARIAN – 3½ CARB CHOICES

Serves: 4 Sodium Per Recipe: 354.11 mg Sodium Per Serving: 88.5 mg

Terrific for picnics, just make sure you keep it chilled. Diabetics, this may be one of those "eat only half a serving" recipes. Exchanging Splenda for sugar offers negligible carbohydrate help.

2 large eggs, hardboiled, cooled and chopped (126 mg)
6 medium Yukon or red potatoes, washed[1], (76.7 mg)
1 medium stalk of celery, chopped (32 mg)
⅓ cup shallots (save 1 tablespoon for the dressing) (about 1 or 2) (6.36 mg)
4 to 6 tablespoons dressing[2] (below)
½ cup nonfat homemade Yo Cheese (Page: 233)(93.1 mg)
¼ teaspoon white pepper (.03 mg)
1 teaspoon granulated onion powder (1.296 mg)
¼ teaspoon paprika (.178 mg)

The Dressing

3 tablespoons red wine vinegar (3.576 mg)
3 tablespoons extra virgin olive oil (.81 mg)
¼ teaspoon dry mustard (.041 mg)
1½ teaspoons sugar or Splenda (trace)
1 tablespoon shallots chopped (Included)

Cover eggs with water, bring to a boil in a small pan, then turn down heat and simmer for 15 minutes. Drain and cool. (Might be a good idea to boil the the day before and refrigerate them for the salad the following day.)

Wash and scrub potatoes, place in pan and cover with water. Cover and bring to a boil. Then turn down heat to a simmer for 15 minutes or until thoroughly cooked but still solid (not soft). Drain and cool. See Tips, next page.

Chop celery and shallots and set aside.

Make the dressing by mixing all the ingredients with a small whisk in a small bowl.

When potatoes are cool or cold, slice into small bite-size pieces, place them in a large salad bowl and sprinkle with white pepper and granulated onion powder. Add the celery and shallots and toss thoroughly.

Add the Dressing and mix again. Fold in Yo Cheese.

Finally add chopped eggs mixing well and sprinkle with paprika if desired.

[1] May peel if you prefer.
[2] To taste or consistency (depending on potato sizes)

Potato Salad Nutrient Data Per Serving: Calories: 395.4, Protein: 12.1 g, Carbohydrate: 59 g, Dietary Fiber: 5.744 g, Total Sugars: 5.385 g, Total Fat: 13.2 g, Saturated Fat: 2.325 g, Monounsaturated Fat: 8.416 g, Polyunsaturated Fat: 1.63 g, Cholesterol: 106.7 mg, Trans Fatty Acids: 0 g, Total Omega-3 FA: .147 g, Total Omega-6 FA: 0 g, Potassium: 1650 mg, Sodium: 88.5 mg, Vitamin K: 18.5 mcg

SPINACH SALAD With PERSIMMON

VEGAN – 1½ CARB CHOICES

Serves 4 Sodium Per Recipe: 110.5 mg Sodium Per Serving: 27.6 mg

This salad is refreshing and easy to make. If persimmons are out of season, use in-season citrus or canned mandarin slices.

4 cups baby spinach (94.8 mg)
½ medium red onion, thinly sliced (2.20 mg)
2 small or medium Fuyu persimmons (hard) (3.36 mg)
4 tablespoons Salad Dressing Extraordinaire (See Page: 232) (10.2 mg)

Wash spinach and pat dry.
Slice onion and peel and slice the Fuji persimmons.
Mix all ingredients and serve with chosen entrée.

Nutrient Data Per Serving: Calories: 129.9, Protein: 1.59 g, Carbohydrate: 22.2 g, Dietary Fiber: 3.918 g, Total Sugars: 15 g, Total Fat: 4.84 g, Saturated Fat: .671 g, Monounsaturated Fat: 3.344 g, Polyunsaturated Fat: .578 g, Cholesterol: 0 mg, Trans Fatty Acids: 0 g, Total Omega-3 FA: .08 g, Total Omega-6 FA: 0 g, Calcium: 42.9 mg, Potassium: 335.7 mg, Sodium: 27.6 mg, Vitamin K: 149.8 mcg

MORE SALAD TIPS

1. For potato salad, Yukon Gold, New Potatoes or Red Potatoes are best.
2. Chill salad plates before serving. This helps keep your salad crisp.
3. When using hot pasta for salads, cool after cooking before adding herbs or other ingredients.
4. For potato salad we often like to marinate the warm potatoes in a little vinegar and oil, or vinegraitte, then chill. This adds more flavor to the finished salad.
5. To prepare iceberg lettuce, remove the core. Wash the lettuce then spin dry or use paper towels. Dry as best as you can and store in zipper lock bags to keep fresh in your fridge for up to 5 or more days.
6. Another ploy I have when eating out is to use fruit juice or lemon juice as a salad dressing. Just use some juice and extra virgin olive oil.

SOUTHWEST CITRUS SALAD

VEGAN - 2 CARB CHOICES

Serves 4 Sodium Per Recipe: 44.8 mg Sodium Per Serving: 11.2 mg

This delicious salad was first introduced to us by Marlene Winger, who worked as a Home Economist for a large public utility company. She later taught school with Maureen.

5 cups loosely packed, shredded Romaine (18.8 mg)
1 cup red onion, sliced, cut into halves (9.2 mg)
1 cup 1½" julienne cut jicama (4.8 mg)
cup chopped cilantro (1.84 mg)

In medium bowl, combine above and set aside.

¼ cup fresh orange juice (.62 mg)
1 teaspoon sugar or 1 packet Splenda (trace)
½ teaspoon cumin (1.764 mg)
1½ tablespoon extra virgin olive oil (trace)
2 cups of orange or mandarin sections (7.8 mg)

In small bowl, combine above, stir together.

Mix salad together in the medium bowl and serve.

Southwest Citrus Salad Nutrient Date Per Serving: Calories: 154.7, Protein: 2.537 g, Carbohydrate: 25.8 g, Dietary Fiber: 5.523 g, Total Sugars: 16.4 g, Total Fat: 5.908 g, Saturated Fat: .854 g, Monounsaturated Fat: 2.641 g, Polyunsaturated Fat: 1.929 g, Cholesterol: 0 mg, Trans Fatty Acids: 0 g, Total Omega-3 FA: .115 g, Total Omega-6 FA: 0 g, Calcium: 77.1 mg, Potassium: 476.8 mg, Sodium: 11.2 mg, Vitamin K: 64.8 mcg

SPICES & RUBS

Spices are our friend, especially when living a no-salt lifestyle. Commercial spice mixes are often good, but more expensive than making up your own. I like to mix my own rubs, which are a combination of spices and herbs. I also like to make spice mixes that work with a variety of dishes.

If you get "into" making a lot of spice mixes and storing them, then a local natural food store might be your best bet for finding fresh bulk spices. Specialty stores might also sell them. The price on the bin might frighten you because many are listed by the pound. But if you grab a cup of one and weigh it you'll quickly see that the fresh bulk prices are a great deal. It really takes a lot of any spice to weigh a pound. In the end you pay about a 1/3 of the cost of commercial mixes.

You can make rubs using a variety of spices or just a few.

With barbecuing, a simple spice/herb mix can work wonders. A mix of onion powder, garlic powder, some paprika or red pepper flakes and black or white pepper, and your baby back ribs will develop a terrific flavor. Same with fowl, and beef cooked in your oven or on the barbecue grill. But it's also nice to add other flavors like sage, coriander, savory, lemon peel, marjoram, oregano, basil and more. If you're new to rubs, please give them a try. You'll learn quickly why we don't need to add salt to any meat dish.

IT'S EASY TO MAKE YOUR OWN

Use a small bowl to mix spices. If you are using fresh seeds and want to grind them down, then use a processor or a coffee grinder, or do it the old fashioned way with a mortar and pestle.

You may want to try some new flavors such as fennel, savory, or lavender.

Want a hot chili mix or Cajun formula to start with? Then mix together paprika, garlic powder, cayenne pepper flakes and black or white pepper. Add other spices as well to offset the heat you've just created, like sage, thyme, coriander, etc. Your measurements of each will be based on what you're searching for. Want it hot? Then start with paprika or cayenne or salt-free chili powder and go from there.

I like a hot chili rub for baby back ribs so I use salt-free Wayzata Bay (hot) chili powder, or dried red chilies we grind ourselves. Add to that other flavors like onion and garlic powder or some cumin (always good).

Mix ingredients together well and store in an airtight jar for up to 6-months.

DON'S HOT BARBECUE SPICE MIX

VEGAN – 0 CARB CHOICES

Makes 5 teaspoons *Sodium Per Teaspoon: .63 mg*

1 teaspoon garlic powder (.728 mg)
1 teaspoon paprika (.714 mg)
1 teaspoon sugar or Splenda (trace)
½ teaspoon allspice (.731 mg)
¼ teaspoon nutmeg (.088 mg)
¼ teaspoon ground cinnamon (.065 mg)
¼ teaspoon onion powder (.324 mg)
¼ teaspoon thyme (.192 mg)
¼ teaspoon sage (.019 mg)
¼ teaspoon black pepper (.231 mg)
⅛ teaspoon cayenne pepper (.067 mg)

Mix together and store in tight container in dry place. Works with fowl, pork and beef with any barbecue method.

Nutrient Data Per Teaspoon: Calories: 8.853, Protein: .218 g, Carbohydrate: 2.033 g, Dietary Fiber: .432 g, Total Sugars: 1.103 g, Total Fat: .139 g, Saturated Fat: .05 g, Monounsaturated Fat: .014 g, Polyunsaturated Fat: .049 g, Cholesterol: 0 mg, Trans Fatty Acids: 0 g, Total Omega-3 FA: .006 g, Total Omega-6 FA: 0 g, Calcium: 6.823 mg, Potassium: 23.3 mg, Sodium: .632 mg, Vitamin K: 2.391 mcg

DON'S CHICKEN RUB

VEGAN – 0 CARB CHOICES

Makes: 7 tablespoons *Sodium Per Tablespoon: 1.314 mg*

3 tablespoons rosemary (4.95 mg)
2 tablespoons sage (.44 mg)
1 tablespoon oregano (.81 mg)
2 teaspoons thyme (1.54 mg)
½ teaspoon black pepper (.462 mg)
½ teaspoon onion powder (.648 mg)
½ teaspoon ground ginger (.288 mg)
½ teaspoon grated lemon peel (.06 mg)

Nutrient Data Per Tablespoon: Calories: 11.4, Protein: .299 g, Carbohydrate: 2.355 g, Dietary Fiber: 1.392 g, Total Sugars: .12 g, Total Fat: .412 g, Saturated Fat: .18 g, Monounsaturated Fat: .063 g, Polyunsaturated Fat: .093 g, Cholesterol: 0 mg, Trans Fatty Acids: 0 g, Total Omega-3 FA: .058 g, Total Omega-6 FA: 0 g, Calcium: 48.9 mg, Potassium: 41.2 mg, Sodium: 1.314 mg, Vitamin K: 21.7 mcg

DON'S ITALIAN SEASONING

VEGAN – 0 CARB CHOICES

Makes 16 tablespoons ***Sodium Per Teaspoon: 1.662 mg***

Italian seasoning works well with all meats, pasta dishes,and pizzas.

2 tablespoons dried rosemary (3.3 mg)
2 tablespoons dried basil (4.59 mg)
2 tablespoons dried marjoram (2.618 mg)
2 teaspoons granulated onion powder (2.592 mg)
1½ tablespoons ground oregano (.405 mg)
2 tablespoons dried parsley (14,5 ng)
2 tablespoons ground thyme (4.732 mg)
2 tablespoons ground sage (4.73 mg)
1 tablespoon lavender[1] (trace)
1 teaspoon dried savory (.336 mg)
¼ teaspoon red pepper flakes (.135 mg)

Combine all the ingredients in a small bowl or container of your food processor with a steel blade and process for about 20 to 30 seconds only.

Place into a tight container (possibly an older spice jar or container) and store in a cool dry place. Date it. Store all your spices no more than 6 months.

[1] Available in natural food sections or stores or in your garden. Optional, but offers a fine European spice flavor. Nutrients unknown but not suspected to alter figures. If not available, try adding a teaspoon or two of savory.

Calories: 6.082, Protein: .239 g, Carbohydrate: 1.36 g, Dietary Fiber: .731 g, Total Sugars: .152 g, Total Fat: .138 g, Saturated Fat: .044 g, Monounsaturated Fat: .02 g, Polyunsaturated Fat: .039 g, Cholesterol: 0 mg, Trans Fatty Acids: 0 g, Total Omega-3 FA: .024 g, Total Omega-6 FA: 0 g, Calcium: 33.5 mg, Potassium: 37.9 mg, Sodium: 1.662 mg, Vitamin K: 18.9 mcg

BASIC ITALIAN SEASONING

VEGAN – 0 CARB CHOICES

Makes 7 teaspoons ***Sodium Per Teaspoon: .356 mg***

2 teaspoons dried basil (.952 mg)
2 teaspoons dried marjoram (.924 mg)
2 teaspoons dried oregano (.54 mg)
1 teaspoon dried sage (.077 mg)

Mix or process together, store in tight jar for up to 6 months.

Nutrient Data Per Teaspoon: Calories: 3.357, Protein: .146 g, Carbohydrate: .74 g, Dietary Fiber: .491 g, Total Sugars: .037 g, Total Fat: .093 g, Saturated Fat: .023 g, Monounsaturated Fat: .009 g, Polyunsaturated Fat: .045 g, Cholesterol: 0 mg, Trans Fatty Acids: 0 g, Total Omega-3 FA: .034 g, Total Omega-6 FA: 0 g, Calcium: 21.6 mg, Potassium: 26 mg, Sodium: .356 mg, Vitamin K: 12.8 mcg

DON'S RIB RUB

VEGAN – 0 CARB CHOICES

Makes 4 ½ tablespoons *Sodium Per Teaspoon: .958 mg*

- **1 teaspoon coriander (.63 mg)**
- **2 teaspoons ground cumin (7.056 mg)**
- **4 teaspoons Splenda (trace)**
- **4 teaspoons paprika (2.856 mg)**
- **½ teaspoon cayenne pepper (.27 mg)**
- **½ teaspoon ground allspice (.731 mg)**
- **1½ teaspoons black pepper (1.386 mg)**

Stir together well. Store in airtight container in dry place.

***Nutrient Data Per Teaspoon:** Calories: 4.354, Protein: .202 g, Carbohydrate: .798 g, Dietary Fiber: .416 g, Total Sugars: .08 g, Total Fat: .199 g, Saturated Fat: .025 g, Monounsaturated Fat: .074 g, Polyunsaturated Fat: .074 g, Cholesterol: 0 mg, Trans Fatty Acids: 0 g, Total Omega-3 FA: .007 g, Total Omega-6 FA: 0 g, Iron: .453 mg, Calcium: 6.527 mg, Potassium: 26.9 mg, Sodium: .958 mg, Vitamin K: .952 mcg*

SOUTHWEST HOT SPICE MIX

VEGAN – 0 CARB CHOICES

Makes: 4 tablespoons *Sodium Per Tablespoon: 2.516*

- **1 tablespoon Wayzata Bay chili powder (trace)**
- **½ teaspoon dry mustard (.082 mg)**
- **½ teaspoon nutmeg (.178 mg)**
- **1 teaspoon ground cumin (3.528 mg)**
- **½ teaspoon black pepper (.462 mg)**
- **2 tablespoons paprika (4.692 mg)**
- **1 teaspoon sugar or Splenda (trace)**
- **½ teaspoon ground thyme (.385 mg)**
- **½ teaspoon ground sage (.038 mg)**
- **½ teaspoon curry powder (.52 mg)**
- **⅓ teaspoon cayenne pepper (.18 mg)**

Combine all ingredients in a small container and shake well. Use with chili con carne, hot chili beans, taco meat sauce, or as a dry rub for a sparerib barbecue. Hot to the lips and tongue.

***Nutrient Data Per Tablespoons:** Calories: 25.8, Protein: .825 g, Carbohydrate: 4.8 g, Dietary Fiber: 1.757 g, Total Sugars: 1.553 g, Total Fat: 1.063 g, Saturated Fat: .182 g, Monounsaturated Fat: .23 g, Polyunsaturated Fat: .353 g, Cholesterol: 0 mg, Trans Fatty Acids: 0 g, Total Omega-3 FA: .048 g, Total Omega-6 FA: 0 g, Calcium: 21 mg, Potassium: 106.6 mg, Sodium: 2.516 mg, Vitamin K: 8.121 mcg*

DON'S SPICY MEAT RUB

VEGAN – 0 CARB CHOICES

Makes: 5.6 tablespoons ***Sodium Per Tablespoon: 2.197 mg***

This rub works with pork, fowl and beef, especially when barbecuing.

- **3 tablespoons paprika (7.038 mg)**
- **1 tablespoon garlic powder (2.184 mg)**
- **1 teaspoon onion powder (1.296 mg)**
- **1 teaspoon black pepper (.924 mg)**
- **½ teaspoon red pepper (.27 mg)**
- **½ teaspoon thyme (.385 mg)**
- **⅓ teaspoon oregano (.09 mg)**
- **⅓ teaspoon nutmeg (.117 mg)**

Nutrient Data Per Tablespoon: Calories: 20, Protein: .932 g, Carbohydrate: 4.044 g, Dietary Fiber: 1.818 g, Total Sugars: .962 g, Total Fat: .602 g, Saturated Fat: .13 g, Monounsaturated Fat: .06 g, Polyunsaturated Fat: .34 g, Cholesterol: 0 mg, Trans Fatty Acids: 0 g, Total Omega-3 FA: .041 g, Total Omega-6 FA: 0 g, Calcium: 15.5 mg, Potassium: 118.4 mg, Sodium: 2.197 mg, Vitamin K: 6.537 mcg

SOUTHERN COMFORT

VEGAN – 0 CARB CHOICES

Makes 8 tablespoons ***Sodium Per Tablespoon: 2.318 mg***

This rub works well with ribs, blackened barbecued bass or other white fish and it will also heat up chicken wings for a hot wings appetizer.

- **3 tablespoons paprika (7.038 mg)**
- **1 tablespoon granulated onion powder (3.726 mg)**
- **1 tablespoon unsalted garlic powder (2.184 mg)**
- **1 tablespoon ground coriander (1.75 mg)**
- **1½ tablespoons dry mustard (.84 mg)**
- **1½ teaspoons red pepper flakes (cayenne) (.81 mg)**
- **¼ teaspoon ground cloves (1.276 mg)**
- **1 teaspoon black pepper (.924 mg)**

Mix together, store in airtight container.

Nutrient Data Per Tablespoon: Calories: 27.6, Protein: 1.32 g, Carbohydrate: 4.38 g, Dietary Fiber: 1.875 g, Total Sugars: 1.009 g, Total Fat: 1.147 g, Saturated Fat: .111 g, Monounsaturated Fat: .548 g, Polyunsaturated Fat: .383 g, Cholesterol: 0 mg, Trans Fatty Acids: 0 g, Total Omega-3 FA: .085 g, Total Omega-6 FA: 0 g, Calcium: 26 mg, Potassium: 113.4 mg, Sodium: 2.318 mg, Vitamin K: 3.02 mcg

CAJUN MEAT RUB

VEGAN – 0 CARB CHOICES

Makes: 12 1/3 Tablespoons ***Sodium Per Tablespoon: 1.759***

A dry rub on baby-back ribs or on any barbecued or oven-baked pork tenderloin can really add a great flavor. Use one of our barbecue sauces to top off the ribs and wow. Great eating. Note, trim all fat off ribs before barbecuing. Baby back ribs are within our reach whereas the larger country ribs have too much fat. I also like this on barbecued bass and catfish.

- **¼ cup paprika (9.384 mg)**
- **1 tablespoon black pepper (2.816 mg)**
- **1 tablespoon unsalted chili powder[1] (3.038 mg)**
- **1 tablespoon garlic powder (2.184 mg)**
- **1 tablespoon onion powder (3.726 mg)**
- **1 teaspoon cayenne (red pepper flakes) (.54 mg)**
- **¼ cup granular Splenda[2] (trace)**

Combine all ingredients in an air-tight container and shake well. Store in cool dry place. Best for barbecued baby-back ribs or mixed in with ground beef for burgers.

[1] Wayzata Bay is unsalted and available from healthyheartmarket.com
[2] Or brown sugar

Calories: 15.2, Protein: .627 g, Carbohydrate: 3.293 g, Dietary Fiber: 1.155 g, Total Sugars: 1.15 g, Total Fat: .355 g, Saturated Fat: .06 g, Monounsaturated Fat: .038 g, Polyunsaturated Fat: .216 g, Cholesterol: 0 mg, Trans Fatty Acids: 0 g, Total Omega-3 FA: .023 g, Total Omega-6 FA: 0 g, Calcium: 9.406 mg, Potassium: 83.6 mg, Sodium: 1.759 mg, Vitamin K: 3.171 mcg

STORING SPICES & RUBS

There's really no mystery concerning the storage of spices. Just remember to store in a dark and cool place in air-tight containers. Loose fitting lids can allow those "pantry" bugs to get into herbs and spices. The following table lists the generally accepted time table for storing spices, mixes and rubs.

Rubs, Seasonings, Mixes – Up to 2 years
Whole Spices – Up to 3 years
Grouind Spices – Up to 3 years
Dried Herbs – Up to 3 years
Extracts – Up to 4 years
Substitutes (includes potassium chloride or preservatives) Up to 4 years

SAUCES

A good sauce can add flavor to many dishes, often exciting our palates in a favorable way. Many sauces can also contribute added nutrients to a meal, but careful, some can add calories.

HOT DIPPING SAUCE

FLEXITARIAN – 0 CARB CHOICES

Makes About 24 Tablespoons (1½ cups)

Sodium Per Recipe: 117.3 mg   Sodium Per Tablespoon: 4.888 mg

4 large cloves garlic, minced (2.04 mg)
⅓ cup finely chopped yellow onion (1.584 mg)
2 tablespoons extra-virgin olive oil (trace)
¼ cup brown sugar, packed[1] (21.5 mg)
2 cups of Zinfandel or non-alcoholic red wine (18.8 mg)
2 tablespoons balsamic vinegar (.30 mg)
1 cup Maureen's Chicken Broth[2] (20.8 mg)
3 tablespoons no-salt-added tomato paste (47 mg)
2 tablespoons unsalted butter (3.124 mg)
white pepper to taste (trace)
1/8 Cayenne Pepper[4] (.067 mg)(Footnotes)

In a medium saucepan over medium-high heat, sauté garlic and onion in oil for 2 to 3 minutes. Add brown sugar and cook until the sugar liquefies and caramelizes the onion and garlic. Add the remaining ingredients, except the unsalted butter and pepper. Reduce the liquid by boiling uncovered, until there are approximately 1½ cups left. Remove pan from heat and whisk in butter one tablespoon at a time until sauce is thickened. Season sparingly with pepper. If you need to heat the sauce at a later time, do so over low heat. Do not boil or sauce will separate.

[1] Or Brown Sugar Twin or Splenda® Brown Sugar substitute

[2] See Page: 231 or use Swanson, Progresson or other unsalted Chicken Broth.

Hot Dipping Sauce Nutrient Data Per Tablespoon: Calories: 50, Protein: .293 g, Carbohydrate: 3.891 g, Dietary Fiber: .171 g, Total Sugars: 2.888 g, Total Fat: 2.183 g, Saturated Fat: .79 g, Monounsaturated Fat: 1.104 g, Polyunsaturated Fat: .179 g, Cholesterol: 3.015 mg, Trans Fatty Acids: 0 g, Total Omega-3 FA: .018 g, Total Omega-6 FA: .026 g, Calcium: 6.959 mg, Potassium: 60.3 mg Sodium: 4.888 mg, Vitamin K: 1.169 mcg

BASIL PESTO

VEGAN – 0 CARB CHOICES

Makes About 1 cup (16 tablespoons)

Sodium Per Recipe: 5.175 mg   Sodium Per Tablespoon: 323 mg

This pesto recipe can be used with pasta, on a sandwich or panini or served spread on barbecued chicken after it's cooked. It's easy to make and has an excellent flavor. We have left out the pine nuts or walnuts to help cut down on calories. The garlic gives it just the right snap.

1 cup basil leaves, packed (1.696 mg)
4 large cloves garlic, peeled (2.04 mg)
⅓ cup extra virgin olive oil (1.439 mg)

Wash one bunch of fresh basil leaves. Towel dry. Trim off stems.

One bunch should pack into a measuring cup after cleaning stems and chopping.

Place all ingredients in your processor and process until right consistency. If it needs more oil add one teaspoon at a time.

Chill in airtight container, may store in refrigerator for a day. Serving suggestions follow.

Pasta

Cook 8-ounces of spaghetti, fettuccini, or linguini noodles. When done, drain and mix pesto into pasta, tossing until well combined. Serve hot. May add grated low-sodium Swiss cheese.

Sandwich

We use pesto on burger or chicken sandwiches. For a turkey burger without spices or salt, use the pesto as a spread on one side, on the other add a thin slice of tomato and a ¼ of avocado spread over the bun. Add lettuce if desired.

Panini

You can get at least 8 panini sandwiches with this recipe.

Using cooked and thinly sliced chicken breast, spread pesto over your bun and place meat on pesto. (Place 1-ounce of sliced low-sodium cheddar, mozzarella, or Swiss on the meat.) Put buns together and grill in panini machine for three to five minutes.

Basil Pesto Nutrient Data Per Serving Pesto: Calories: 41.5, Protein: .131 g, Carbohydrate: .318 g, Dietary Fiber: .058 g, Total Sugars: .015 g, Total Fat: 4.516 g, Saturated Fat: .622 g, Monounsaturated Fat: 3.282 g, Polyunsaturated Fat: .485 g, Cholesterol: 0 mg, Trans Fatty Acids: 0 g, Total Omega-3 FA: .043 g, Total Omega-6 FA: 0 g, Calcium: 6.093 mg, Potassium: 10.9 mg, Sodium: .323 mg, Vitamin K: 13.7 mcg

HOT AND SWEET BBQ SAUCE

VEGAN – ½ CARB CHOICES

Makes: Approximately 3½ cups or 56 tablespoons

Sodium Per Recipe: 213.8 mg Sodium Per Tablespoon: 3.818 mg

- **1 tablespoon extra virgin olive oil (.27 mg)**
- **1 medium onion, diced fine (4.4 mg)**
- **2 garlic cloves, minced (1.02 mg)**
- **2 tablespoons lemon peel, grated (.72 mg)**
- **1 cup packed brown sugar (61.6 mg)**
- **½ teaspoon no-salt chili powder (trace)**
- **½ teaspoon cayenne pepper (.27 mg)**
- **¼ teaspoon onion powder (.324 mg)**
- **¼ teaspoon freshly ground black pepper (.231 mg)**
- **¼ cup no-salt added tomato paste[1] (64.2 mg)**
- **2 8-ounce cans no-salt-added tomato sauce (53.7 mg)**
- **½ cup apple cider vinegar (5.975 mg)**
- **2 tablespoons Homemade Worcestershire sauce[2] (8 mg)**

In a medium sauce pan over medium heat, heat oil. Sauté onions, garlic and lemon peel until onions become translucent, but not brown. Add sugar and cook for three to four more minutes, stirring often. Add remaining ingredients, bring to boil and then reduce heat to simmer and cook uncovered or partially covered to prevent spattering, for 30 minutes. Mixture will be thick.

[1] Various brands produce plain canned tomato paste without salt. Our favorite is Contadina. Check ingredients.

[2] See page 259. Exchange with 2 tablespoons rice vinegar if you prefer.

Hot and Sweet BBQ Sauce Nutrient Data Per Tablespoon: Calories: 23.7, Protein: .207 g, Carbohydrate: 5.215 g, Dietary Fiber: .252 g, Total Sugars: 4.432 g, Total Fat: .274 g, Saturated Fat: .039 g, Monounsaturated Fat: .181 g, Polyunsaturated Fat: .038 g, Cholesterol: 0 mg, Trans Fatty Acids: 0 g, Total Omega-3 FA: .003 g, Total Omega-6 FA: 0 g, Calcium: 6.155 mg, Potassium: 55.6 mg, Sodium: 3.818 mg, Vitamin K: .001 mcg, Vitamin K: .646 mcg

HOT MUSTARD SAUCE

VEGAN – 0 CARB CHOICES

Makes Approximately 9 tablespoons *Sodium Per Tablespoon: 2.861 mg*

- **4 ounces[1] Mendocino, Grey Poupon, Hain Stone Ground Mustard or other very low sodium honey mustard[2] (10 mg)**
- **½ tablespoon low sodium molasses (7.5 mg)**
- **2 teaspoons minced shallot (.8 mg)**
- **¼ teaspoon Tabasco Pepper Sauce (7.438 mg)**

Combine and stir ingredients together. Use with fish when barbecuing or grilling. Works exceptionally well with catfish, orange roughy and cod. May store in sealed container in refrigerator for about two weeks. You may double this recipe.

[1] Approximately 6⅓ level tablespoons

[2] FDA labels may read "0 mg," but the listed serving size may also be very low.

Hot Mustard Sauce Nutrient Data Per Tablespoon: Calories: 5.437, Protein: .131 g, Carbohydrate: 1.07 g, Dietary Fiber: .001 g, Total Sugars: .778 g, Total Fat: .113 g, Saturated Fat: 0 g, Monounsaturated Fat: 0 g, Polyunsaturated Fat: .001 g, Cholesterol: 0 mg, Trans Fatty Acids: 0 g, Total Omega-3 FA: 0 g, Total Omega-6 FA: 0 g, Calcium: .289 mg, Potassium: 2.639 mg, Sodium: 2.86 mg, Vitamin K: 0 mcg

SWEET AND SOUR MUSTARD SAUCE

LACTO OVO – ½ CARB CHOICES

Makes: About 8 tablespoons ***Sodium Per Tablespoon: .575 mg***

Works well with salmon, trout, steelhead and other pink fish. Also works well when barbecuing beef steaks or roasts.

- **2 tablespoons white wine vinegar (2.384 mg)**
- **2 tablespoons Grey Poupon, East Shore, Hain or Mendocino honey mustard (20 mg)**
- **2 tablespoons sweet honey (1.68 mg)**
- **2 tablespoons extra virgin olive oil (.54 mg)**

Combine all ingredients and whisk together until well blended. Whisk again, just before serving. May replace honey with one packet Splenda.

Sweet and Sour Mustard SauceNutrient Data Per Tablespoon: Calories: 46.5, Protein: .017 g, Carbohydrate: 6.586 g, Dietary Fiber: .01 g, Total Sugars: 5.811 g, Total Fat: 3.375 g, Saturated Fat: .466 g, Monounsaturated Fat: 2.462 g, Polyunsaturated Fat: .355 g, Cholesterol: 0 mg, Trans Fatty Acids: 0 g, Total Omega-3 FA: .026 g, Total Omega-6 FA: 0 g, Calcium: .572 mg, Potassium: 4.216 mg, Sodium: .575 mg, Vitamin K: 2.032 mcg

FRESH TOMATO MARINARA

VEGAN – 0 CARB CHOICES

Makes 1 cup

Sodium Per Recipe: 52.9 mg Sodium Per Tablespoon: 3.31 mg

With Garlic & Mushrooms this version of marinara can be made with or without meat. Freeze or refrigerate some for future use.

4 large fresh tomatoes, diced (36.4 mg)
2 tablespoons extra virgin olive oil (.54 mg)
1 medium onion, sautéed (3.3 mg)
4 garlic cloves, minced (2.04 mg)
8 ounces mushrooms, sliced (7.2 mg)
¾ cup filtered water (trace)
1 teaspoon oregano (.27 mg)
1 teaspoon basil (.476 mg)
¼ teaspoon ground cloves (1.276 mg) .069 mg)
1 bay leaf, removed after cooking (.138 mg)
pepper to taste (.011 mg)
1 tablespoon fresh lemon juice (.153 mg)

Remove skins of tomatoes by lowering them into a boiling pot of water for a few minutes. Their skins will begin to crack making them easy to peel.

Heat olive oil in large fry pan. Chop onions and garlic and sauté for only a few minutes. Add mushrooms. Sauté until they begin to lose juice.

Add tomatoes, rest of ingredients except for lemon juice. Cook uncovered for an hour until sauce reduces and thickens.

Before serving, remove bay leaf and add lemon juice.

Fresh Tomato Marinara Nutrient Data Per Tablespoon: Calories: 30, Protein: .835 g, Carbohydrate: 3.226 g, Dietary Fiber: .878 g, Total Sugars: 1.674 g, Total Fat: 1.845 g, Saturated Fat: .259 g, Monounsaturated Fat: 1.249 g, Polyunsaturated Fat: .242 g, Cholesterol: 0 mg, Trans Fatty Acids: 0 g, Total Omega-3 FA: .022 g, Total Omega-6 FA: 0 g, Calcium: 12 mg, Potassium: 156.2 mg, Sodium: 3.306 mg, Vitamin K: 6.899 mcg

WILD BLACKBERRY SAUCE

VEGAN – 0 CARB CHOICES

Makes 2-cups Sodium Per Tablespoon: .095 mg

2 cups of fresh, washed crushed domestic berries or 2 cups of wild blackberry juice[1] (2.88 mg)
½ cup granulated sugar[2] (trace)
1 teaspoon fresh lemon juice (.153 mg)
½ cup filtered water (trace)

Over medium heat, bring water to the boiling point. Add sugar and stir until it's dissolved. Add berries and stir for a minute, then simmer uncovered for an hour stirring occasionally.

Remove from heat and let cool for ten minutes. Pour into storage container or bowl, cover and chill for serving later. (We use empty syrup bottles and store in the refrigerator.) Heat before serving or serve cold.

[1] If using Splenda instead, add only 1/3 cup after cooking. Stir in until dissolved and then pour into jars or containers for storage or use.

[2] Crushed domestic berries will take approx 2½ to 3 cups of fresh berries. Wild Black berries will take about 6 cups of fresh berries to make 2 cups of juice. Wild loganberries, gooseberries, etc. will vary as well.

Wild Blackberry Sauce Nutrient Data Per Tablespoon (Sugar): Calories: 16.1, Protein: .127 g, Carbohydrate: 4.03 g, Dietary Fiber: .479 g, Total Sugars: 3.573 g, Total Fat: .044 g, Saturated Fat: .001 g, Monounsaturated Fat: .004 g, Polyunsaturated Fat: .025 g, Cholesterol: 0 mg, Trans Fatty Acids: 0 g, Total Omega-3 FA: .008 g, Total Omega-6 FA: 0 g, Calcium: 2.675 mg, Potassium: 15.2 mg, Sodium: .095 mg, Vitamin K: 1.782 mcg

Nutrient Data Per Tablespoon (Splenda): Calories: 7.299, Protein: .127 g, Carbohydrate: 1.806 g, Dietary Fiber: .479 g, Total Sugars: 1.254 g, Total Fat: .044 g, Saturated Fat: .001 g, Monounsaturated Fat: .004 g, Polyunsaturated Fat: .025 g, Cholesterol: 0 mg, Trans Fatty Acids: 0 g, Total Omega-3 FA: .008 g, Total Omega-6 FA: 0 g, Calcium: 2.643 mg, Potassium: 15.2 mg, Sodium: .095 mg, Vitamin K: 1.782 mcg

SPECIAL DRESSING

VEGAN – 0 CARB CHOICES

Makes 1 cup (18 tablespoons)

Sodium Per Recipe: 40.5 mg   Sodium Per Tablespoon: 2.252 mg

Use with lettuce wrap sandwiches, salads and even as a barbecue sauce for burger meat or pork.

½ cup white balsamic vinegar (29.3 mg)
½ cup extra virgin olive oil (2.16 mg)
2 tablespoons brown sugar (7.728 mg)
2 cloves garlic, minced (1.02 mg)
2 tablespoon fresh lemon juice (.305 mg)

Place into tight container and shake well. Use on sandwiches, salads and even as a barbecue sauce for burgers.

Nutrient Data Per Tablespoon:Calories: 66, Protein: .064 g, Carbohydrate: 2.967 g, Dietary Fiber: .014 g, Total Sugars: 2.591 g, Total Fat: 6.002 g, Saturated Fat: .829 g, Monounsaturated Fat: 4.378 g, Polyunsaturated Fat: .632 g, Cholesterol: 0 mg, Trans Fatty Acids: 0 g, Total Omega-3 FA: .046 g, Total Omega-6 FA: 0 g, Calcium: 3.967 mg, Potassium: 13.5 mg, Sodium: 2.252 mg, Vitamin K: 3.618 mcg

CHEESE SAUCE

LACTO OVO – 0 CARB CHOICES

Makes 1¼ Cups Sodium Per Tablespoon: 6.38 mg

Great over fresh steamed broccoli and an essential when making Mac 'n Cheese

- **1 teaspoon extra virgin olive oil (trace)**
- **2 tablespoons finely chopped onion (.8 mg)**
- **1 tablespoon of all-purpose flour (.156 mg)**
- **1 cup nonfat milk with vitamin A (102.9 mg)**
- **3 ounces (1-cup grated) low-sodium cheddar (23.7 mg)**
- **⅛ teaspoon white pepper (.015 mg)**

Heat olive oil in small pan over medium heat. Sauté onion until translucent. Remove onion from pan. Remove pan from heat and pour in milk. Whisk flour with milk until smooth. Return to heat and bring to boil stirring continually while mixture thickens.

Add grated cheese and stir until melted. Add cooked onion and white pepper. Stir until thoroughly blended.

Serve hot over fresh vegetables, baked potato, and pasta.

Cheese Sauce Nutrient Data Per Tablespoon: Calories: 28.5, Protein: 1.842 g, Carbohydrate: 1.117 g, Dietary Fiber: .031 g, Total Sugars: .695 g, Total Fat: 1.858 g, Saturated Fat: 1.181 g, Monounsaturated Fat: .522 g, Polyunsaturated Fat: .057 g, Cholesterol: 5.895 mg, Trans Fatty Acids: 0 g, Total Omega-3 FA: .021 g, Total Omega-6 FA: 0 g, Calcium: 55.4 mg, Potassium: 27.3 mg, Sodium: 6.38 mg, Vitamin K: .158 mcg

SOY SAUCE REPLACMENT[1]

VEGAN – 0 CARB CHOICES

Makes 1 Cup Sodium Per Recipe: 28.4 mg Sodium Per Tablespoon: 1.775 mg

- **¾ cup rice vinegar[2] (1.8 mg)**
- **1 clove garlic, crushed in garlic press (.51 mg)**
- **3 tablespoons Grandma's molasses (22.2 mg)**
- **3 teaspoons onion powder (3.888 mg)**

Combine all ingredients in a small jar. Tighten lid and shake well. Store in refrigerator. Use as needed.

[1] Borrowed from *The No Salt, Lowest Sodium International Cookbook*

[2] Not seasoned

Soy Sauce Replacement Nutrient Data Per Tablespoon: Calories: 14.3, Protein: .057 g, Carbohydrate: 3.891 g, Dietary Fiber: .03 g, Total Sugars: 2.906 g, Total Fat: .009 g, Saturated Fat: .002 g, Monounsaturated Fat: .002 g, Polyunsaturated Fat: .004 g, Cholesterol: 0 mg, Trans Fatty Acids: 0 g, Total Omega-3 FA: 0 g, Total Omega-6 FA: 0 g, Potassium: 71.1 mg, Sodium: 1.775 mg, Vitamin K: .021 mcg, Folic Acid: 0 mcg

EGGLESS MAYONNAISE

LACTO OVO – 0 CARB CHOICES

Serves 2 Sodium Per Recipe: 23.8 mg Sodium Per Serving: 11.9 mg

Commercial mayonnaise is high in sodium at 104.5 mg sodium and nearly 5 grams of total fats per serving. So, we came up with another use for our Yo-Cheese recipe. This works well, especially with sandwiches and potato salad.

2 tablespoons homemade Yo-Cheese (23.3 mg)
¼ teaspoon dill weed (.53 mg)
½ packet Splenda or 1/8 teaspoon sugar (trace)

Mix together and use or store in sealed container in refrigerator for up to 4 days. May double, triple, etc. Great for salad dressings, sandwiches and sauces. Use less Splenda or sugar if you want it a bit more tart.

Nutrient Data For Eggless Mayonnaise per Tablespoon Using Sugar: Calories: 13.6, Protein: 1.219 g, Carbohydrate: 2.112 g, Dietary Fiber: .017 g, Total Sugars: .402 g, Total Fat: .036 g, Saturated Fat: .015 g, Monounsaturated Fat: .009 g, Polyunsaturated Fat: .001 g, Cholesterol: .459 mg, Trans Fatty Acids: 0 g, Total Omega-3 FA: 0 g, Total Omega-6 FA: 0 g, Calcium: 32.7 mg, Potassium: 43.2 mg, Sodium: 11.9 mg, Vitamin K: 0 mcg

FRESH SALSA

VEGAN – 0 CARB CHOICES

Makes: 2 cups Sodium Per Tablespoon: 1.058 mg

2 small cloves garlic, minced (1.02 mg)
6 tablespoons finely chopped onion (2.4 mg)
3 large ripe tomatoes, seeds removed, chopped (27.3 mg)
2 -3 tablespoons minced cilantro (trace)
½ medium green or red bell pepper (2.38 mg)
2 tablespoons lime juice (.616 mg)
For Hot Salsa add: 1 or 2 Jalapeno chile peppers, seeded and finely chopped[1] (.14 mg)

Peel garlic and onion, wash tomatoes and bell pepper, chop and toss together with lime juice in a medium bowl. Refrigerate in bowl tightly sealed with stretch plastic for a few hours before serving.

[1]Handle with care when cleaning and chopping. Chili oils can get on your skin and burn for a long time. Nutrient Data is based on one pepper. Replaces Bell pepper. May use red pepper flakes instead.

Nutrient Data Per Tablespoon: Calories: 5.424, Protein: .23 g, Carbohydrate: 1.181 g, Dietary Fiber: .296 g, Total Sugars: .64 g, Total Fat: .046 g, Saturated Fat: .007 g, Monounsaturated Fat: .006 g, Polyunsaturated Fat: .018 g, Cholesterol: 0 mg, Trans Fatty Acids: 0 g, Total Omega-3 FA: .001 g, Total Omega-6 FA: 0 g, Calcium: 2.786 mg, Potassium: 49.9 mg, Sodium: 1.058 mg, Vitamin K: 1.498 mcg

DON'S WORCESTERSHIRE SAUCE

FLEXITARIAN – 1 CARB CHOICES

Makes about 2 cups

Sodium Per Recipe: 224.5 mg Sodium Per tablespoon: 7.074 mg

Works well with beef, especially barbecued and broiled beef.

2 tablespoons extra virgin olive oil (trace)
2 large sweet onions, roughly chopped (9 mg)
¼ cup filtered water (trace)
1 tablespoon Grandma's Chili powder (trace)
¼ teaspoon mint sauce or 2-fresh mint leaves[2] (trace)
2 tablespoons minced garlic (2.89 mg)
2 tablespoons minced ginger (1.56 mg)
1 jalapeno, seeds removed and minced (.14 mg)
¼ cup tomato paste (64.2 mg)
¼ teaspoon ground cloves (5.103 mg)
2 tablespoons freshly ground or cracked black pepper (5.632 mg)
½ cup honey (6.78 mg)
2¼ cups filtered water (trace)
1 cup Grandma's Molasses (112 mg)
3 cups white wine vinegar (7.2 mg)
1 cup fresh orange juice, not from concentrate (trace)
2 lemons or limes, thinly sliced (6.48 mg)

In a large saucepan, heat the olive oil and sauté the onion until translucent. Add the ¼-cup water, chili powder, mint sauce (or leaves), garlic, ginger, jalapeno, and 1/4 cup of water and stir for about 3 to 5 minutes over low-medium heat. Add the rest of the ingredients and stir to a boil over medium to medium high heat. Reduce and simmer, stirring occasionally for about 2 hours or until thickened.

Strain sauce into a glass bottle and refrigerate. Throw out debris. Bring to room temperature and gently shake before using.

[1] Most of the carbohydrates are in the molasses (256 g) and the honey (139.7 g)

[2] Instead of mint leaves you can use lemon or lime juice mixed with a touch of brown sugar. Use 2-tablespoons of lemon juice with a 1/8 teaspoon of brown sugar.

Worcestershire Sauce Nutrient Data Per tablespoon: Calories: 66.8, Protein: .414 g, Carbohydrate: 17.2 g, Dietary Fiber: .731 g, Total Sugars: 12.1 g, Total Fat: .951 g, Saturated Fat: .134 g, Monounsaturated Fat: .625 g, Polyunsaturated Fat: .117 g, Cholesterol: 0 mg, Trans Fatty Acids: 0 g, Total Omega-3 FA: .012 g, Total Omega-6 FA: 0 g, Calcium: 33.5 mg, Potassium: 226.3 mg, Sodium: 7.017 mg,
Vitamin K: 1.578 mcg

MUSHROOM SAUCE

LACTO OVO – ½ CARB CHOICES

Serves 4 Sodium Per Recipe: 123.7 Sodium Per Serving: 30.9 mg

We love mushrooms as accents for soups, stews, salads and marinara sauces. I also like to put lightly sauteed mushrooms in hamburgers. This sauce works especially well with pasta or rice, and it works well if you like add meat like chicken, pork or beef. This recipe also works well with wild game from duck to venison. You'll really enjoy it.

2 tablespoons extra virgin olive oil (trace)
1 cup chopped onion (6.4 mg)
1 pound mushrooms, use any variety, sliced (21 mg)
½ cup dry white wine[1] (trace)
½ cup sour cream (92 mg)
2 tablespoons chopped fresh parsley (4.256 mg)
white pepper to taste (trace)

Heat 1-tablespoon olive oil in 12" or larger fry pan.

Sauté onion until translucent. Push to one side and add the other tablespoon of olive oil to open area. Add mushrooms and sauté, turning regularly until musroom are softened and releas their juices.

Add wine and pepper and simmer for 8 to 10 minutes.

Stir in sour cream and parsley and heat.

Serve over fettucini or linguini noodles or rice.

To make a complete entree serve with cooked broccoli. I you enjoy meat, add one cup of chopped cooked chicken at same time you add sour cream.

[1] Or white non alcoholic wine

Mushroom Sauce Nutrient Data Per Serving: Calories: 181.3, Protein: 4.373 g, Carbohydrate: 8.836 g, Dietary Fiber: 1.834 g, Total Sugars: 4.451 g, Total Fat: 13.1 g, Saturated Fat: 4.379 g, Monounsaturated Fat: 4.831 g, Polyunsaturated Fat: 2.71 g, Cholesterol: 14.9 mg, Trans Fatty Acids: 0 g, Total Omega-3 FA: .085 g, Total Omega-6 FA: .005 g, Calcium: 47 mg, Potassium: 443.5 mg, Sodium: 30.9 mg, Vitamin K: 33.3 mcg

COOKIES & CRACKERS

Here are some tips for making excellent cookies (especially chocolate chip) from your own recipe. Our recipes have already taken the below into consideration.

Never use margarine, lard or hydrogenated shortening. Use either real unsalted butter, real unsalted peanut butter, some of the newer non trans fatty acids shortenings. Some cookie recipes can also use oil. For some, using applesauce works well, too. We use applesauce in our oatmeal cookies.

Double the amount of pure vanilla extract called for. Don't use imitation vanilla or vanillin. Vanilla extract works well and it's healthier, however, we also like to use Cook's powdered vanilla. It has a flavorful punch to it.

Always melt cold butter slowly. You can use your microwave defrost button for a minute or less. Just watch it like a hawk. Don't over-soften or melt it; don't burn it. (You can also dissolve your hard block of brown sugar much the same way in the microwave. Stir immediately after taking out.) Again, not too long or you might find molasses where the sugar used to be.

For chocolate chip recipes add 1 or 2 tablespoons of milk. This will make the cookies less "crunchy" and softer than many local bakery chocolate chip cookies. (Or add two tablespoons of sour cream for the same results.) If you prefer them less soft, try adding a little extra flour to the basic recipe instead.

When converting your favorite "family" chocolate chip recipe, why not leave out one or two tablespoons of the sugar called for? They'll still be sweet but lower in calories and carbohydrates. Always use semi-sweet chocolate chips and remember that butterscotch chips are higher in sodium.

Chill your batter before baking. When baking, put batter back into refrigerator while first batches cook. Use only cold dough on a room temperature cookie sheet. Always bring your cookie sheet to room temperature or use more than one to bake a single recipe. Don't put cold dough on a hot sheet you've just baked on. This will cause the outer edges of the cookie to slightly melt before baking and that part will then burn.

To cool a baking/cookie sheet (jelly roll pan) you can run the bottom of the sheet under cold tap water for a few moments and then wipe dry.

We recommend using parchment paper on the jelly roll pan or cookie sheet. If not using parchment paper, then lightly oil the surface. A product known as Silpat is also available to cover the cooking sheet. Silpat, the original silicon coated baking sheet is a nonstick and it fits perfectly into a jelly roll pan. These are reusable and you don't have to grease them.

Mix the dough thoroughly but don't over-mix it.

Good cookies will not look done in the oven or when you take them out. Let them cool on the sheet for one or two minutes, then move to a rack. After they cool, they'll be perfect.

Featherweight Baking Powder should be mixed into your batter last and placed into hot oven immediately with most baked products. **However,** if you use **Ener-g Baking Powder** (and baking soda) then you can either mix it in at the end or when sifting dry ingredients. Ener-g has been able to produce a double-acting baking powder that is as efficient as the potassium based Featherweight. I have had success mixing an entire batch with the Ener-g baking powder and putting it on hold in the refrigerator between baking times or even overnight.

When baking cookies with Featherwieght or Ener-G, you'll have to press down on the cookie to make the shape you want. Another method with some cookie recipes is to roll the batter into a ball and set that on the cooking surface Then press down with the back of a spoon. Cookies that work best this way are indicated in our recipes.

BUTTERSCOTCH & CHOCOLATE CHIP COOKIE

LACTO-OVO VEGETARIAN – 1½ CARB CHOICES

Makes 32 2" cookies

Sodium Per Recipe: 233.2 mg Sodium Per Cookie: 7.288

A nicely flavored cookie using a minimal number of butterscotch chips, which are higher in sodium than semi-sweet chocolate chips. Freezes well.

Beat Together

½ cup white granulated sugar (trace)
½ cup (packed) brown sugar (30.8 mg)
½ cup (1 stick) softened unsalted butter (12.4 mg)
2 large eggs (140 mg)
1½ teaspoons vanilla extract (.567 mg)

Add In

1 cup white, unbleached all-purpose flour (2.5 mg)
1 teaspoon cinnamon (.26 mg)
1 pinch ground cloves (.255 mg)
½ cup Nestle Butterscotch morsels (75.7 mg)
½ cup semi-sweet chocolate chips (9.24 mg)
1 cup (1 package) black seedless raisins (18.1 mg)
2¾ cups quick oatmeal (13.4 mg)
1 tablespoon (level) Ener-G Baking Soda (2.88 mg)

Preheat oven to 350° F.

Prepare two baking sheets with parchment paper. (Jelly roll pan size.)

Using a hand or countertop beater combine the first five ingredients in a medium or large size mixing bowl until smooth.

Using a spoon, add the rest of the ingredients holding off on the baking soda until just before forming cookies and baking them.

Make balls and place on cooking sheet. Press down in the center of the ball with a spoon to form the cookie.

Bake on lower third rack for 10 to 12 minutes or until they just begin to turn color.

Cool on rack.

Butterscotch Chocolate Chip Cookies Nutrient Values per Cookie: Calories: 136.4, Protein: 1.88 g, Carbohydrate: 21.8 g, Dietary Fiber: 1.198 g, Total Sugars: 12.8 g, Total Fat: 5.096 g, Saturated Fat: 3.055 g, Monounsaturated Fat: 1.268 g, Polyunsaturated Fat: .36 g, Cholesterol: 14.2 mg, Trans Fatty Acids: 0 g, Total Omega-3 FA: .034 g, Total Omega-6 FA: .077 g, Calcium: 24.3 mg, Potassium: 87.5 mg, Sodium: 7.288 mg, Vitamin K: .933 mcg

WALNUT BISCOTTI

LACTO-OVO VEGETARIAN – 1 CARB CHOICES

Makes 24 Sodium Per Recipe: 187 mg Sodium Per Biscotti: 10.3 mg

This recipe makes a thin biscotti cookie. Serve with scoop of ice cream or our Yo Cheese Raspberry Swirl.

- **½ cup granulated sugar (trace)**
- **1 tablespoon softened unsalted butter[1] (1.562 mg)**
- **1¼ cups unbleached all-purpose flour (3.125 mg)**
- **⅓ cup seedless golden raisins (6.593 mg)**
- **¾ cup unsalted walnuts (1.755 mg)**
- **2 teaspoons Ener-G baking powder (trace)**
- **2 medium or 1-large egg and 1-large egg white (123.2 mg)**
- **1 tablespoon filtered water[2] (trace)**
- **¾ teaspoon almond extract (.283 mg)**
- **1 large egg white for basting (54.8 mg)**

Preheat oven to 350° F.

Line jelly roll pan or baking sheet with parchment paper. In a medium size bowl knead butter and sugar together. Stir in flour, baking powder, golden raisins, and walnuts.

In a smaller bowl mix together the 2-eggs with water and almond extract.

Using a large spoon, slowly add the wet mix to the dry mix. If mixing becomes too dry, wet hands with water and knead with your hands.

Roll dough out onto parchment paper on baking sheet. Wet hands again and roll into a log about 12" long x 4" wide and a half inch thick.

Place egg white into small bowl, whisk with a dash of water. Baste this on log. Bake 25 to 30 minutes (browning should just begin). When done, leave oven on and move baking sheet to countertop.

Slide parchment paper to cutting board with cookie on it. Cool 5-minutes. Using a serrated knife in a sawing motion, slice about ¼ to ⅓ inch thick. (A ½-inch cut will produce about 16 cookies.) Lay on baking sheet sliced side down and bake about ten minutes. Turn each piece over and bake another 5 to ten minutes or until dry. Cool on rack. Store in airtight container.

[1] Or non-trans fatty acid shortening

[2] May use orange or fresh lemon juice for an extra kick to the flavor. I use fresh lemon juice.

Almond Biscotti Nutrient Data Per Cookie: Calories: 81.8, Protein: 2.073 g, Carbohydrate: 11.5 g, Dietary Fiber: .512 g, Total Sugars: 5.696 g, Total Fat: 3.308 g, Saturated Fat: .655 g, Monounsaturated Fat: .597 g, Polyunsaturated Fat: 1.823 g, Cholesterol: 16.8 mg, Trans Fatty Acids: 0 g, Total Omega-3 FA: .341 g, Total Omega-6 FA: .013 g, Calcium: 8.107 mg, Potassium: 50 mg, Sodium: 10.3 mg, Vitamin K: .251 mcg

PISTACHIO BISCOTTI

LACTO-OVO VEGETARIAN – ½ CARB CHOICES

Makes 24

Sodium Per Recipe: 138.8 mg Sodium Per Biscotti: 5.783 mg

This recipe was contributed by Cheryl Colbert, who manages a pistachio orchard in Paso Robles, California. The uniqueness of course is that the cookie is using unsalted pistachio nuts instead of the normally used almonds. We think you'll like this one. You can add cranberries, or golden raisins.

Dry Mix

1¼ cups unbleached all-purpose flour (3.125 mg)
⅓ cup granulated sugar or Splenda (trace)
1 tablespoon grated orange peel (.18 mg)
⅓ cup dried cranberries[1] (1.8 mg)
¾ cup fresh unsalted pistachios (9.225 mg)
2 teaspoons Ener-G baking powder (trace)

Wet Mix

1 large egg (63 mg)
1 large egg white (54.8 mg)
1 tablespoon orange juice (trace)
¾ teaspoon vanilla (.378 mg)

Preheat oven to 350° F.

Line jelly roll pan or baking sheet with parchment paper.

Put dry mix in a large mixing bowl. In a smaller bowl mix together the egg, egg white, orange juice, and vanilla.

Using a large spoon, slowly add the wet mix to the dry mix. If mixing becomes too hard, wet hands with water and mix with your hands.

Roll dough out onto parchment paper on baking sheet. Wet hands again and pat out to a 7-inch by 11-inch rectangle, about 1/2" thick. Bake about 25 minutes or until golden brown. Cool 10-minutes, peel off parchment paper carefully.

Using a serrated knife in a sawing motion, slice about ¼ to 1/3 inch thick. Lay on baking sheet sliced side down and bake 10 minutes. Turn each piece over and bake another 5 minutes.

[1] or golden raisins, currants or chopped dates.

Pistachio Biscotti Nutrient Data Per Cookie: Calories: 57.1, Protein: 1.91 g, Carbohydrate: 8.034 g, Dietary Fiber: .693 g, Total Sugars: 1.968 g, Total Fat: 2.064 g, Saturated Fat: .29 g, Monounsaturated Fat: 1.019 g, Polyunsaturated Fat: .601 g, Cholesterol: 8.812 mg, Trans Fatty Acids: 0 g, Total Omega-3 FA: .014 g, Total Omega-6 FA: 0 g, Calcium: 6.994 mg, Potassium: 53.5 mg, Sodium: 5.783 mg, Vitamin K: .596 mcg

DON'S FRUIT BARS

LACTO-OVO VEGETARIAN – 1 CARB CHOICES[2]

Makes 54 1 ½" by 1 ½" Bars or Makes 24 2" x 3" Bars

Sodium Per Recipe: 408.4 mg

Sodium Per Fruit Bar (54): 7.563 mg Sodium Per Fruit Bar (24): 17 mg

This could become a popular bar or cookie for you and your friends.

Batter

2 cups sifted all-purpose flour (5 mg)
1 teaspoon Ener-G baking soda (trace)
2 teaspoons Ener-G Baking Powder (trace)
¾ teaspoon mace (1.02 mg)
½ teaspoon cinnamon (.13 mg)
1 stick unsalted butter[1] (12.4 mg)
1 cup white granulated sugar or Splenda (trace)
1 cup dark Brown sugar firmly packed[2] (61.6 mg)
4 large eggs (280 mg)
1 tablespoon nonfat milk with vitamin A (6.483 mg)
1 tablespoon Grandma's Robust Molasses (15 mg)

Add Fruit & Nuts

½ cup unsalted walnuts, lightly chopped (1.17 mg)
¾ cup dried apricots, chopped (9.75 mg)
½ cup seedless black raisins, packed (9.075 mg)

Let butter stand in room temperature for a few hours. Preheat oven to 350° F. Prepare jelly roll pan with parchment (cooking) paper or grease the pan and dust it with flour. We prefer the parchment paper, which we find can be used two or three times.

Chop fruit, mix together and set aside in a small bowl.

Sift flour, Ener-G baking soda and Ener-G baking powder and mace and cinnamon together and set aside.

In a medium size mixing bowl beat together the softened butter with the white and brown sugar. Add eggs as needed for beating until you add all four eggs. Add molasses. Add flour mix and beat until smooth.

When done, pour all fruits and nuts into batter, stir with a large spoon.

Spread immediately onto the jelly roll pan. If using cooking paper you'll have to hold the paper down while you spread and flatten the batter with a large spatula. There will be enough batter here to cover the entire pan.

Put into oven immediately and bake for 25 to 30 minutes.

Remove from oven when done. Slice into 54 1½ inch by 1½ inch squares or into 24 2" x 3" pieces. If using paper, slide onto cooling rack. If baking on the metal pan then lift off pan with large pancake turner and place on cooling racks.

When cookies cool, store in zipper lock bags. These will freeze for a few months. Good for snacks, picnics or traveling.

[1] Or 8-level tablespoons non-trans-fat Crisco or other non trans fat shortening (We have found other brands in stores like Whole Foods Market, Trader Joe's, etc.) Add 1/8 teaspoon of ground cinnamon to recipe if using non-trans-fat shortening. Note biggest change is with saturated fats and the Omega-3 and Omega-6. Cholesterol also drops as does Vitamin K.

[2] Diabetics, you can use 1/2 cup Splenda Brown Sugar Blend to help lower carbohydrates instead of a cup of dark brown sugar. For more information see: http://www.splenda.com/products/brown-sugar-blend. Also found in the glossary. The first and third nutrient tables below reflect the 1 Carb Choices rating below the title.

Don's Fruit Bars Nutrient Data Per Bar (54) Carb Choices 1: Calories: 84.5, Protein: 1.252 g, Carbohydrate: 14.1 g, Dietary Fiber: .407 g, Total Sugars: 9.867 g, Total Fat: 2.842 g, Saturated Fat: 1.267 g, Monounsaturated Fat: .687 g, Polyunsaturated Fat: .647 g, Cholesterol: 20.2 mg, Trans Fatty Acids: 0 g, Total Omega-3 FA: .115 g, Total Omega-6 FA: .045 g, Calcium: 16.1 mg, Potassium: 67.8 mg, Sodium: 7.563 mg, Vitamin K: .318 mcg

Don's Fruit Bars Nutrient Data Per Bar (24) Carb Choices 2: Calories: 190.1, Protein: 2.818 g, Carbohydrate: 31.8 g, Dietary Fiber: .915 g, Total Sugars: 22.2 g, Total Fat: 6.395 g, Saturated Fat: 2.851 g, Monounsaturated Fat: 1.545 g, Polyunsaturated Fat: 1.457 g, Cholesterol: 45.4 mg, Trans Fatty Acids: 0 g, Total Omega-3 FA: .26 g, Total Omega-6 FA: .102 g, Calcium: 36.2 mg, Potassium: 152.5 mg, Sodium: 17 mg, Vitamin K: .715 mcg

Using Splenda also Helps lower calories.

Don's Fruit Bars Nutrient Data Per Bar (24) Splenda Version: Carb Choices 1: Calories: 145.4, Protein: 2.812 g, Carbohydrate: 20 g, Dietary Fiber: .915 g, Total Sugars: 10.6 g, Total Fat: 6.395 g, Saturated Fat: 2.851 g, Monounsaturated Fat: 1.545 g, Polyunsaturated Fat: 1.457 g, Cholesterol: 45.4 mg, Trans Fatty Acids: 0 g, Total Omega-3 FA: .26 g, Total Omega-6 FA: .102 g, Calcium: 36.2 mg, Potassium: 146.3 mg, Sodium: 15.7 mg, Vitamin K: .715 mcg

TIPS FOR BAKERS

1. When measuring molasses or corn syrup with a measuring spoon, spray it first with oil. When the molasses or syrup are then added to the recipe they will easily slip off the spoon, leaving it clean.
2. Spray the top of your oven with water just before baking crackers, some cookies and for bread when you want a crisp crust.

PECAN ROCA

LACTO OVO – 1 CARB CHOICES

Makes 16 to 24 pieces Sodium Per Recipe: 79.1 mg
Sodium Per Serving (16): 4.946 Sodium Per Serving (24): 3.297

Here's a treat that I make only during the Christmas holidays. I think you'll enjoy it.

1 stick of unsalted butter (12.4 mg)
¾ cup packed brown sugar (46.2 mg)
1 cup chopped unsalted pecans (1.1 mg)
1 teaspoon vanilla extract (.378 mg)
1 cup Nestle or other semi-sweet chocolate bits or chips (19 mg)

Grease an 8 x 8 or 9 x 9 baking dish (preferably Pyrex).

Evenly spread the unsalted pecans over the bottom of the baking dish.

Set chocolate chips aside.

In a medium size pan over medium heat bring butter and sugar to a boil, stirring constantly. When at a boil, stir for another 6 minutes. Stir vanilla in at last few seconds.

Quickly pour the boiling mix evenly over the chopped pecans. Evenly spread the chocolate chips over the hot mix.

After about 20 minutes of cooling, evenly spread the chocolate chips with an oiled pancake turner or a dinner knife until flat.

Cool for about an hour. Remove and turn dish upside down onto a cutting board. If it doesn't drop out, use the pancake turner to pry it out. It will come out easily. Cut or break into edible pieces. Serve. Will store in zipper lock bags.

Pecan Roll Nutrient Values Per Piece (24): Calories: 127.5, Protein: .773 g, Carbohydrate: 11.9 g, Dietary Fiber: .846 g, Total Sugars: 6.877 g, Total Fat: 9.408 g, Saturated Fat: 4.014 g, Monounsaturated Fat: 3.583 g, Polyunsaturated Fat: 1.293 g, Cholesterol: 10.1 mg, Trans Fatty Acids: 0 g, Total Omega-3 FA: .077 g, Total Omega-6 FA: .102 g, Calcium: 12.2 mg, Potassium: 54.8 mg, Sodium: 3.297 mg, Vitamin K: .33 mcg

Pecan Roll Nutrient Data Per Piece (16): Calories: 191.3, Protein: 1.159 g, Carbohydrate: 17.9 g, Dietary Fiber: 1.269 g, Total Sugars: 10.3 g, Total Fat: 14.1 g, Saturated Fat: 6.021 g, Monounsaturated Fat: 5.375 g, Polyunsaturated Fat: 1.939 g, Cholesterol: 15.2 mg, Trans Fatty Acids: 0 g, Total Omega-3 FA: .115 g, Total Omega-6 FA: .153 g, Calcium: 18.3 mg, Potassium: 82.2 mg, Sodium: 4.946 mg, Vitamin K: .494 mcg

GRAHAM CRACKERS

FLEXITARIAN – 1 CARB CHOICES

Makes 24 to 36 Crackers Sodium Per Recipe: 163.8 mg
Sodium Per Cracker (24): 6.898 mg Sodium Per Cracker (36): 4.598 mg

These will taste like they just came out of a box from your market. Delicious and useful for cheesecakes, any cream pies and as a tasty snack.

½ cup all-purpose flour (1.25 mg)
1¾ cups whole-wheat graham flour[1] (10.5 mg)
½ cup brown sugar (trace)
¼ teaspoon ground cinnamon (.065 mg)
1 teaspoon Ener-G baking soda (trace)
2 teaspoons Ener-G Baking Powder[2] (mg)
2 tablespoons cold unsalted butter, cut into 1/2 inch cubes (3.124 mg)
5 tablespoons expeller pressed canola oil[3] (trace)
2 tablespoons honey (1.68 mg)
2 tablespoons Grandma's or B'rer Rabbit molasses (or other molasses without added salt) (14 mg)
1 tablespoon light corn syrup (13.6 mg)
5 tablespoons cold filtered water[4] (trace)
1 teaspoon vanilla extract (.378 mg)

For prep, clear a shelf in your fridge to hold the baking sheet for 45 minutes.

In a food processor, mix together the flours, brown sugar, Ener-G baking powder, Ener-G baking soda, and cinnamon. Add the cold butter and oil and process until the mixture resembles coarse meal, about 30 seconds or so. Add the honey, corns syrup, molasses, milk, and vanilla. Mix until the batter starts to come together in a ball in about 30 seconds. Scrape dough out of the mixer.

Roll the dough to about ⅛-inch thick between 2 sheets of waxed or parchment paper. Chill for at least 45 minutes to an hour, or until firm.

Preheat oven to 350° F. With a sharp knife or pizza cutter, cut into 24 3-inch squares or 36 2" squares. Arrange the crackers on parchment lined jelly roll pans or sizeable baking sheets. (You can put 12 crackers on each sheet, separated about an inch or more.) With a toothpick or larger skewer prick several holes in each cracker.

Bake for 12 to 17 minutes, or until lightly browned at the edges.

Remove from the oven and let cool on the pan for about five minutes.

Remove to cooling rack.

[1] Check online for Graham flour at bobsredmill.com or at megaheart.com/where-tobuy.html or at www.healthyheartmarket.com

[2] Featherweight will not work with this recipe.

[3] May exchange oil for five tablespoons cold butter making cold butter a total of 7-tablespoons. See nutrient data below for crackers using only the butter.

[4] Might need a tablespoon more. Don't let batter get sticky, but just wet enough to spread with a rolling pin. Can also use milk instead of water.

Graham Cracker Nutrient Data Per Graham Cracker (24) (3" squares): Calories: 102.5, Protein: 1.484 g, Calories: 102.5, Protein: 1.484 g, Carbohydrate: 16 g, Dietary Fiber: 1.156 g, Total Sugars: 6.925 g, Total Fat: 4.07 g, Saturated Fat: .855 g, Monounsaturated Fat: 2.117 g, Polyunsaturated Fat: .937 g, Cholesterol: 2.544 mg, Trans Fatty Acids: .012 g, Total Omega-3 FA: .544 g, Total Omega-6 FA: .569 g, Calcium: 16.9 mg, Potassium: 64.3 mg, Sodium: 6.898 mg, Vitamin K: 2.345 mcg

Graham Cracker Nutrient Data Per Graham Cracker (36) (2" squares): Calories: 68.3, Protein: .99 g, Carbohydrate: 10.7 g, Dietary Fiber: .771 g, Total Sugars: 4.616 g, Total Fat: 2.713 g, Saturated Fat: .57 g, Monounsaturated Fat: 1.411 g, Polyunsaturated Fat: .624 g, Cholesterol: 1.696 mg, Trans Fatty Acids: .008 g, Total Omega-3 FA: .363 g, Total Omega-6 FA: .38 g, Calcium: 11.3 mg, Potassium: 42.9 mg, Sodium: 4.598 mg, Vitamin K: 1.563 mcg

Graham Cracker Nutrient Data Per Graham Cracker (24) using butter instead of oil: Calories: 97.9, Protein: 1.509 g, Carbohydrate: 16 g, Dietary Fiber: 1.156 g, Total Sugars: 6.926 g, Total Fat: 3.552 g, Saturated Fat: 2.16 g, Monounsaturated Fat: .893 g, Polyunsaturated Fat: .206 g, Cholesterol: 8.905 mg, Trans Fatty Acids: 0 g, Total Omega-3 FA: .03 g, Total Omega-6 FA: .09 g, Calcium: 17.6 mg, Potassium: 65 mg, Sodium: 7.223 mg, Vitamin K: .472 mcg

PUMPKIN OATMEAL COOKIES

LACTO OVO– 1 CARB CHOICES

Makes 36 cookies

Sodium Per Recipe: 302.4 mg   Sodium Per Cookie: 8.399 mg

These cookies came about because I had to scramble something up quickly for arriving grandchildren. They loved them and so will you. Enjoy!

- **1 cup Libby's canned (unsalted) pumpkin (12.2 mg)**
- **½ cup (one stick of unsalted butter) (12.5 mg) or expeller pressed canola oil (trace)**
- **1 cup firmly packed brown sugar (61.6 mg)**
- **½ cup granulated sugar (trace)**
- **2 large eggs (140 mg)**
- **1 teaspoon vanilla (.378 mg)**
- **¼ teaspoon ground cloves (1.276 mg)**
- **¼ teaspoon ground ginger (.144 mg)**
- **1 teaspoon ground cinnamon (.26 mg)**
- **1½ cups white unbleached all-purpose flour (3.75 mg)**
- **1 tablespoon Ener-G Baking soda (trace)**
- **3 cups Quick Quaker oats (28.1 mg)**
- **1 cup Nestle or other chocolate chips (24 mg)**
- **1 cup not packed black seedless raisins (18.1 mg)**

Preheat oven to 350° F.

In a large bowl beat unsalted butter and sugars until creamy. Add eggs and vanilla and pumpkin, continue beating until blended. Mix in flour, Ener-G baking soda, spices and stir well with wooden or large metal spoon. Stir in the oats, chips and raisins.

Drop by tablespoonfuls onto a lightly greased cookie sheet and press down with spoon to flatten cookie slightly. Bake for 12 minutes. Cool on sheet for a minute then place on wire rack.

Pumpkin Oatmeal Cookies Nutrient Data Per cookie: Calories: 124.1, Protein: 1.804 g, Carbohydrate: 19.6 g, Dietary Fiber: 1.051 g, Total Sugars: 11.5 g, Total Fat: 4.542 g, Saturated Fat: 2.621 g, Monounsaturated Fat: 1.23 g, Polyunsaturated Fat: .385 g, Cholesterol: 18.5 mg, Trans Fatty Acids: 0 g, Total Omega-3 FA: .032 g, Total Omega-6 FA: .174 g, Calcium: 16.4 mg, Potassium: 97.5 mg, Sodium: 8.399 mg, Vitamin K: 1.596 mcg

OYSTER CRACKERS

VEGAN – 0 CARB CHOICES[1]

Makes 160 or more 1/2" Crackers

Sodium Per Recipe: 9.608 mg   Sodium Per Cracker: .06 mg

Serve with any soup or stew. Great snacks as well.

- **¾ cup filtered water (trace)**
- **1 tablespoon white wine vinegar (.745 mg)**
- **¼ cup extra virgin olive oil (.068 mg)**
- **3 cups white unbleached flour (7.5 mg)**
- **1 tablespoon plus ½ teaspoon white granulated sugar or Splenda (trace)**
- **2 tablespoons Ener-G Baking Soda (trace)**
- **¼ teaspoon ascorbic acid (trace)**
- **1 teaspoon onion powder (1.296 mg)**

Place ingredients into bread machine in order listed and set for dough. Watch kneading for about 5 minutes to make sure you don't need more water or don't have too much. This will depend on your flour. When kneading cycle ends, roll dough onto floured breadboard. You are using the machine only to knead, not to rise. Of course, if you prefer, you can knead this one with your hands.

Preheat oven to 375° F. Slice dough in half and work with first half. Roll out as thin as you can, about 1/16".

You can use two parchment-paper-covered jelly roll pans at the same time for this recipe if you like. Using a ½-inch to 1-inch cutter or homemade cutter, cut out discs and place on baking sheet.

Using a four prong fork, poke holes into each cracker. Spray a coat of water on the top of your oven and bake crackers at 375° F for about 10 to 12 minutes. When 5 minutes are up, reach in and pull sheet out and turn crackers over using a wide pancake flipper. Cook for 5 to 8 minutes more or until they begin to turn golden.

They'll bubble just like your favorite oyster crackers. Don't overcook them. You may lightly toast these to warm them before serving. May freeze and use later.

[1] Six crackers will equal 1 Carb Choices.

Oyster Crackers Nutrient Data Per Cracker: Calories: 9.094, Protein: .244 g, Carbohydrate: 1.88 g, Dietary Fiber: .064 g, Total Sugars: .091 g, Total Fat: .044 g, Saturated Fat: .007 g, Monounsaturated Fat: .017 g, Polyunsaturated Fat: .012 g, Cholesterol: 0 mg, Trans Fatty Acids: 0 g, Total Omega-3 FA: .001 g, Total Omega-6 FA: 0 g, Calcium: 4.539 mg, Potassium: 2.719 mg, Sodium: .06 mg, Vitamin K: .02 mcg

SEEDED CRACKERS

LACTO-OVO VEGETARIAN – ½ CARB CHOICES

Makes: 24

Sodium Per Recipe: 43 mg Sodium Per Cracker: 1.791 mg

This very good recipe was sent to us by Cheryl Colbert, who owns and manages a pistachio farm in Paso Robles, California, as well as a grape vineyard where she produces red wine vinegar and other products.

- **½ egg white[1] (27.4 mg)**
- **1½ cup unbleached all-purpose flour (3.75 mg)**
- **½ cup white whole wheat flour (3 mg)**
- **½ cup filtered water (trace)**
- **3 tablespoons extra virgin olive oil (trace)**
- **1½ teaspoons granulated onion powder (1.944 mg)**

Seed Mix

- **1 tablespoon + 1 teaspoon sesame seeds (5.076 mg)**
- **2 teaspoon poppy seeds (1.456 mg)**
- **1 teaspoon caraway seeds (.357 mg)**

Set oven rack to middle or bottom third. Preheat oven to 450° F.

Whisk egg white with dash of water, set aside for basting.

Mix next five ingredients together and knead until well combined. Divide into halves. Working with half the dough, roll out between two lightly floured wax or parchment paper sheets. When ready, pull away the top layer of paper.

Baste top of dough with egg white mix.

Top with a quarter of the seed mix. Replace top layer of paper and carefully place dough seed-side down on jelly roll pan. Brush other side with egg white and sprinkle with one-quarter of the seeds. Using a pizza roller, cut out two-inch crackers. You may have some dough left over. Add this to the other half. Repeat process with other half.

Hand form last of the crackers with with any left over dough.

Spray water n the top of your oven. Bake at 450° F for about 10 minutes or just as they begin to turn golden brown. Watch closely since they can quickly get too dark. Remove from pan to cool on rack.

[1] Data based on using only half the egg white.

Seeded Crackers Nutrient Data Per Oyster Cracker: Calories: 57.6, Protein: 1.391 g, Carbohydrate: 8.064 g, Dietary Fiber: .655 g, Total Sugars: .099 g, Total Fat: 2.261 g, Saturated Fat: .324 g, Monounsaturated Fat: .981 g, Polyunsaturated Fat: .815 g, Cholesterol: 0 mg, Trans Fatty Acids: 0 g, Total Omega-3 FA: .013 g, Total Omega-6 FA: 0 g, Sodium: 1.791 mg, Vitamin K: .445 mcg

BASIC CRACKER RECIPE

LACTO OVO – 1 CARB CHOICES[1]

Makes: 70 2" Crackers ***Sodium Per Cracker: 1.228 mg***

You can turn this into a cheese cracker by spreading grated low-sodium *cheddar over half the rolled out dough, then folding it over and rolling it out again*[2].

- **2 cups of all-purpose flour (5 mg)**
- **½ teaspoon onion powder (.648 mg)**
- **1 teaspoon Ener-G Baking Powder (trace)**
- **2 tablespoons unsalted butter, softened (3.124 mg)**
- **¾ cup of nonfat milk with Vitamin A (77.2 mg)**

Preheat oven to 350'F.

Lightly grease two jelly roll baking sheets (12" x 17").

Sift flour, onion powder and baking powder into a medium size mixing bowl. Cut butter in with fork or with your hands until dough is crumbly.

Slowly stir in milk until dough is soft but not sticky. If it gets sticky, just add a bit more flour while working it. Divide dough in half[3]. On a lightly floured breadboard roll dough until it's very thin.

Use a 2" cookie cutter to make round crackers. Place each cracker on pan. A jelly roll pan will hold up to 42 cookies, however we use two pans with 35 each. They may be placed closely together but not touching. Using a fork, poke each cracker a few times, making multiple holes.

Spray a light coat of water on the top of your oven. Bake until crisp, about 15 to 20 minutes. Allow to cool on the tray and then store in an air tight container for up to a week. Crackers will only turn slightly golden at edges.

You can alter this recipe easily by adding low-sodium cheese, or carraway, sesame, or poppy seeds before rolling out to bake or before freezing. Enjoy with soups, salads, tea or serve at parties topped with red chili jam or a very thin layer of low sodium cheese and chili jam. A dash of cream cheese and the chili jam for guests will really bring you kudos.

[1] 5 crackers will equal 1 Carb Choice.

[2] If you make this into a cheese cracker, go light on the cheese and bake at 300° F for about 25 minutes.

[3] You can roll this dough into a log, freeze it, then bake later after allowing it to thaw partially. At that time, slice very thin round crackers and set on jelly roll pan.

Basic Cracker Nutrient Data Per Cracker: Calories: 16.9 Protein: .463 g, Carbohydrate: 2.87 g, Dietary Fiber: .097 g, Total Sugars: .15 g, Total Fat: .366 g, Saturated Fat: .215 g, Monounsaturated Fat: .089 g, Polyunsaturated Fat: .027 g, Cholesterol: .925 mg, Trans Fatty Acids: 0 g, Total Omega-3 FA: .003 g, Total Omega-6 FA: .009 g, Calcium: 3.977 mg, Potassium: 8.175 mg, Sodium: 1.228 mg, Vitamin K: .04 mcg

DESSERTS

When it comes to desserts, many of us have to watch our waistline as well as our sodium intake. We can get the sodium way down below standard recipes but cutting the calories is often difficult, yet necessary. In many dishes from meat to desserts, the flavor is in the fat, one reason restaurant meat generally contains a lot of fat.

Another challenge for diabetics is to cut or lower the carbohydrates in their diet and that includes desserts. For instance, check out the carbs in our low sodium apple pie on the next page. The shell has 104 grams of carbs, the apples have 251 grams, the two sugars total close to 200 grams and the flour for the topping hits 108 grams. The resultant pie slice ends up with 83.8 grams of carbohydrates and 554 calories, but the sodium is only 8.5 mg. So, how do we deal with the high level of calories and carbohydrates?

We can lower calories a bit by exchanging the sugar with Splenda Granulated. But this particular pie uses a "crumble" crust, which contains more shortening and quite a bit of brown sugar. Even if we exchange those items with substitutes, we come out with a high carbohydrate dessert.

So, if we've done everything we can to lower the ingredients but we can't get low enough per serving, then we suggest eating just a quarter or a half of a serving.

With some of our recipes we have provided a second nutrition data bar with the "half-serving" nutrient information. Other recipes might have a second nutrition panel because we've exchanged sugar or some other ingredient with a substitute like Splenda.

When using Splenda Granulated, cut the measurement in half. That is, if a recipe calls for a cup of sugar, use only 1/2 cup of Splenda Granulated even though the Splenda package states measurement for measurement. You might also want to consider using Splenda Sugar Blend. Caution: Splenda has so many substitutes now that it can get confusing when figuring nutrient data. We used Splenda Granulated for most of our exchange data throughout this book. You can learn more about Splenda in the glossary. This information was furnished to us by McNeil Nutritionals, LLC, makers of Splenda

CRISPY APPLE PIE

LACTO OVO – ½ = 3 CARB CHOICES

Serves 8 ***Sodium Per Recipe: 67.8 mg*** ***Sodium Per Slice 8.475 mg***

If you replace sugars with Splenda, you cut carbs down low enough to make a half-serving 2½ carb choices. See Nutrient data bottom Page: 276.

1 8 or 9" single layer pie shell (See Page 284) (2.498 mg)
10 Pippin or Granny Smith apples, with skin (18.2 mg)
1 teaspoon of lemon juice (.153 mg)
½ cup granulated sugar (trace)
1 teaspoon cinnamon (.26 mg)
¼ tablespoon nutmeg (.088 mg)
1 tablespoon cornstarch (.749 mg)

Crumble Topping

1 1 cup flour (2.5 mg)
½ cup packed brown sugar (30.8 mg)
1 1 stick (8 tablespoons) unsalted butter (12.4 mg)

Pre heat oven to 350° F. Prepare your pie shell in 9" pie baking dish.

Wash, core and thinly slice apples. Combine sugar or Splenda Granulated, cinnamon, nutmeg and mixed cornstarch. In a large bowl toss the apples with the lemon juice and spice/sugar mix. Stir until completely mixed.

Place apple mix into pie shell.

For topping, cut unsalted butter into thin slices. Combine butter, flour and sugar in medium bowl and using fork mix together until it's either crumbly or a loose mixture. You may also use a hand beater for this step.

Sprinkle topping over the top of the apple mix in the pie shell.

Place pie on cookie sheet and bake in preheated standard oven at 350° F for 50 to 60 minutes.

***Note**: See page 278 for nutrient data when using Splenda.*

Crispy Apple Pie Nutrient Data Per Serving (8 slices): Calories: 553.7, Protein: 3.984 g, Carbohydrate: 83.7 g, Dietary Fiber: 6.509 g, Total Sugars: 50.7 g, Total Fat: 24.2 g, Saturated Fat: 10.4 g, Monounsaturated Fat: 8.015 g, Polyunsaturated Fat: 4.676 g, Cholesterol: 30.4 mg, Trans Fatty Acids: 0 g, Total Omega-3 FA: .116 g, Total Omega-6 FA: .306 g, Calcium: 36.8 mg, Potassium: 303.1 mg, Sodium: 8.462 mg, Vitamin K: 6.189 mcg

Crispy Apple Pie Half-Serving (16 slices) - 3 Carb Choices: Calories: 276.8, Protein: 1.992 g, Carbohydrate: 41.9 g, Dietary Fiber: 3.254 g, Total Sugars: 25.3 g, Total Fat: 12.1 g, Saturated Fat: 5.194 g, Monounsaturated Fat: 4.008 g, Polyunsaturated Fat: 2.338 g, Cholesterol: 15.2 mg, Trans Fatty Acids: 0 g, Total Omega-3 FA: .058 g, Total Omega-6 FA: .153 g, Calcium: 18.4 mg, Potassium: 151.6 mg, Sodium: 4.231 mg, Vitamin K: 3.094 mcg

WILD BLACKBERRY COBBLER

LACTO OVO– 3 CARB CHOICESS[1]

Serves 10 Sodium Per Recipe: 67.1 mg Sodium Per Serving: 6.715 mg

Pie Filling

6 - 8 cups fresh wild blackberries (11.5 mg)
1½ cups granulated sugar[1] (trace)
3 level tablespoons cornstarch (2.154 mg)
¼ teaspoon ground cinnamon (.065 mg)
2 tablespoons fresh squeezed lemon juice (.305 mg)

Topping

1¼ cups flour (3.125 mg)
⅔ cup packed brown sugar (40.7 mg)
1 stick unsalted butter (9.323 mg)

Preheat oven to 400° F.

Prepare a 9 x 13-inch baking pan by very lightly greasing the bottom and sides of the pan.

For topping, cut unsalted butter into thin slices. Combine butter, flour and sugar in medium bowl and mix until crumbly. You may use beater, pastry blender or fork. Set aside.

For pie filling, wash berries, place in bowl and add lemon juice. Mix dry ingredients and stir them into berries. Pour berries into prepared 9 x 13 baking pan, include any juice that remains in bowl. Sprinkle on topping.

Bake for 20 to 25 minutes. Serve warm with whipped cream or low-sodium vanilla ice cream.

[1]Diabetics, the sugar in this recipe has 300 grams carbohydrates and the berries themselves have 109 grams of carbs. Brown sugar has 14.1 grams carbs per serving. You can lower carbohydrates by using Splenda or Splenda Brown Sugar Blend. See data below for Splenda Granulated. See Splenda in our glossary, page 330.

Blackberry Cobbler Nutrient Data Per Serving (Sugar): Calories: 348.5, Protein: 3.325 g, Carbohydrate: 69.7 g, Dietary Fiber: 6.596 g, Total Sugars: 49.8 g, Total Fat: 7.594 g, Saturated Fat: 4.394 g, Monounsaturated Fat: 1.85 g, Polyunsaturated Fat: .646 g, Cholesterol: 18.2 mg, Trans Fatty Acids: 0 g, Total Omega-3 FA: .165 g, Total Omega-6 FA: .184 g, Calcium: 51.1 mg, Potassium: 229.4 mg, Sodium: 6.715 mg, Vitamin K: 23.5 mcg

Diabetics: Blackberry Cobbler Nutrient Data Per Serving (Splenda ®Granulated) Carb Choices 2½: Calories: 244.3, Protein: 3.325 g, Carbohydrate: 43 g, Dietary Fiber: 6.596 g, Total Sugars: 22.7 g, Total Fat: 7.594 g, Saturated Fat: 4.394 g, Monounsaturated Fat: 1.85 g, Polyunsaturated Fat: .646 g, Cholesterol: 18.2 mg, Trans Fatty Acids: 0 g, Total Omega-3 FA: .165 g, Total Omega-6 FA: .184 g, Calcium: 50.8 mg, Potassium: 229 mg, Sodium: 6.715 mg, Vitamin K: 23.5 mcg

LEMON CHEESECAKE

LACTO-OVO VEGETARIAN – 1 CARB CHOICES[1]

Serves 14 Sodium Per Recipe: 477.1 mg Sodium Per Serving: 34.1 mg

Requires Springform Pan

- **1½ cups homemade graham cracker crumbs[2] (15.3 mg)**
- **1 cup granulated sugar or Splenda (trace)**
- **1 cup or 8-ounces of firm unsalted tofu (9.48 mg)**
- **2 cups of our nonfat Yo Cheese (185.2 mg**
- **2 level tablespoons cornstarch (1.44 mg)**
- **2 level tablespoons grated lemon peel (.72 mg)**
- **½ teaspoon vanilla extract (.189 mg)**
- **3 large eggs (210 mg)**
- **⅓ cup light or low-fat sour cream (52.3 mg)**

Make your homemade graham crackers from our Graham Cracker recipe[2]. Crumble about 6 to 10 of the crackers in a food processor that uses a steel blade. Spread the cracker crumbs across the bottom of a 9" springform pan evenly. Press down. Spray the crackers and the sides of the pan with a very light coating of oil.

Preheat your oven to 300° F.

Beat together the Yo Cheese, tofu, cornstarch, sugar, lemon peel and vanilla extract. Continue beating adding the eggs one at a time. When mix is fluffy, pour over the cracker crumbs in the springform pan. Smooth top.

Bake for 1-hour plus about 10-minutes or until center is lightly firm to the touch. Let cool for about an hour. Spread "light" or low-fat sour cream or your glaze over the top, return to oven for ten minutes, then cook and then chill in the refrigerator for about 4 hours before serving.

[1]Diabetics, 1 carb choices based on using Splenda instead of sugar. There's room here to use half Splenda and half sugar if you like.

[2]See Page: 261

[3] For the taste of a New York cheesecake, you can stir in a bit of sugar or Splenda and a dash of lemon to the sour cream before spreading on cheesecake.

Cheesecake Nutrient Data Per Serving (sugar) (2 Carb Choices): Calories: 151.7, Protein: 5.077 g, Carbohydrate: 25.4 g, Dietary Fiber: .917 g, Total Sugars: 17.7 g, Total Fat: 3.744 g, Saturated Fat: .885 g, Monounsaturated Fat: 1.531 g, Polyunsaturated Fat: 1.033 g, Cholesterol: 47.7 mg, Trans Fatty Acids: 0 g, Total Omega-3 FA: .135 g, Total Omega-6 FA: 0 g, Calcium: 85.5 mg, Potassium: 120.3 mg, Sodium: 34.1 mg, Vitamin K: 1.661 mcg

Cheesecake Nutrient Data Per Serving (Splenda) (1 Carb Choices): Calories: 101.2, Protein: 5.051 g, Carbohydrate: 12.3 g, Dietary Fiber: .735 g, Total Sugars: 4.723 g, Total Fat: 3.739 g, Saturated Fat: .884 g, Monounsaturated Fat: 1.531 g, Polyunsaturated Fat: 1.031 g, Cholesterol: 47.7 mg, Trans Fatty Acids: 0 g, Total Omega-3 FA: .134 g, Total Omega-6 FA: 0 g, Calcium: 83.1 mg, Potassium: 117.3 mg, Sodium: 34 mg, Vitamin K: 1.661 mcg

BERRY SORBET

VEGAN – 1 CARB CHOICES[1]

Makes 8 ½-cups Sodium Per Recipe: 9.08 Sodium Per ½-Cup: 1.135 mg

This makes a wonderful sorbet. An ice cream machine helps but if you don't have one, you can freeze overnight in your freezer. Why not teach the youngsters in your family how we used to do it.

4 cups fresh berries[2] (6.64 mg)
1 cup sugar or Splenda Granulated[3] (trace)
1 cup filtered water (trace)
1 tablespoon fresh lemon juice[4] (2.44 mg)

In a small saucepan, bring water and sugar to a boil, reduce heat and simmer until sugar is completely dissolved. About three to five minutes. Allow cooling time before using to make sorbet.

In a processor, purée the berries with 1/4 cup of the sugar/water mix until smooth. Pour in one cup of the sugar/water mix and the lemon juice and stir until smooth. (If you have any sugar/water mix left over, it will store in your refrigerator for a couple of weeks.)

Pour into an ice cream maker or machine and freeze according to manufacturer's instructions. If you don't have an ice cream machine, place into freezable container and freeze overnight in your freezer. Works well either way.

Serve.

[1] One-Carb Choice when using Splenda. When using sugar: 3 Carb Choices

[2] Strawberries, blackberries, blueberries, raspberries and even peaches. May use frozen unsweetened berries. Nutrient data based on strawberries. Other berries a closely similar.

[3] If fruit is really ripe, use only ½ cup of sugar/water mix where one cup is called for. When using Splenda Granulated, use 1/2 cup instead of one.

[4] If you like your sorbet really sweet, then use 2 tablespoons of orange juice instead of the lemon juice.

Sorbet Nutrient Data Per Serving Using Sugar: Calories: 130.9, Protein: .672 g, Carbohydrate: 34 g, Dietary Fiber: 1.782 g, Total Sugars: 29.8 g, Total Fat: .249 g, Saturated Fat: .012 g, Monounsaturated Fat: .036 g, Polyunsaturated Fat: .129 g, Cholesterol: 0 mg, Trans Fatty Acids: 0 g, Total Omega-3 FA: .054 g, Total Omega-6 FA: 0 g, Calcium: 15.7 mg, Potassium: 165.3 mg, Sodium: 1.135 mg, Vitamin K: 1.826 mcg

Sorbet Nutrient Data Per Serving Using Splenda: Calories: 44.1, Protein: .672 g, Carbohydrate: 11.7 g, Dietary Fiber: 1.782 g, Total Sugars: 7.201 g, Total Fat: .249 g, Saturated Fat: .012 g, Monounsaturated Fat: .036 g, Polyunsaturated Fat: .129 g, Cholesterol: 0 mg, Trans Fatty Acids: 0 g, Total Omega-3 FA: .054 g, Total Omega-6 FA: 0 g, Calcium: 15.4 mg, Potassium: 164.9 mg, Sodium: 1.135 mg, Vitamin K: 1.826 mcg

DECADENT CREAM PUFFS

LACTO-OVO VEGETARIAN – 1 CARB CHOICES[1]

Makes 12 Sodium Per Recipe: 307.1 mg Sodium Per Puff 25.6 mg

Sodium Per puff Whipped Cream: 32.5 mg

Sodium Per Puff Italian Filling 56.4 mg

The cream puff originated in Italy. Apparently it was created by a chap named Poelini, who served as chef for Catherine de Medici. It was exported from there to France in the 16th century. In the U.S. it debuted at the Wisconsin State Fair in 1924. I first met the cream puff while standing on the tips of my toes peering like a Norman Rockwell youngster might into the long drawer of goodies that the Helms Bakery man pulled out to do exactly what it did: get my fifteen cents for his cream puff. I've been a fan ever since, but these days they are very occasional and with a lot less sodium and fat. We offer you two versions here.

The Shell

1 cup filtered low-sodium water (trace)
1 stick unsalted butter (12.4 mg)
1 cup white unbleached flour (2.5 mg)
1 tablespoon cider vinegar (.15 mg)
½ teaspoon vanilla extract (.189 mg)
4 large eggs (280 mg)

Filling: Whipped Cream Version

1 small container (cup) light Whipping Cream[1] (81.3 mg)
¼ cup unsifted Confectioner's sugar (.3 mg)
1 teaspoon Cook's powdered vanilla (.378 mg)
2 teaspoons cornstarch (.461 mg)

Whip cream at high speed in a chilled bowl, add sugar, vanilla and cornstarch after cream begins to form. Whip until stiff but not too long or else it will turn into butter.

Filling: Italian Version

1 cup white granulated sugar or Splenda® (trace)
⅓ cup cornstarch (3.802 mg)
1 large egg, lightly beaten (70 mg)
2 cups scalded 1% milk with added Vit. A (214.7 mg)
1 teaspoon powdered vanilla (.378 mg)

Preheat your standard oven to 400° F or your convection oven to 375° F. Crack eggs and place into a bowl. Set aside.

Heat water and butter in a medium pan until they boil. Using a wooden spoon, stir in the flour, stirring steadily over a low to medium heat for about a minute or until the batter becomes one smooth ball. Remove this from the heat and using beaters, beat in the vinegar, vanilla, and 4 eggs all at the same time. Beat until smooth.

On large cookie sheet covered with parchment paper, spoon or scoop about a ¼ cup of dough setting them about three inches apart. (I use a ¼ cup measuring cup. This forms a very nice round well shaped "puff.") You can also shape into elongated puffs.

Bake on middle rack for about 35 to 40 minutes or until golden brown. Test with a toothpick. Cool on rack for about 10 to 20 minutes.

Cut in half. Dig a bit of the dough out. Fill with whipped cream filling. If on a low fat diet you may use light whipping cream. We have included two choices: one with the whipping cream and the other with the original Italian filling. The whipping cream version is easier to make and is lower in calories than the Italian version.

[1] May exchange for Light Whipping Cream. Add 2-tablespoons of confectioner's sugar and 1 teaspoon of cornstarch if you do. Calories remain about the same, about 4 calories fewer per cream puff.

Cream Puff Nutrient Data, Puff Only: Calories: 134, Protein: 3.253 g, Carbohydrate: 8.29 g, Dietary Fiber: .281 g, Total Sugars: .264 g, Total Fat: 9.397 g, Saturated Fat: 5.37 g, Monounsaturated Fat: 2.624 g, Polyunsaturated Fat: .557 g, Cholesterol: 90.7 mg, Trans Fatty Acids: 0 g, Total Omega-3 FA: .074 g, Total Omega-6 FA: .204 g, Calcium: 14.1 mg, Potassium: 50.5 mg, Sodium: 25.6 mg, Vitamin K: .74 mcg

[1]Cream Puff Nutrient Data, Puff with Whipped Cream Filling: Calories: 204.5, Protein: 3.686 g, Carbohydrate: 11.8 g, Dietary Fiber: .285 g, Total Sugars: 2.778 g, Total Fat: 15.6 g, Saturated Fat: 9.222 g, Monounsaturated Fat: 4.435 g, Polyunsaturated Fat: .734 g, Cholesterol: 112.9 mg, Trans Fatty Acids: 0 g, Total Omega-3 FA: .127 g, Total Omega-6 FA: .204 g, Calcium: 27.9 mg, Potassium: 70.4 mg, Sodium: 32.5 mg, Vitamin K: 1.278 mcg

[1]Cream Puff Nutrient Data, Puff with Italian Filling (Splenda): Calories: 236.2, Protein: 5.589 g, Carbohydrate: 16 g, Dietary Fiber: .313 g, Total Sugars: 4.083 g, Total Fat: 16.4 g, Saturated Fat: 9.608 g, Monounsaturated Fat: 4.707 g, Polyunsaturated Fat: .805 g, Cholesterol: 132.5 mg, Trans Fatty Acids: 0 g, Total Omega-3 FA: .133 g, Total Omega-6 FA: .215 g, Calcium: 78.5 mg, Potassium: 137.1 mg, Sodium: 56.4 mg, Vitamin K: 1.331 mcg

Cream Puff Nutrient Data, Puff with Italian Filling (sugar): Calories: 294.1, Protein: 5.589 g, Carbohydrate: 30.9 g, Dietary Fiber: .313 g, Total Sugars: 19.1 g, Total Fat: 16.4 g, Saturated Fat: 9.608 g, Monounsaturated Fat: 4.707 g, Polyunsaturated Fat: .805 g, Cholesterol: 132.5 mg, Trans Fatty Acids: 0 g, Total Omega-3 FA: .133 g, Total Omega-6 FA: .215 g, Calcium: 78.7 mg, Potassium: 137.4 mg, Sodium: 56.4 mg, Vitamin K: 1.331 mcg

YO CHEESE MOUSSE

LACTO OVO – 1 CARB CHOICES[1]

Serves 4 Sodium Per Recipe: 93.8 mg Sodium Per Serving: 23.5 mg

With wild or fresh berry sauce

8 tablespoons homemade yo cheese (93.1 mg)
8 tablespoons fresh berry sauce made from fresh wild or domestic berries[1] (.72 mg)

Prepare your Yo Cheese a day or two earlier.

In four ramekins or similar size serving dish, spoon in 2 tablespoons of Yo Cheese, then top with 2 tablespoons of your homemade chilled berry sauce.

With skewer swirl together once. Top with a tablespoon of canned nonfat or light whipped cream if you like.[2] Recipe may be doubled.

Serve cold for dessert.

[1] Nutrient Data based on wild and domestic blackberries. See Don's Wild Blackberry Sauce in ths book. Sugar carbs are in the sauce.

[2] Optional ingredient: 1-tablespoon light or nonfat whipped cream from can as topping. Adds 5 mg of sodium per serving and 7.5 calories per serving.

Yo Cheese Mousse Nutrient Data Per Serving (with sugar): Calories: 55.2, Protein: 2.639 g, Carbohydrate: 11.2 g, Dietary Fiber: .954 g, Total Sugars: 7.123 g, Total Fat: .15 g, Saturated Fat: .032 g, Monounsaturated Fat: .026 g, Polyunsaturated Fat: .053 g, Cholesterol: .919 mg, Trans Fatty Acids: 0 g, Total Omega-3 FA: .017 g, Total Omega-6 FA: 0 g, Calcium: 66.2 mg, Potassium: 107.4 mg, Sodium: 23.5 mg, Vitamin K: 3.564 mcg

LEMON MERINGUE PIE

LACTO OVO – 2½ CARB CHOICES[1]

Serves 8 Sodium Per Recipe: 211.3 mg Sodium Per Serving: 26.4 mg

We've worked on this recipe to keep the sodium, calorie and carbohydrate levels down. If it's still too high for you, try having a half-slice. It's easy to make and for lemon lovers, it's delicious.

1 one-crust pie shell (12.3 mg)
1⅓ cups sugar (trace)
5 tablespoons cornstarch (3.15 mg)
1½ cups filtered water (trace)
3 tablespoons unsalted butter (4.686 mg)
½ cup fresh squeezed lemon juice (1.22 mg)
1 tablespoon finely grated lemon zest (.36 mg)
3 large egg yolks (24.5 mg)
3 large egg whites (164.3 mg)
½ teaspoon cream of tartar (.78 mg)
5 tablespoons sugar (trace)

Prepare one-crust pie shell, cooked. (See Page: 276)

Separate eggs cleanly, saving both yolks and whites. Beat yolks with a fork.

Mix sugar, cornstarch and water in a medium sized sauce pan. Cook over medium high heat stirring continuously until mixture comes to a boil.

Remove mixture from heat and add egg yolks, blending until smooth. Work quickly or eggs may begin to clump.

Continue to cook for an additional 5-minutes while sitrring. Mixture will thicken. Remove from stove, stir in zest, juice, and butter until it melts. Pour into crust and smooth with spatula blade. Allow to cool.

Set oven temperature to 350° F.

To make meringue, beat the egg whites with the cream of tartar at slow speed for about ten to fifteen seconds, then at high speed until peaks form. While beating at high speed gradually add 5 tablespoons of sugar until the whites have increased to about five to six times the volume and are glossy and firm. (The whites will make pointed peaks when pulled up with the beaters.) Spread the meringue over the filling to touch the edge of the crust. Bake until the meringue is golden brown – 10 to 15 minutes. Cool on wire rack.

Baker's Tip: Add cream of tartar to egg whites at the beginning. Don't worry about it clumping. It won't. Egg whites need an acid to bind and hold them together. Either lemon juice or vinegar work, but add a distinct flavor while Cream of Tartar doesn't. Use beaten egg whites immediately.

[1] Diabetics, this pie is adaptable by using Splenda or eating only a half slice, which provides 25.6 grams carbs, or 2 carb choices.

Lemon Meringue Pie Nutrient Data Per Serving (sugar) 3½ Carb Choices: Calories: 379.5, Protein: 4.191 g, Carbohydrate: 59 g, Dietary Fiber: .602 g, Total Sugars: 41.7 g, Total Fat: 14.8 g, Saturated Fat: 8.84 g, Monounsaturated Fat: 4.121 g, Polyunsaturated Fat: .82 g, Cholesterol: 113 mg, Trans Fatty Acids: 0 g, Total Omega-3 FA: .119 g, Total Omega-6 FA: .346 g, Calcium: 17.9 mg, Potassium: 100.5 mg, Sodium: 26.4 mg, Vitamin K: 1.21 mcg

[1]Lemon Meringue Pie Nutrient Data Per Serving (Splenda Granular) 2½ Carb Choices: Calories: 290.9, Protein: 4.191 g, Carbohydrate: 36.2 g, Dietary Fiber: .602 g, Total Sugars: 18.7 g, Total Fat: 14.8 g, Saturated Fat: 8.84 g, Monounsaturated Fat: 4.121 g, Polyunsaturated Fat: .82 g, Cholesterol: 113 mg, Trans Fatty Acids: 0 g, Total Omega-3 FA: .119 g, Total Omega-6 FA: .346 g, Potassium: 100 mg, Sodium: 26.4 mg, Vitamin K: 1.21 mcg

SINGLE LAYER PIE SHELL

VEGAN – 1 CARB CHOICES

Serves 8 Sodium Per Recipe: 2.652 mg Sodium Per Slice (8): .332 mg

Use for single pie shell recipes.

1 cup unbleached white flour (2.5 mg)
1 tablespoon lemon juice (.053 mg)
2 teaspoons granulated sugar (trace)
8 tablespoons non transfat shortening[1] (trace)
3 to 4 tablespoons cold filtered water (trace)

Combine the flour, lemon juice, and sugar in a mixing bowl.

Cut in the shortening with a pastry blender or with two knives until the mixture is the consistency of coarse cornmeal or small peas.

Sprinkle the cold water, 1 tablespoon at a time, tossing and stirring. Each time, add a tablespoon of water to the driest part of the mixture. The dough should be moist enough to hold together when pressed gently with a fork. Don't let it get sticky.

Shape the dough into a smooth ball with your hands and roll it out by hand or with a rolling pin. Refrigerate for about 45-minutes. Roll out after that.

This recipe makes enough crust for one 8-inch or 1-9 inch pie shell.

[1]There are currently a variety of non stransfatty acid shortenings on the market today including Crisco and a popular brand from Whole Foods.

Single Layer Pie Shell Nutritional Data Per Serving: Calories: 171.4, Protein: 1.621 g, Carbohydrate: 13.1 g, Dietary Fiber: .43 g, Total Sugars: 1.137 g, Total Fat: 12.2 g, Saturated Fat: 3.024 g, Monounsaturated Fat: 5.014 g, Polyunsaturated Fat: 4.065 g, Cholesterol: 0 mg, Trans Fatty Acids: 0 g, Total Omega-3 FA: .003 g, Total Omega-6 FA: 0 g, Calcium: 2.488 mg, Potassium: 19.1 mg, Sodium: .332 mg, Vitamin K: .047 mcg

Crispy Apple Pie Using Splenda, Page 268

Crispy Apple Pie Nutrient Data When Made With Splenda, based on half a serving: : Calories: 237.8, Protein: 1.989 g, Carbohydrate: 31.8 g, Dietary Fiber: 3.337 g, Total Sugars: 15.2 g, Total Fat: 12.1 g, Saturated Fat: 5.194 g, Monounsaturated Fat: 4.008 g, Polyunsaturated Fat: 2.338 g, Cholesterol: 15.2 mg, Trans Fatty Acids: 0 g, Total Omega-3 FA: .058 g, Total Omega-6 FA: .153 g, Calcium: 16.1 mg, Potassium: 144.9 mg, Sodium: 2.947 mg, Vitamin K: 3.145 mcg

ADDED RECIPES

This book has been credited with having helped thousands of Heart, Meniere's, Diabetic, Nephorotic and other patients since its iniitial publication. The original publication had a few typos and we hope those are now fixed. The first edition also had 134 terrific recipes, but now it has nearly 200.

When we first published this book we promised updates and that new recipes would be added.

From breakfast to dinner to salads and jams and jellies, this bonus section is chock full of great new recipes, each designed for no-salt and low-sodium eaters and each calculated for diebetic carbohydrate choices and listed for Vegans as well.

As always, if you have any questions, feel free to write us at arrohead@wavecable.com. If that address changes, simply visit us at megaheart.com/contact.html and we'll get back to you.

And now, for the first time, I'd like list my favorite recipes in each of the five books we have. If you'll email me your favorites, we'll post them online along with your name but not your email address.

The No Salt, Lowest Sodium Cookbook
Chicken Enchiladas, page 112
Charlotte's Potatoes, 286
Fettuccine Alfredo, page 152

The No Salt, Lowest Sodium Baking Book
Walnut Raisin Bread, page 74
Almond Meringue Cookies, page 168
Whole Wheat Scones, page 116

The No Salt, Lowest Sodium Light Meals Book
Spicy Thai Soup, page 33
Maureen's Special Enchilada Soup, page 19
Musketeer Salad, page 150

The No Salt, Lowest Sodium International Cookbook
Ethiopian Spice Bread, 180
Chicken Cordon Bleu, page 77
Soy Sauce Replacement, page 37

CREPES with APPLESAUCE

LACTO OVO – **2** CARB CHOICES

Serves 2

Sodium Per Crepe Recipe: 111.4 mg   Sodium Per Crepe 27.9 mg
Sodium Per Sauce Recipe: 1.4 mg   Sodium PerSauce Serving: .358 mg
Sodium Per Crepe with Applesauce: 28.2 mg

*Top with a dash of sour cream or natural maple syrup. Recipe may be doubled. Also can top with Greek yogurt or our Yo Cheese (**See Page 225**).*

The Crepe

1 **medium to large egg (70 mg)**
6 **tablespoons nonfat milk with Vitamin A & D (39.1 mg)**
1 **teaspoon fresh lemon juice (.153 mg)**
¼ **cup unbleached, all -purpose flour (.625 mg)**
1 **tablespoon unsalted butter (melted) (1.562 mg)**

Combine the eggs, milk, flour, lemon juice and butter in a medium size mixing bowl or blender bowl and beat together on high speed for about a minute or until smooth. It should not be lumpy.

Set aside in regrigerator while you make the applesauce below.

The Crepe

1 cooking apples, with skin[1] (1.25 mg)
¼ **teaspoon of lemon juice (..076 mg)**
1 teaspoon granulated sugar (trace)
¼ **teaspoon cinnamon (.065 mg)**
⅛ **teaspoon nutmeg (.044 mg)**
6 - 7 tablespoons water (trace)

Wash, core and thinly slice apples. Combine sugar or Splenda Granulated, cinnamon and nutmeg. In a small stovetop pan toss the apples with the lemon juice and spice/sugar mix. Stir until completely mixed. Add water. Cover pot.

Over low heat, cook the applesauce, stirring a few times. When apples soften from cooking, remove lid and let cook another few minutes so that liquid turns into a syrup. When crepes are cooked, place apples in center of each crepe, roll and drizzle with the apple syrup. Serve hot.

Crepes with Applesauce Nutrient Data Per Serving :Calories: 102.2, Protein: 3.307 g, Carbohydrate: 13.2 g, Dietary Fiber: 1.084 g, Total Sugars: 5.76 g, Total Fat: 4.297 g, Saturated Fat: 2.262 g, Monounsaturated Fat: 1.239 g, Polyunsaturated Fat: .327 g, Cholesterol: 61 mg, Trans Fatty Acids: 0 g, Total Omega-3 FA: .036 g, Total Omega-6 FA: .077 g, Calcium: 41.8 mg, Potassium: 103.8 mg, Sodium: 28.2 mg, Vitamin K: 1.048 mcg

LOW SUGAR WILD BLACKBERRY JAM

VEGAN — ½ CARB CHOICES
Makes 6 cups, 96 Tablespoons
Sodium Per Recipe: 107.4 mg   Sodium Per Tablespoon: 1.119 mg

4 total cups of juice from wild blackberries(7.2 mg)
1 cup wild blackberries crushed (includes juice)
6 drops of fresh lemon juice (.117 mg)
4 cups of white granulated sugar (trace)
1 package of pectin (100 mg)[1]
Optional: 1/3 teaspoon unsalted butter(.133 mg)[2]

Takes approximately 9 cups fresh wild blackberries.

Press berries or mash with potato masher. Pull one cup of mashed berries (and their juice) and set aside. Mash balance of berries some more then setting a tightly woven sieve on a large bowl pour the berries into the sieve and press down. We use the sieve exclusively, but you can also use cheesecloth. Wrap berries in the cloth and squeeze it tightly until all juice has been extracted. We also place a one gallon jug of water on top of the sieve after our "human" efforts are complete and always get one or two more cups of juice that way.

Once juice is extracted, measure 4-cups into large pot and add the crushed berries with their juice that you set aside. Add the pectin. Bring to a rolling boil and add the sugar.

Stir until a rolling boil and boil for one minute only. Remove from heat.

Ladle into prepared canning jars (we use pint and half-pint jars).

Wipe jar top edge with wet towel, place lid on, cap it down tightly and finish other jars. Set into steamer and cover. Steam for ten minutes. Remove to countertop let cook for an our so before storing. If you prefer, you can let the jars stand without the steaming and within an hour the lids shouyld "pop," meaning they are sealed.

[1]Or 6 tablespoons of pectin purchased in bulk containers

[2] Butter helps keep the jam from foaming. If you prefer to not use it, then you'll have to skim the foam before pouring into canning jars.

Low Sugar Wild Blackberry Jam Nutrient Data Per Tablespoon: Calories: 37.3, Protein: .106 g, Carbohydrate: 9.53 g, Dietary Fiber: .443 g, Total Sugars: 8.694 g, Total Fat: .052 g, Saturated Fat: .01 g, Monounsaturated Fat: .007 g, Polyunsaturated Fat: .022 g, Cholesterol: .035 mg, Trans Fatty Acids: 0 g, Total Omega-3 FA: .007 g, Total Omega-6 FA: 0 g, Calcium: 2.304 mg, Potassium: 12.5 mg, Sodium: 1.119 mg, Vitamin K: 1.486 mcg

BAKING MIX

VEGAN – 1 CARB CHOICES

Makes 7-cups Sodium: 56 mg Vitamin K: 136.3 mcg

A no-salt replacement for commercial baking mixes such as Bisquick..

6 cups white, all-purpose flour (15 mg)
3 tablespoons white granulated sugar (0 mg)
⅓ cup Ener-g Baking Powder (24 mg)
1 cup expeller pressed canola oil (trace)

Sift dry ingredients together a couple of times. Using a pastry blender add the oil slowly and mix/blend until texture of corn meal or similar.

Store in refrigerator in airtight container for up to a month.

Baking Mix Nutrient Data per 1/4 cup: Calories: 282.8, Protein: 17 g, Carbohydrate: 16.5 g, Dietary Fiber: 4.934 g, Total Sugars: 8.959 g, Total Fat: 17.6 g, Saturated Fat: 2.635 g, Monounsaturated Fat: 8.365 g, Polyunsaturated Fat: 5.348 g, Cholesterol: 34.2 mg, Trans Fatty Acids: .015 g, Total Omega-3 FA: .247 g, Total Omega-6 FA: .002 g, Calcium: 77.5 mg, Potassium: 924.6 mg

COWBOY COOKIES

LACTO OVO – 2 CARB CHOICES[1]

Makes (18) 4-inch cookies or (24) 3-inch cookies
Sodium Per Recipe: 262.9 mg
Sodium (18) 4.789 mg Sodium Per Cookie (24) 3.592 mg

This is my second version of a popular cookie known as the "Cowboy Cookie." There are plenty of versions of a cowboy cookie, but this is the one I finally settled on for a good no-salt, very low-sodium treat and one that salt eaters also like. You can increase the cinnamon by a half-teaspoon or add one-quarter teaspoon ground cloves for an added kick.

1 cup softened unsalted butter (25 mg) or trans fat free shortening such as Crisco (trace)
¾ cup brown sugar, packed (46.2 mg)
¾ cup white granulated sugar or Splenda for baking (trace)
2 large eggs (140 mg)
1 teaspoon vanilla extract (.378 mg)
2 cups white unbleached all-purpose flour (5 mg)
2 cups Quaker Quick oats or unsalted rolled oats (4.8 g)
2 teaspoons Ener-g Baking Soda[2] (trace)
2 teaspoons Ener-g Baking Powder (9 mg)
1 teaspoon ground cinnamon (.26 mg)
¼ teaspoon granulated onion powder (.324 mg)
¾ cup unsalted walnuts, chopped 1.755 mg)
1 cup (6-oz package) semi-sweet chocolate chips (18.5 mg)

Preheat oven to 350° F.

We're going to bake two sheets of cookies at the same time. Place one oven rack in the top third of your oven, and one oven rack in the bottom third.

Line two baking sheets with parchment paper.

In a large bowl, beat the shortening or unsalted butter with the sugars until creamy — about two to three minutes. Add the eggs while beating one at a time. Add the vanilla extract a beat another thirty seconds or so.

In a separate bowl, whisk together the flour, baking soda, baking powder, granulated onion powder, and cinnamon. Add the dry mixture to the creamed mixture and beat just until combined. Stir in the unsalted walnuts, oats and chocolate chips.

Form dough into balls, using ¼ measuring. A quarter cup equal 4 level tablespoons. To make your cookies a bit smaller and bring the total from 18 to 24, use 3 tablespoons instead.

(Continued next page)

Place six balls of dough on each baking sheet. With moistened hands gently flatten each ball of dough into a ½-inch thick cookie.

Bake the cookies for about 15 to 20 minutes. Depending on ovens, this could take up to about 22 minutes.

When cookies are a golden brown around the edges the centers should be soft or not quite set. Remove from oven and let the cookies cool a few minutes on the baking sheet before transferring them to a wire rack to cool.[3]

Will store for up to a few days in an airtight zipper lock bag or in the freezer for up to three months.

Footnotes:

[1] 2 Carb Choices per cookie when making 24, 3 Carb Choices when making 18.

[2] Or two-teaspoons cream of tartar if you don't have Ener-G baking soda. (We recommend the Ener-G for best results, however.)

[3] While baking the first batch we put together two more baking sheets with parchment paper. If you don't have four sheets, then prepare the next batch after cookies cool on sheet as described below.

Cowboy Cookies Nutrient Data Per Cookie (24) 3" cookies: Calories: 245, Protein: 2.856 g, Carbohydrate: 30.7 g, Dietary Fiber: 1.634 g, Total Sugars: 17 g, Total Fat: 13 g, Saturated Fat: 3.557 g, Monounsaturated Fat: 4.499 g, Polyunsaturated Fat: 4.656 g, Cholesterol: 0 mg, Trans Fatty Acids: 0 g, Total Omega-3 FA: .346 g, Total Omega-6 FA: 0 g, Calcium: 49.3 mg, Potassium: 129 mg, Sodium: 3.592 mg, Vitamin K: .77 mcg

Cowboy Cookies Nutrient Data Per 4" Cookie (18): Calories: 326.7, Protein: 3.808 g, Carbohydrate: 41 g, Dietary Fiber: 2.179 g, Total Sugars: 22.6 g, Total Fat: 17.4 g, Saturated Fat: 4.743 g, Monounsaturated Fat: 5.999 g, Polyunsaturated Fat: 6.208 g, Cholesterol: 0 mg, Trans Fatty Acids: 0 g, Total Omega-3 FA: .461 g, Total Omega-6 FA: 0 g, Calcium: 65.7 mg, Potassium: 172 mg, Sodium: 4.789 mg, Vitamin K: 1.027 mcg

10 GRAIN WHOLE WHEAT BREAD

LACTO-OVO – 1 CARB CHOICES

Bread Machine Recipe

Makes One Loaf (14 slices)

Sodium Per Recipe: 81.8 mg Sodium Per Slice 6.006 mg

We were asked to reduce our 10-Grain Bread, found in The No Salt, Lowest Sodium Baking Book to a 1.3 pound loaf. Since bread recipes can't be remodeled by just cutting them in half, we worked this formula out and it's quite good. We use a white whole-wheat flour. You can replace the egg white if you like with a teaspoon of vinegar. If after it has kneaded for five minutes you find the dough not quite in a ball, you might want to add another teaspoon to a tablespoon of water. If you don't care for the flavor of lemon or orange juice, exchange that with one-tablespoon of water and 1/3 a teaspoon of ascorbic acid or one crushed 500 mg vitamin C tablet.

- **¾ cup filtered, warmed water (about 105° F) (trace)**
- **2 tablespoons red wine vinegar (5 mg)**
- **2 tablespoons extra virgin olive oil (trace)**
- **1 tablespoon lemon juice (.54 mg)**
- **1 large egg white (54.8 mg)**
- **1 cup whole wheat flour, red or white (6 mg)**
- **1 cup white, unbleached bread flour (2.5 mg)**
- **1 tablespoon vital wheat gluten (2.25 mg)**
- **¼ teaspoon granulated onion powder (.324 mg)**
- **½ cup 10-grain cereal (10 mg)**
- **1 tablespoon plus 1 teaspoon white granulated sugar (trace)**
- **2½ teaspoons bread machine yeast (5 mg)**

Add ingredients to bread machine in order or in your manufacturer's suggested order. Set for whole wheat, medium or light crust. This will make a 1/3 pound to ½ pound loaf.

Cool on rack for about ten minutes before slicing.

10-Grain Whole Wheat Nutrient Data Per Slice: Calories: 127.4, Protein: 3.908 g, Carbohydrate: 18.9 g, Dietary Fiber: 2.162 g, Total Sugars: 1.342 g, Total Fat: 4.223 g, Saturated Fat: .599 g, Monounsaturated Fat: 2.414 g, Polyunsaturated Fat: .968 g, Cholesterol: 0 mg Trans Fatty Acids: 0 g, Total Omega-3 FA: .029 g, Total Omega-6 FA: 0 g, Calcium: 5.343 mg, Potassium: 66.4 mg, Sodium: 6.006 mg, Vitamin K: 1.772 mcg

AVOCADO RANCH DRESSING

VEGAN – 0 CARB CHOICES

Makes 1-cup (16 tablespoons)

Sodium Per Recipe: 87.3 mg Sodium Per Tablespoon 5.454 mg

Easy to make, delicious on salads

¼ cup ripe California avocado (4.6 mg)
¼ cup (plain) Greek yogurt or our Yo Cheese (28.2 mg)
¼ cup sour cream (46 mg)
⅓ teaspoon dried dill weed (.693 mg)
1 tablespoon nonfat milk with Vitamin A (6.426 mg)
¼ teaspoon fresh lemon juice (.076 mg)
1½ teaspoons red wine vinegar (.6 mg)
⅛ teaspoon dried parsley (.282 mg)
¼ teaspoon onion powder (.324 mg)
⅛ teaspoon granulated garlic powder (.091 mg)

In a small mixing bowl, mash the avocado and stir in the yogurt, sour cream and dill week. Stir in the nonfat milk and lemon juice and vinegar. Stir in the parsley, onion powder and garlic powder. Chill before serving.

Avocado Ranch Dressing Nutrient Data Per Tablespoon:Calories: 16.1, Protein: .324 g, Carbohydrate: .742 g, Dietary Fiber: .255 g, Total Sugars: .394 g, Total Fat: 1.39 g, Saturated Fat: .571 g, Monounsaturated Fat: .569 g, Polyunsaturated Fat: .099 g, Cholesterol: 2.386 mg.Trans Fatty Acids: 0 g, Total Omega-3 FA: .016 g, Total Omega-6 FA: .001 g, Calcium: 10.9 mg, Magnesium: 2.175 mg, Potassium: 32.9 mg, Sodium: 5.454 mg, Vitamin K: .882 mcg

GLAZED NUTS

VEGAN – 1 CARB CHOICES
Bread Machine Recipe

Makes About 2-Cups
Sodium Per Recipe: 4.52 mg   Sodium Per 1/4-Cup: .565 mg

We use these for topping salads, ice cream, pies and some muffins or cakes. Wonderful flavor with health benefits from walnuts and pecans. We have not tried this recipe with Splenda yet.

¼ cup filtered water (trace)
¼ cup white granulated sugar (trace)
2 teaspoons Chinese five-spice (ground) (.52 mg)
2 cups unsalted walnuts or pecans (4 mg)[1]

Preheat oven to 375o F. Use parchment paper.

Use a small, heavy saucepan to bring water, sugar and Chinese 5-spice to a boil. Stir in the nuts and simmer, stirring for about a minute. Immediately pour glazed nuts onto the parchment paper and spread nuts into a single layer use a metal (pancake turner 'spatula') to spread.

Bake nuts on center rack in oven for eight-minutes or until they turn a darker color and most of the liquid is gone. Transfer nuts to clean piece of parchment paper making sure they are in a single layer. Cool to room temperature. May store in airtight container for up to two weeks. Use wax paper for layers so that they don't stick together.

[1]2 cups pecans contain 2.2 mg sodium

Glazed Nuts Nutritional Data Per Slice: Calories: 189.3, Protein: 3.833 g, Carbohydrate: 10.2 g, Dietary Fiber: 2.02 g, Total Sugars: 6.911 g, Total Fat: 16.3 g, Saturated Fat: 1.534 g, Monounsaturated Fat: 2.235 g, Polyunsaturated Fat: 11.8 g, Cholesterol: 0 mg, Trans Fatty Acids: 0 g, Total Omega-3 FA: 2.27 g, Total Omega-6 FA: 0 g, Calcium: 31.1 mg, Potassium: 113.2 mg, Sodium: .565 mg, Vitamin K: .878 mcg

SHORTBREAD COOKIES

VEGAN – 1 CARB CHOICES

Makes 16 Sodium Per Recipe: 16.5 mg Sodium Per Cookie: 1.179 mg

When a Megaheart visitor wrote and asked about adjusting a recipe he had for shortbreads, we took a look at it and came up with this cookie. Our visitor said they were to place on a holiday table for guests. Of course we had to "test" them and we have to say, "Yummy." Caution, they do have calories.

1 cup unbleached all-purpose flour (2.5 mg)
½ cup unsalted butter, slightly chilled and sliced (12.5 mg)[1]
¼ cup sugar (trace)
¼ teaspoon, scant, granulated onion powder (.324 mg)
⅓ cup dried cranberries (Craisins)[2] (1.2 mg)

Line a cookie sheet with parchment paper.

Using a food processor, mix the flour, butter, sugar and granulated onion powder for 20 seconds. Add the Craisins or sweetened dried cranberries and pulse until chopped (about 20 seconds). Another way is to place into a deep bowl and mix with hand mixer until crumbly, then roll into ball with your hands. Food processors are nice, but I prefer doing a lot of baking using my hands only.

Place mixture onto a flour dusted work surface and using your hands gather into a smooth, compact ball. Using your hands or a rolling pin, form the dough into a 7 by 9 inch rectangle (approximately), about 1/4 inch thick. Lightly dust with white granulated sugar.

Cut into 14 rectangles. Prick each cookie 3 times with a fork. Using a spatula (pancake turner), place the cookies about 1 inch apart on the prepared cookie sheet and refrigerate for 20 minutes.

Bake until light golden brown (30 minutes). Let cool for 10 minutes before transferring to a rack to cool completely.

[1]Unsalted butter can be replace by using a non-trans fat shortening like Crisco.
[2]May also use dried cherries, blueberries, or raspberries.

Shortbread Cookies Nutritional Data Per Serving: Calories: 113.4, Protein: .998 g, Carbohydrate: 12.8 g, Dietary Fiber: .406 g, Total Sugars: 5.47 g, Total Fat: 6.703 g, Saturated Fat: 4.181 g, Monounsaturated Fat: 1.718 g, Polyunsaturated Fat: .303 g, Cholesterol: 17.4 mg, Trans Fatty Acids: 0 g, Total Omega-3 FA: .054 g, Total Omega-6 FA: .176 g, Calcium: 3.762 mg, Magnesium: 2.322 mg, Potassium: 13.1 mg, Sodium: 1.179 mg, Vitamin K: .705 mcg

FRESH SANDWICH BREAD

VEGAN – 2 CARB CHOICES

Bread Machine Recipe

Makes 1 Loaf (16 slices)

Sodium Per Recipe: 77.5 mg Sodium Per Slice: 4.483 mg

Extra tasty fresh bread is dangerous. My joke around here is take it out of the bread machine run away for a while, think it through and then return, wrap it and pass it along to neighbor. This bread will knock your socks off.

- 1 **cup warmed not from concentrate orange juice (2.48 mg)**
- 2 **tablespoons expeller pressed canola oil (trace)**
- 2 **tablespoons red wine vinegar (2.384 mg)**
- 3 **cups white unbleached bread flour (7.5 mg)**
- 1 **tablespoon vital wheat g, luten (2.958 mg)**
- 3 **vitamin C tablets, crushed (trace)**
- ¼ **teaspoon g, round cinnamon (.065 mg)**
- 3 **tablespoons white g, ranulated sugar (trace)**
- ¼ **teaspoon g, ranulated onion powder (.324 mg)**
- 1 **tablespoon bread machine yeast (6 mg)**

After Kneading

egg white (whisked) (54.8 mg)

tablespoon sesame seeds (.99 mg)

Place all ingredients in bread pan as listed or per manufacturers suggestion. Set machine to 2 pound loaf, medium crust, white bread.

When machine is finished kneading, open lid, and using your hands shape dough evenly in pan for a g, ood rise.

Brush dough with whisked egg white (whisked with a ¼ teaspoon of filtered water). Evenly spread sesame seeds over loaf. Close lid and let machine do the rest.

When done, roll out onto a cooling rack. Slice after ten minutes using a bread knife.

Sandwich Bread Nutritional Data Per Slice: Calories: 126.3, Protein: 3.627, Carbohydrate: 22.4 g, Dietary Fiber: .915 g, Total Sugars: 3.756 g, Total Fat: 2.341 g, Saturated Fat: .226 g, Monounsaturated Fat: 1.176 g, Polyunsaturated Fat: .74 g, Cholesterol: 0 mg, Trans Fatty Acids: .006 g, Total Omega-3 FA: .212 g, Total Omega-6 FA: .402 g, Calcium: 12.9 mg, Magnesium: 10.1 mg, Potassium: 79 mg, Sodium: 4.843 mg, Vitamin K: .839 mcg

THAI BONANZA

FLEXITARIAN – 4.5 CARB CHOICES

Serves 2

Sodium Per Recipe: 299.3 mg Sodium Per Serving: 144.2 mg

You can adjust the flavor of this by cutting back on the vinegar or adding to it.

2 cups cooked fettuccini[1] (6 mg)
2 tablespoons cider or red wine vinegar) (2.384 mg)
½ cup orange juice (1.24 mg)
2 teaspoons brown sugar (2.576 mg)
1 teaspoon cornstarch (.749 mg)
1 tablespoon sesame oil (trace)
6 ounces cooked chicken, cut into bite size pieces[2] (153.4 mg)
2 cloves garlic, minced (1.02 mg)
1 tablespoon fresh ginger, minced (.78 mg)
½ teaspoon red pepper flakes (.27 mg)
2 celery stalks (64 mg)
2 medium carrots (42.1 mg)
2 broccoli florets (7.26 mg)
12 snow peas (1.632 mg)
6 asparagus stalks, cut bite size (1.92 mg)
3 medium mushrooms (about 3 tablespoons) (2.7 mg)
1 tablespoon toasted sliced unsalted almonds (.284 mg)

Mix first 4 ingredients in a small bowl and set aside.

Heat sesame oil in 12-inch fry pan over medium heat and add garlic and ginger. Stir-fry for a minute or until aromatic. Add celery, carrots, broccoli and asparagus. Stir-fry until vegetables turn bright but still crisp. Add mushrooms and snow peas and stir-fry for another 2 minutes.

Remove all vegetables from heat and place in bowl. Then add chicken and rice to same pan and reheat.

When rice and chicken are warm, add vegetables to chicken and rice and reheat if necessary. You may use any fresh vegetables that you enjoy in place of those recommended.

[1]or 1 cup cooked brown rice (1.95 mg) (boil or steam)

[2]Equals about 8-ounces raw chicken (white breast meat)

Nutritional Data on bottom of Next Page

DRIED TOMATO GARNISH

VEGAN - 0 CARB CHOICES

This easy to make garnish offers great flavors for barbecued meats as well as broiled in the oven meat. It also finds its way into burgers or mixed into ground meat before barbecuing burgers. Recipe may be halved or doubled.

Makes 6 Tablespoons

Sodium Per Recipe:7 4 mg   Sodium Per Tablespoon: 12.3 mg

8 dried tomatoes (oil packed)1 (7.36 mg)
3 cloves raw garlic, minced (1.53 mg)
½ small onion, chopped (1.4 mg)
8 button mushrooms, loosely chopped (7.2 mg)
1 tablespoon extra virgin olive oil (trace)

If using dry dried tomatoes then soak in warm water for an hour before using. If using oil packed, then drain the oil from the mushrooms you are using or keep the oil that clicks to the tomatoes and don't use the oil listed above. Chop tomatoes loosely, that is into about 6 chunks for each tomato.

Combine all ingredients and saute together for medium heat for about three to four minutes. Reheat to use and spoon over beef, pork or mix iinto ground turkey or ground beef before cooking patties.

[1]If you can find dried tomatoes not in oil, make sure to check the sodium level. Many non oil packed dried tomatoes are very high in sodium, as much as 45 mg per tomato. Oil-packed are generally smaller and each tomato has about 8 mg of sodium.
Dried Tomato Garnish Nutritional Data per tablespoon: Calories: 39, Protein: 1.104 g, Carbohydrate: 2.761 g, Dietary Fiber: .603 g, Total Sugars: .658 g, Total Fat: 2.991 g, Saturated Fat: .425 g, Monounsaturated Fat: 1.468 g, Polyunsaturated Fat: .891 g, Cholesterol: 0 mg, Trans Fatty Acids: 0 g, Total Omega-3 FA: .014 g, Total Omega-6 FA: 0 g, Calcium: 6.657 mg, Potassium: 153.5 mg, Sodium: 12.3 mg, Vitamin K: .539 mcg

---

Thai Bonanza Nutritional Data per serving with noodles: ***Calories: 603.7, Protein: 41.5 g, Carbohydrate: 69.4 g, Dietary Fiber: 5.668 g, Total Sugars: 15 g, Total Fat: 17.2 g, Saturated Fat: 2.038 g, Monounsaturated Fat: 7.887 g, Polyunsaturated Fat: 5.186 g, Cholesterol: 68.4 mg, Trans Fatty Acids: .029 g, Total Omega-3 FA: .089 g, Total Omega-6 FA: 0 g, Calcium: 121.2 mg, Potassium: 1036 mg, Sodium: 144.2 mg, Vitamin K: 53.6 mcg***

Thai Bonanza Nutritional Data per serving with brown rice: ***Calories: 502.9, Protein: 36.7 g, Carbohydrate: 51.4 g, Dietary Fiber: 7.423 g, Total Sugars: 15 g, Total Fat: 17.2 g, Saturated Fat: 2.199 g, Monounsaturated Fat: 8.18 g, Polyunsaturated Fat: 5.474 g, Cholesterol: 68.4 mg, Trans Fatty Acids: .029 g, Total Omega-3 FA: .102 g, Total Omega-6 FA: 0 g, Calcium: 131 mg, Potassium: 1113 mg, Sodium: 142.1 mg, Vitamin K: 53.6 mcg***

MINT SAUCE

VEGAN – 1 CARB CHOICES
Bread Machine Recipe

Makes 4 servings

Sodium Per Recipe: 160.9 mg   Sodium Per Tablespoon: 1.675 mg

If you want to flavor lamb without using mint jelly, then try this mint sauce. This sauce is a bit different than commercial sauces. Some mint sauces add white pepper, cumin and other spices in order to generate a stronger flavor. This sauce is excellent for lamb because the mint is fresh and you'll taste that more than you will spices. You can replace the vinegar if you like with one tablespoon of fresh lemon juice.

1 cup chopped fresh mint leaves (about one large bunch of fresh mint leaves without stems) (3.98 mg)
2 tablespoons granulated sugar or Splenda Granulated (trace)
1 clove fresh garlic, minced (.51 mg)
1 teaspoon fresh lemon juice[1] (.305 mg)
4 tablespoons red wine vinegar (4.768 mg)
1 cup water (trace)

Wash mint leaves thoroughly. Chop finely.

Put in a medium size stovetop pan with water, vinegar, garlic, sugar. Bring to quick boil, turn heat down to simmer. Add sugar and lemon juice and stir. Let simmer for about ten to twenty minutes until a thick syrupy texture. Add more sugar if you think the sauce is too biting and stir. Let simmer for another minute or two.

Drain through sieve or serve with leaves.

Serve hot or cold with roasted lamb. Works well with other meat roasts such as prime beef or pork tenderloin.

[1]In a pinch, you can use Real Lemon.

Mint Sauce Nutritional Data Per Serving: Calories: 32.5 , Protein: .203 g, Carbohydrate: 7.721 g, Dietary Fiber: .302 g, Total Sugars: 6.485 g, Total Fat: .034 g, Saturated Fat: .009 g, Monounsaturated Fat: .001 g, Polyunsaturated Fat: .018 g, Cholesterol: 0 mg, Trans Fatty Acids: 0 g, Total Omega-3 FA: .014 g, Total Omega-6 FA: 0 g, Calcium: 10.6 mg, Potassium: 36.6 mg, Sodium: 2.388 mg, Vitamin K: .013 mcg

MINT JELLY

VEGAN – 1 CARB CHOICES
Bread Machine Recipe

Makes 6-cups (96 tablespoons)
Sodium Per Recipe: 160.9 mg Sodium Per Tablespoon: 1.675 mg

One of our favorite meat dishes, especially during holidays and birthdays, is leg of lamb. Roasted potatoes, fresh string beans, yams, our Parker House rolls, and a great salad make for a great meal. And, let's not forget the home made mint jelly, a favorite to serve along with the lamb.

2-cups fresh mint leaves, chopped, packed (15.9 mg)

Wash mint leaves and chop, the finer the better. When ready follow instructions below.

4½ cups pure apple juice, unsweetened (44.6 mg)*
8 drops of fresh lemon juice (.117 mg)
1 package of pectin (100 mg)[1]
Optional: 1/3 teaspoon unsalted butter(.133 mg)[2]
4 cups of white granulated sugar[3] (trace)
11 drops green Food Coloring Dye (trace)

Place apple juice into medium size pan with chopped mint leaves. Bring to boil, remove from heat, cover and let stand for ten minutes.

When ready, place sieve over medium to large size bowl, pour contents (mint/apple juice) through sieve. Once liquid has drained, measure 4½-cups into large pot.

Stir in the lemon juice and pectin and unsalted butter. Add 11 drops green food dye at this point and stir. Bring to a rolling boil and add the sugar.

Stir until a rolling boil and boil for one minute only. Remove from heat.

Ladle into prepared half-pint (one cup) canning jars.

Wipe jar top edge with wet towel, place lid on, cap it down tightly and finish other jars. Set aside or into steamer and cover. (Steaming for about ten minutes ensure a very tight seal. Remove and set on countertop for about an hour or so before storing or using.

[1]When using unsweetened apple juice. If you use water instead, then carbohydrates drop enough to place this into a ½ Carb Choices rating.

[2] Butter helps keep the jelly from foaming.

[3] May cut 1 cup of sugar out to reduce calories and carbohydrates.

Mint Jelly Nutritional Data Per Tablespoon: Calories: 39.8, Protein: .034 g, Carbohydrate: 10.2 g, Dietary Fiber: .111 g, Total Sugars: 9.447 g, Total Fat: .032 g, Saturated Fat: .011 g, Monounsaturated Fat: .004 g, Polyunsaturated Fat: .008 g, Cholesterol: .027 mg, Trans Fatty Acids: 0 g, Total Omega-3 FA: .003 g, Total Omega-6 FA: 0 g, Calcium: 2.357 mg, Magnesium: 1.021 mg, Potassium: 15.1 mg, Sodium: 1.675 mg, Vitamin K: .001 mcg

DIPPED STRAWBERRIES

LACTO OVO – 1/2 CARB CHOICES

Makes 24

Sodium Per Recipe: 28.9 mg   Sodium Per Strawberry: 1.205 mg

The easiest way to make chocolate dipped strawberries is to use fresh, juicy strawberries with melted chocolate chips. Yes, it's that easy. You just have to have an audience who wants to help you eat them. Although strawberries by themselves are low in calories, chocolate chips aren't. I like to dip strawberries for guests and grandchildren, but when it's for us, the chocolate coating is kept as thin as it can be, yet still be a treat to eat.

8 ounces semisweet chocolate chips (24.9 mg)
2 tablespoons unsalted butter or non-transfat shortening (trace)[1]
24 medium to large strawberries with stems (3.96 mg)

Prepare with a large Styrofoam sponge or a series of them (like those used for flowers in vases) on hand. We want a toothpick to be able to stick into the sponge to hold the strawberries after dipping.

By stems we mean the star shaped foliage at the top of the strawberry. Stick a toothpick into each berry at the stem.

Melt chocolate chips and unsalted butter or shortening in a double boiler. Stir occasionally or until smooth.

Dip strawberries by holding them with their toothpick. You might discover that the best way to dip these berries, since we aren't creating a bucket full of melted chocolate, is to use a large spoon to scoop chocolate up. Then quickly roll the strawberry in the spoon and insert toothpick into the Styrofoam..

[1]Figures based on non transfat Crisco. Unsalted butter will have 3.124 mg sodium.

Strawberries, Chocolate Dipped, Nutritional Data Per Strawberry using butter:Calories: 90.4, Protein: .944 g, Carbohydrate: 12.8 g, Dietary Fiber: .245 g, Total Sugars: 6.985 g, Total Fat: 4.056 g, Saturated Fat: 2.487 g, Monounsaturated Fat: 1.055 g, Polyunsaturated Fat: .196 g, Cholesterol: 16 mg, Trans Fatty Acids: 0 g, Total Omega-3 FA: .034 g, Total Omega-6 FA: .102 g, Calcium: 10.1 mg, Magnesium: 7.815 mg, Potassium: 48.1 mg, Sodium: 4.028 mg, Vitamin K: .441 mcg

Stawberries, Choclate Dipped, Nutriitonal Data Per Strawberry non transfat shortenting: Calories: 59.7, Protein: .507 g, Carbohydrate: 7.23 g, Dietary Fiber: .888 g, Total Sugars: 5.957 g, Total Fat: 3.885 g, Saturated Fat: 1.93 g, Monounsaturated Fat: 1.366 g, Polyunsaturated Fat: .45 g, Cholesterol: 0 mg, Trans Fatty Acids: 0 g, Total Omega-3 FA: .017 g, Total Omega-6 FA: 0 g, Calcium: 5.664 mg, Potassium: 59.7 mg, Sodium: 1.205 mg, Vitamin K: .892 mcg

MOLASSES COOKIES

LACTO OVO – 1 CARB CHOICES

Makes About 30 to 36 Cookies

Sodium Per Recipe: 145 mg   Sodium Per Cookie: 4.833 mg

This cookie goes back a long way as a favorite. However, the molasses cookies we used to eat had about thirty-six times more sodium in them than these. I've also cut the sugar down. These Molasses cookies have 15.4 carbs (1 Carb Choices) instead of a commercial molasses cookie, which is rated at 23 carbohydrates (2 Carb Choices).

¾ cup unsalted butter, melted (18.7 mg)
½ cup white sugar (trace)
¼ cup packed brown sugar (15.4 mg)
1 large egg (70 mg)
¼ cup molasses (31.2 mg)
2 cups all-purpose flour (5 mg)
4 teaspoons Ener-g baking soda (trace)
1 teaspoon ground cinnamon (.26 mg)
¾ teaspoon ground cloves (3.827 mg)
½ teaspoon ground ginger (.288 mg)
¼ granulated onion powder (.324)
¼ cup white sugar (trace)

In a medium bowl, mix together the melted margarine, 1/2 cup white sugar and ¼ cup brown sugar, and egg until smooth. Stir in the molasses. Set aside the last ingredient in small bowl – the quarter cup of white sugar.

Sift together the flour, baking soda, cinnamon, cloves, and ginger; blend into the molasses mixture. Cover, and chill dough for 1 hour.

Preheat oven to 375° F (190° C). Roll dough into walnut sized balls then roll in the small bowl of sugar, place 2 or 3-inches apart on parchment paper covered cooking sheet and flatten with your hands or the bottom of a measuring cup.

Bake for 8 to 10 minutes in the preheated oven.

Cool on wire racks.

Molasses Cookies Nutritional Data Per Cookies (30): Calories: 108.4, Protein: 1.132 g, Carbohydrate: 15.4 g, Dietary Fiber: .294 g, Total Sugars: 8.383 g, Total Fat: 4.867 g, Saturated Fat: 2.984 g, Monounsaturated Fat: 1.266 g, Polyunsaturated Fat: .236 g, Cholesterol: 19.3 mg, Trans Fatty Acids: 0 g, Total Omega-3 FA: .041 g, Total Omega-6 FA: .123 g, Calcium: 12.1 mg, Magnesium: 9.378 mg, Potassium: 57.7 mg, Sodium: 4.833 mg, Vitamin K: .53 mcg

Molasses Cookies Nutritional Data Per Cookies (36):Calories: 90.4, Protein: .944 g, Carbohydrate: 12.8 g, Dietary Fiber: .245 g, Total Sugars: 6.985 g, Total Fat: 4.056 g, Saturated Fat: 2.487 g, Monounsaturated Fat: 1.055 g, Polyunsaturated Fat: .196 g, Cholesterol: 16 mg, Trans Fatty Acids: 0 g, Total Omega-3 FA: .034 g, Total Omega-6 FA: .102 g, Calcium: 10.1 mg, Magnesium: 7.815 mg, Potassium: 48.1 mg, Sodium: 4.028 mg, Vitamin K: .441 mcg

REAL GOOD PANCAKES

VEGAN[1] – 1 CARB CHOICES

Makes 10

Sodium Per Recipe: 191.2 mg   Sodium Per Strawberry: 23.9 mg

Maureen and I have fooled around with pancake recipes for years. I think you'll like this one. Easy to make, tasty and with no salt and very little sodium.

1 cup all-purpose flour (2.5 mg)
1 cup warmed nonfat milk vitamin A (103 mg)
¼ lemon, juice only (.117 mg)
2 teaspoons Ener-G Baking Powder (9 mg)
1 teaspoon Ener-G Baking Soda (4.5)
1 tablespoon soft unsalted butter (1.562 mg)
1 large egg (70 mg)
⅓ teaspoon granulated onion powder (.432 mg)
½ teaspoon vanilla extract (.189 mg)

Place all ingredients into a small or medium size mixing bowl. Beat together with hand mixer for about two minutes.

Use either a griddle or fry pan over medium to medium-high heat.

If using a cast iron or similar pan or griddle use a spray oil or a dash of extra virgin olive oil or expeller pressed canola oil to grease the surface.

To pour batter for pancake, scoop a full ¼ measuring cup and pour batter over surface. If using a pan with a handle tilt the pan in circle motion to get the batter to expand across the surface. Replace on heat. When bubbles form, flip pancake over and cook for about thirty seconds to a minute.

If using a griddle or other stationary surface, pour the batter our in a circular motion starting with the center and working it outward like a pinwheel.

Serve hot. Top with warmed real maple syrup (not the Log Cabin types, which are high in sodium) and fresh berries like strawberries, blueberries or raspberries. Some like a spoon of sour cream.

1 Vegetarians can replace butter with trans-fat free shortening or 1 tablespoon expeller pressed canola oil.

Real Good Pancakes, Nutriitonal Data Per Pancake: Calories: 92.2, Protein: 3.465 g, Carbohydrate: 14.6 g, Dietary Fiber: .475 g, Total Sugars: 1.754 g, Total Fat: 2.247 g, Saturated Fat: 1.147 g, Monounsaturated Fat: .632 g, Polyunsaturated Fat: .207 g, Cholesterol: 30.9 mg, Trans Fatty Acids: 0 g, Total Omega-3 FA: .02 g, Total Omega-6 FA: .038 g, Calcium: 126.1 mg, Magnesium: 8.377 mg, Potassium: 265.8 mg, Sodium: 23.9 mg, Vitamin K: .194 mcg

PIZZA KIT

LACTO OVO – 1 CARB CHOICES

Makes 8 Servings

Sodium Per Recipe: 300.4 mg Sodium Per Slice: 37.6 mg

This marvelous pizza kit makes eating pizza fun again. It contains the flour mix for the pizza dough and low sodium, no salt added pizza sauce that tastes incredibly like an original Italian sauce. We love it.

The Crust

1 Healthy Heart Market[3] Pizza Kit Package (252 mg)

The Suggested Topping

1 teaspooon extra virgin olive oil (trace)
cup chopped onions, lightly sauteed with garlic
½ (below) (3.2 mg)
cloves garlic, minced (1.53 mg)
3 cup sliced mushrooms (may use more) (2.625 mg)
¾ fresh, thinly sliced tomato (4.55 mg)
1 ounces fresh no-salt mozzarella packed in fresh
4 water[1] (17.9 mg)
small zucchini, thinly sliced (11.8 mg)
1

Follow instructions included with the pizza kit. After making dough you can place on cookie sheet, pizza pan or in an 8 to 9-inch round cake pan. Place dough on parchment paper (highly recommended) and bake for about 5 to ten minutes at package heat. This will ensure that your dough is cooked through after you cook with topping.

Saute onions and garlic in nonstick pan with 1 teaspoon of extra virgin olive oil over medium heat. Saute for only two minutes.

Spread sauce that comes with the kit over the dough. You can sprinkle any spices you like over the sauce at this time.

Layer with vegetables, then spread cheese over top.

Bake at recommended level for time suggested in the kit.

[1]For meat eaters, about 8-ounces of ground meat will work with 4 servings.

[2]Or low sodium cheddar or low-fat, lower sodium Sergento Swiss cheese. Low Sodium cheddar often doesn't cook well. We prefer the mozzarella.

[3]www.healthyheartmarket.com

Pizza Kit Nutritional Data Per Serving (8): Calories: 132.4, Protein: 7.617 g, Carbohydrate: 19.5 g, Dietary Fiber: 2.823 g, Total Sugars: 3.333 g, Total Fat: 2.706 g, Saturated Fat: 1.493 g, Monounsaturated Fat: .667 g, Polyunsaturated Fat: .126 g, Cholesterol: 7.29 mg, Trans Fatty Acids: 0 g, Total Omega-3 FA: .03 g, Total Omega-6 FA: 0 g, Calcium: 106.8 mg, Potassium: 170.8 mg, Sodium: 37.6 mg, Vitamin K: 3.308 mcg

RHUBARB CRISP

VEGAN – 3 CARB CHOICES

Makes 8 Servings

Sodium Per Recipe: 56.6 mg   Sodium Per Tablespoon: 7.073 mg

If you like rhubarb then here's a terrific a flexible dessert. Flexible since you can use any berry fruit you like and even add chopped unsalted walnuts to the topping if you like.

5 cups rhubarb cut into 1" pieces (24.4 mg)
2 cups berries strawberries[1] (3.04 mg)
2/3 cup granulated sugar (trace)
¾ cup water (trace)

Place 4 cups of rhubarb and the berries in a 7x11 or 9" square Pyrex casserole and sprinkle with 1/3 cup of the sugar.

Mix the remaining 1/3 cup sugar with the water in a small pan and cook until the sugar dissolves. Add the remaining cup of rhubarb and cook for about 10 minutes or until the rhubarb can be stirred into a sauce. Remove from heat and cool.

4 tablespoons unsalted butter (softened)[3] (6.248 mg)
1/3 cup brown sugar, packed (15.4 mg)
1/3 cup oats (1.8 mg)
1/3 cup all purpose flour (1.25 mg)
2-3 teaspoons ground cinnamon (.78 mg)[2]

Mix all the ingredients in a small bowl using a pastry blender, fork, or clean hands until well blended.

Pour the sauce evenly over the fresh rhubarb and berries. Sprinkle the topping over all.

Bake at 350° F for 45-55 minutes.

Serve warm or cold. Excellent with whipped cream or vanilla ice cream.

Footnotes:

[1]Exchange with blueberries, raspberries, or cranberries.

[2]Based on 3 teaspoons.

[3] May use trans fat free vegetable shortening for topping.

Nutrient Data Per Serving: Calories: 214, Protein: 2.132 g, Carbohydrate: 39.4 g, Dietary Fiber: 3.165 g, Total Sugars: 28.2 g, Total Fat: 6.363 g, Saturated Fat: 3.749 g, Monounsaturated Fat: 1.625 g, Polyunsaturated Fat: .464 g, Cholesterol: 15.3 mg, Trans Fatty Acids: 0 g, Total Omega-3 FA: .075 g, Total Omega-6 FA: .154 g, Calcium: 93.5 mg, Magnesium: 27.6 mg, Potassium: 315.9 mg, Sodium: 7.073 mg, Vitamin K: 24.1 mcg

SCOTT'S PEACH COBBLER

LACTO OVO – 3 1/2 CARB CHOICES

Serves 6

Sodium Per Recipe: 37.3 mg *Sodium Per Serving: 6.212 mg*

Chef Scott Domeny contributed this no salt, low sodium recipe to Megaheart.com. Scott is a professional chef who also teaches cooking in a local high school. This is one of the best cobblers I've tasted in a very long time.

Peaches

- **4 fresh peaches, pitted and sliced (with skin) (trace)[1]**
- **1 tablespoon cornstarch (.72 mg)**
- **1 tablespoon fresh lemon juice (.153 mg)**
- **¼ cup brown sugar, packed (15.4 mg)**
- **½ teaspoon ground cinnamon (.13 mg)**

Topping

- **1 cup white, unbleached all-purpose flour (2.5 mg)**
- **½ cup white granulated sugar (trace)**
- **2 teaspoons Ener-G Baking Powder (9 mg)**
- **6 tablespoons (¾ stick) unsalted butter (9.372 mg)**
- **¼ cup hot water (about 120° F) (trace)**

In a medium size bowl toss peaches, cornstarch, brown sugar, cinnamon, and lemon juice. Place into 8" x 8" baking dish, (Pyrex or other).

Bake in 425° F oven for ten minutes. Remove, set aside or add topping per instructions below.

Topping

While peaches bake, mix flour, sugar, and baking powder in medium size bowl. Cutin softened butter, mix together with the hot water.

Spoon topping onto peaches and bake in 425° F oven for 25 minutes or until golden brown.

Enjoy!

[1] USDA lists "0" sodium for peaches without skin. They do not list peaches with skin.

Peach Cobbler Nutritional Data Per Serving: Calories: 323.8, Protein: 3.217 g, Carbohydrate: 53.5 g, Dietary Fiber: 2.236 g, Total Sugars: 34.1 g, Total Fat: 12 g, Saturated Fat: 7.348 g, Monounsaturated Fat: 3.071 g, Polyunsaturated Fat: .607 g, Cholesterol: 30.5 mg, Trans Fatty Acids: 0 g, Total Omega-3 FA: .097 g, Total Omega-6 FA: .308 g, Calcium: 94.9 mg, Potassium: 400.7 mg, Sodium: 6.212 mg, Vitamin K: 3.724 mcg

PEANUT BUTTER CUPS

VEGAN – 2 1/2 CARB CHOICES

Makes 24 Cups

Sodium Per Recipe: 101.2 mg   Sodium Per Tablespoon: 4.212 mg

An easy to make replacement for commercial varietis. Works well on Halloween night, too.

24 paper muffin cups
1 1½ pound (24-ounces) milk chocolate chips (74.8 mg)
2 tablespoons unsalted butter (3.124 mg)
½ cup unsalted peanut butter (21.9 mg)
1 cup powdered sugar, not packed (1.2 mg)

Use a mini-muffin pan with mini-muffin cups. The pan's cups should measure about 1.5 to 2" at the top.

Melt 1/2 of the chocolate chips in your microwave. Heat for about one and a half minutes (if you feel more comfortable using a double-boiler then that works well, too). Once chips are soft enough, use an oiled spoon and line the paper cup with chocolate, leaving a bot at the bottom for a think but stronger bottom layer. We're building a wall along the paper cup to hold the peanut butter in. Place cups into the muffin pan. Do this with all the cups for the 24 count pan or if halving this recipe for a twelve-count pan. When done, chill in the refrigerator for about thirty minutes or more.

After the chocolate in the refrigerator has hardened, combine the unsalted peanut butter and unsalted butter and powedered sugar. Heat in microwave for about 30-seconds, or until it's manageble with a spoon. This will not take too much heat. It will not melt, but will become pliable to form using your fingers.

Spoon or using your fingers place an equal amount of the peanut butter mix into each chocolate coated cup. Save room for the top layer of melted chocolate after we harden the peanut butter mix in the fridge for half and hour or more.

After the peanut butter hardens, melt the second half of chocolate and use a spoon to spread it evenly across the top of the peanut butter cups.

Chill the cups one more time to set the chocolate.

Peanut Butter Cup Nutritional Data Per Cup: Calories: 195.3, Protein: 2.549 g, Carbohydrate: 23.9 g, Dietary Fiber: 1.995 g, Total Sugars: 20.8 g, Total Fat: 12.2 g, Saturated Fat: 6.194 g, Monounsaturated Fat: 4.35 g, Polyunsaturated Fat: 1.058 g, Cholesterol: 2.544 mg, Trans Fatty Acids: 0 g, Total Omega-3 FA: .031 g, Total Omega-6 FA: .026 g, Calcium: 11.7 mg, Potassium: 138.7 mg, Sodium: 4.212 mg, Vitamin K: 1.703 mcg

WHOLE WHEAT with ORANGE

VEGAN – 1 CARB CHOICES

Bread Machine Recipe

Makes One Loaf (16 slices)

Sodium Per Recipe: 76.2 mg   Sodium Per Tablespoon: 4.761 mg

This bread is made in the bread machine. It 's exceptionally tasty and since white whole wheat as the same nutrient values as red whole wheat, it's just as nutritious, but easier to bake.

1 cup filtered, warm water (about 105° F) (trace)
2 tablespoons extra virgin olive oil (trace)
2 table spoons apple cider vinegar (1.49 mg)
½ orange, diced (1.59 mg)
½ orange peel, grated (included above)
2¾ cups white whole wheat flour (16.5 mg)
3 tablespoons vital wheat gluten (6.75 mg)
½ teaspoon granulated onion powder (.389 mg)
½ teaspoon ascorbic acid (trace)
2 tablespoons granulated sugar[1] (trace)
1 tablespoon bread machine yeast (6 mg)

Place ingredients into bread pan in the order your manual calls for. Bake on medium crust, two pound loaf setting. Remove to rack, let cool for about ten minutes before slicing. Store in zip lock bag or other airtight container. Will freeze for up to a month, if you don't eat it all the first day. ☺

[1]For this bread you can use the half/half mix of Splenda Granulated/granulated white sugar

White Whole Wheat Bread Per Slice:Calories: 102.4, Protein: 4.26 g, Carbohydrate: 17.9 g, Dietary Fiber: 2.9 g, Total Sugars: 1.682 g, Total Fat: 2.147 g, Saturated Fat: .306 g, Mono-unsaturated Fat: 1.301 g, Polyunsaturated Fat: .341 g, Cholesterol: 0 mg, Trans Fatty Acids: 0 g, Total Omega-3 FA: .021 g, Total Omega-6 FA: 0 g, Calcium: 11.3 mg, Potassium: 110.1 mg, Sodium: 2.079 mg, Vitamin K: 1.41 mcg

AROMATIC TOMATO RICE SOUP

VEGAN – 1 CARB CHOICES

Serves 8

Sodium Per Recipe: 140.3 mg   Sodium Per Tablespoon: 17.5 mg

Another excellent soup from Maureen. This makes a pot full of soup that keeps well in the refrigerator. For us it equals four dinners. Great when you want to take a week off from preparing evening meals, and especially good when tomatoes are plentiful in season.

1 tablespoon extra virgin olive oil (trace)
½ cup garlic cloves, chopped[1] (11.6 mg)
1 small onion, chopped (2.8 mg)
2½ cups fresh, seeded tomatoes (22.5 mg)
4 cups Maureen's Chicken Broth[4] (91.2 mg)
⅓ cup long grain rice, raw (4.312 mg)
3 tablespoons fresh parsley, chopped (6.384 mg)
½ teaspoon dried oregano (.075 mg)[2]
½ teaspoon ground thyme or savory (.275 mg)
1 tablespoon red wine vinegar (1.192 mg)
¼ cup red wine (trace)[3]

In a medium size soup pot, sauté onion and garlic.

Add tomatoes and broth, bring to a boil.

Add rice and fresh parsely and dried herbs. Turn down to a simmer, cover and cook for 15-minutes.

Remove cover, add vinegar and wine and cook for another 5-minutes.

Serve hot. If you like, serve a dollop of sour cream or a sprinkle of low sodium cheese and a few drops of fresh lemon juice.

[1] Measured before mincing. Approximately 3 medium size garlic flowers.

[2] Or use 1½ teaspoons of fresh chopped oregano.

[3] Either with or without alcohol (alcohol will burn off during cooking).

[4] Or use Swanson Unsalted Chicken Broth or other brands of unsalted chicken broth available to you. Add 12 mg sodium per serving.

Tomato Rice Soup Nutritional Data Per Serving: Calories: 99, Protein: 3.134 g, Carbohydrate: 13.7 g, Dietary Fiber: 1.714 g, Total Sugars: 2.648 g, Total Fat: 3.122 g, Saturated Fat: .602 g, Monounsaturated Fat: 1.331 g, Polyunsaturated Fat: .945 g, Cholesterol: 5.648 mg, Trans Fatty Acids: 0 g, Total Omega-3 FA: .03 g, Total Omega-6 FA: 0 g, Calcium: 35.5 mg, Magnesium: 24.4 mg, Potassium: 258.1 mg, Sodium: 17.5 mg, Vitamin K: 31.8 mcg

WEEDEATER SALAD

VEGAN – CARB CHOICES
Bread Machine Recipe
Serves 2 to 4
Sodium Per Recipe: 63 mg Sodium Per Serving (2): 31.5 mg

Before heart failure I had a large piece of property I cared for in my "spare" time. I owned 3 weed-eaters - each one different for a specific type of weed. The grass would fly along with the bushes, brush and weeds. Piles of this stuff would be stacked for hauling away. After about twenty years of this, my wife started showing up at home with these small plastic bags of pre-washed salad makings. We used to buy lettuce, now we were getting all this weird looking stuff that reminded me of what I weeded every week. But looks aren't everything as they say. Softer greens with a mixed variety of various names and appearances from stringy to purple arrived at my dinner each night. The bags had names like "Palm Beach," "Pacific Paradise," etc. At first it was tough to dive into it. I joked "What's this? A weed-eater salad?" Well, here it is for you, too. Why should I be the only one to enjoy this delicious treat.

3 cups of mixed greens for salad (41.9 mg)
2 tablespoons raspberry vinegar (.3 mg)
1 tablespoon extra virgin olive oil (trace)
½ teaspoon white granulated sugar (or to taste) (.021 mg)
½ California Avocado (or whole if small), sliced[1] (20.8 mg)

Don't trust the pre-wash in the salad mix bag. Wash it again and spin dry it. Wash the avocado skin, peel the avocado and slice it length wise getting about 4 to 5 slices per quarter.

Combine the vinegar, oil and sugar and dribble over the mixed greens. Toss the salad. Chill or serve immediately.

[1]Optional. Also works with fresh mandarin slices, papaya, or mango.
[2] We have calculated the fiber in the recipe into the Carb Choices.

Weedeater Salad Nutritional Data Per Serving (2): Calories: 233.1, Protein: 3.152 g, Carbohydrate: 10.4 g, Dietary Fiber: 5.641 g, Total Sugars: 1.039 g, Total Fat: 21.9 g, Saturated Fat: 3.179 g, Monounsaturated Fat: 14.7 g, Polyunsaturated Fat: 2.435 g, Cholesterol: 0 mg, Calcium: 55.6 mg, Potassium: 824.8 mg, Sodium: 31.5 mg, Vitamin K: 3.308 mcg, Folate: 152 mcg

Weedeater Salad Nutritional Data Per Serving (4):Calories: 116.6, Protein: 1.576 g, Carbohydrate: 5.177 g, Dietary Fiber: 2.821 g, Total Sugars: .52 g, Total Fat: 11 g, Saturated Fat: 1.589 g, Monounsaturated Fat: 7.34 g, Polyunsaturated Fat: 1.217 g, Cholesterol: 0 mg, Calcium: 27.8 mg, Potassium: 412.4 mg, Sodium: 15.7 mg, Vitamin K: 1.654 mcg

CREATIVE SALAD DRESSING

VEGAN – ½ CARB CHOICES
Bread Machine Recipe

Makes 16 tablespoons

Sodium Per Recipe: 50.7 mg   Sodium Per Tablespoon: 3.171 mg

This is one you can play with. Adjust the quantities of each or all of the ingredients until you get to the flavor you like the best. Works well with any lettuce salad. Add walnuts or raisins or onion slices to make it even more exciting.

½ cup white balsamic vinegar (1.2 mg)
½ cup extra virgin olive oil (trace)
¼ cup packed brown sugar (15.4 5mg)
1 tablespoon fresh rosemary (.442 mg)
4 cloves garlic, minced (2.04 mg)
1 fresh lemon, juice from (.47 mg)
¼ cup cranberry raisins (.3 mg)

Blend together in a food processor, store in refrigerator.

Creative Salad Dressing Nutritional Data Per Tablespoon:Calfories: 87.5, Protein: .107 g, Carbohydrate: 6.797 g, Dietary Fiber: .149 g, Total Sugars: 5.823 g, Total Fat: 6.786 g, Saturated Fat: .938 g, Monounsaturated Fat: 4.93 g, Polyunsaturated Fat: .725 g, Cholesterol: 0 mg, Trans Fatty Acids: 0 g, Total Omega-3 FA: .053 g, Total Omega-6 FA: 0 g, Calcium: 7.16 mg, Potassium: 21.7 mg, Sodium: 3.171 mg, Vitamin K: 4.148 mcg

DON'S APPLE PIE

VEGAN[1] – 2 ½CARB CHOICES

Serves 8

Sodium Per Recipe: 72.97 mg Sodium Per Serving: 9.113 mg

This is a variation of my Apple Pie Supreme. I like the grated lemon peel and have posted this without it and with it. Now, I suggest it's optional, but please give it a try. The lemon peel adds the zest that salt once gave.

1 - 9" uncooked 2 - crust pie shell (next page) (24 mg)
6 to 8 large apples, unpeeled (0 mg)
2 tablespoons fresh lemon juice (.305 mg)
1 teaspoon lemon peel, grated (.12 mg)
½ unpacked cup brown sugar (28.3 mg)
1½ teaspoons cinnamon (1 mg)
⅓ teaspoon nutmeg (.117 mg)
¼ teaspoon ground cloves (1.276 mg)
1 tablespoon cornstarch (.72 mg)
1 teaspoon sugar (trace)
1 tablespoon nonfat milk (7.879 mg)

Core and thinly slice apples. Toss with lemon juice and grated lemon peel if using it. Mix in sugar, cornstarch and spices. Toss with apples to coat.

Roll half of dough into a round and fit into a 9" pie pan. Fill shell with apple mixture. (Roll remaining dough into a round large enough to cover top of apples. Roll up on roller, then unroll over pie filling carefully. Crimp edges of crusts together. Make slits in top crust to vent. Mix teaspoon of sugar with a dash of cinnamon and brush top of crust with tablespoon of milk and sprinkle lightly with cinnamon sugar.

Bake at 450° F for 10 minutes. Reduce heat to 375° F and bake an additional 20-30 minutes. To prevent black or burned edge crust, cut out 1" inch strips of aluminum foil, link together and lightly grease. Wrap this longer strip around the pie for the first 20 minutes. Remove last 20 minutes and continue to cook.

Don's Apple Pie Nutritional Data Per Slice:Calories: 391.8, Protein: 3.837 g, Carbohydrate: 56.7 g, Dietary Fiber: 3.826 g, Total Sugars: 27.2 g, Total Fat: 17.8 g, Saturated Fat: 11 g, Monounsaturated Fat: 4.514 g, Polyunsaturated Fat: .838 g, Cholesterol: 45.8 mg, Trans Fatty Acids: 0 g, Total Omega-3 FA: .154 g, Total Omega-6 FA: .461 g, Calcium: 36.5 mg, Potassium: 189.5 mg, Sodium: 9.113 mg, Vitamin K: 4.227 mcg

2 - CRUST PIE SHELLS

VEGAN – **2** CARB CHOICES

Serves 8

Sodium Per Recipe: 24 mg   Sodium Per Tablespoon: 3.004 mg

Sodium for this crust recipe is already included in the apple pie figures.

- **2 cups white, unbleached all purpose flour (5 mg)**
- **¾ cup unsalted butter (room temperature)* (18.7mg)**
- **1 tablespoon sugar (trace)**
- **2 tablespoons lemon juice (.3mg)**
- **½ cup lukewarm water (0mg)**

In a medium or large bowl, combine the flour and butter. Stir in the water with a fork until all is mixed. If too sticky afterwards, add a bit of flour. Roll up with your hands until just right. Set in refrigerator while preparing apple pie mix. If you want a cooked shell, bake at 425oF for about 10 minutes.

Roll out the dough on your board until it will fit into the pie pan. Use glass pie pan, not metal. Roll crust up on roller, lay over the pan and unroll it to fit. Crimp the edges. Pour pie ingredients into shell until brimming at edges. (If any left over, you can roll out the remaining shell dough and make smaller tarts in your kitchen counter baker oven). Sprinkle individual recipe's topping over the top of the pie. Roll second crust, crimp edges around pie and bake according to individual recipe's instructions.

[1]Vegans may exchange transfat free shortening for butter (in crust) and water for the milk in the pie. If using the butter, then recipe is classifed Lacto Vegetarian.

2 Crust Pie Shells Nutritional Data Per Serving (8):Calories: 273.4, Protein: 3.424 g, Carbohydrate: 25.8 g, Dietary Fiber: .859 g, Total Sugars: 1.762 g, Total Fat: 17.6 g, Saturated Fat: 11 g, Monounsaturated Fat: 4.501 g, Polyunsaturated Fat: .777 g, Cholesterol: 45.8 mg, Trans Fatty Acids: 0 g, Total Omega-3 FA: .141 g, Total Omega-6 FA: .461 g, Calcium: 10.1 mg, Potassium: 43.3 mg, Sodium: 3.004 mg, Vitamin K: 1.583 mcg

MUSTARD & GARLIC COATED PORK TENDERLOINS

FLEXITARIAN – 0 CARB CHOICES

Serves 8

Sodium Per Recipe: 451 mg   Sodium Per Serving: 56.4mg

This southern recipe came to me from a Nashville friend. It's easy to prepare, punches up the palate with mustard and garlic to make it one of the tastiest pork meals you'll ever enjoy. Tenderloins usually come two to a package. If you want to cook only one and freeze one, then this recipe may be cut in half.

2 pork tenderloins, up to about 1 pound each (446.4 mg)
1 teaspoon extra virgin olive oil (trace)
3 tablespoons Westbrae Natural Stoneground Mustard[1] (1.12 mg)
5 cloves garlic, finely minced (2.55 mg)
1 teaspoon dried savory (.336 mg)
1 teaspoon dried thyme leaves (.55 mg)
1 Pinch of white pepper (trace)

Preheat oven to 375°.

Line a 13 x 9 inch baking pan with parchment paper.

In a small bowl, stir together the olive oil, mustard, garlic, savory, thyme and pepper. Using a basting brush, spread the mix over the two tenderloins covering all sides (top, sides, bottom).

Roast for 45 to 55 minutes. A meat thermometer inserted in thickest part of loin should read 155° F or higher.

Serve hot.

[1] Available at Healthy Heart Market online. No Salt Added mustard. http://healthyheartmarket.com/westbraenaturalstonegroundmustard.aspx

Mustard & Garlic Coated Pork Tenderloins Nutritional Data Per Serving:Calories: 155.5, Protein: 23 g, Carbohydrate: 1.811 g, Dietary Fiber: .582 g, Total Sugars: .211 g, Total Fat: 5.748 g, Saturated Fat: 1.479 g, Monounsaturated Fat: 2.457 g, Polyunsaturated Fat: 1.229 g, Cholesterol: 69.8 mg, Trans Fatty Acids: .039 g, Total Omega-3 FA: .114 g, Total Omega-6 FA: .512 g, Calcium: 30.6 mg, Potassium: 451.2 mg, Sodium: 56.4 mg, Vitamin K: 2.479 mcg

APPLESAUCE ala CROCKPOT

VEGAN[1] – 2 CARB CHOICES

Serves 10

Sodium Per Recipe: 18.7 mg   Sodium Per Serving: 1.868 mg

Here's an idea that works. Applesauce in a crockpot. No stirring, no hot burner involved, no pots and pans to clean up, yet a great side dish for meals, especially when serving barbecued ribs or a pork roast or chops. Want it done when you come home from work?

Well try our wall mounted timer to turn your pot on for the three to four hours needed. Time it for your arrival. Applesauce stores well in the fridge and can easily be canned (Mason jars).

10 fresh medium (3") Granny Smith, Fuji, crisp Golden Delicious or your favorite sauce apples, cored, sliced into bite size pieces, skin on (18.2 mg)
½ cup plus 2-tablespoons white granulated sugar (trace)
1½ teaspoons ground cinnnamon[1] (.325 mg)
½ cup filtered water[2] (trace)
1 teaspoon fresh lemon juice (.153 mg)

Place into Crockpot and turn on high. Should be ready in three to four hours.

For Saucepan Cooking

In a medium to large saucepan, combine apples, sugar, and cinnamon, and "toss." Add only ½ cup water and start cooking with medium heat. Stir occasionally. If ½ cup of water works well (apples will release water when cooking) then don't add the rest. If you need more, add it slowly.

Increase heat to medium high and bring to a boil, stirring about every two or three minutes. When apples boil, stir for one minute and turn heat off. Let sit for a few minutes then pour into bowl and let cool.

[1] More if you like a lot of cinnamon.

[2] Juicy apples will need only the ½ cup. Drier apples might need a bit more.

Crockpot Applesauce Nutritional Data Per Slice: Calories: 134.5, Protein: .492 g, Carbohydrate: 35.5 g, Dietary Fiber: 4.547 g, Total Sugars: 28.9 g, Total Fat: .313 g, Saturated Fat: .052 g, Monounsaturated Fat: .014 g, Polyunsaturated Fat: .093 g, Cholesterol: 0 mg, Trans Fatty Acids: 0 g, Total Omega-3 FA: .016 g, Total Omega-6 FA: 0 g, Calcium: 14.4 mg, Potassium: 198.2 mg, Sodium: 1.868 mg, Vitamin K: 4.105 mcg

MUSHROOM SAUCE

LACTO OVO – 0 CARB CHOICES

Makes 1 3/4 Cups

Sodium Per Recipe: 227.6 mg   Sodium Per Tablespoon: 9.48 mg

Sometimes a good crockpot recipe calls for a good sauce. In this caes the sauce is "great." Maureen came up with this after days of experimenting with an uncomplaining crockpot. She wanted a sauce that would not curdle while spending a day with check thighs or pork. The sauce is made quickly and the dinner late in the day proves its value. Also very tasty with pasta such as fettuccini or spaghetti

.

The Sauce

1 tablespoon olive oil (trace)
6–8 ounces sliced crimini mushrooms (10 mg)
1 tablespoon unsalted butter (1.562 mg)
1 tablespoon flour (.156 mg)
¼ cup nonfat milk (25.7 mg)
¼ cup Maureen's Chicken broth or, other unsalted broth or filtered water, or white cooking wine[1]. (7 mg)[2]

Use Below Just Before Adding Meat

1 cup of sour cream (184 mg)
2 tablespoons flour (.312 mg)

Heat oil in saucepan (low to medium heat). Add mushrooms and stir until they begin to lose their raw color. Place lid on pan and turn down heat if necessary. The juice from the mushrooms will release inabout 3-5 minutes.

Melt butter in another small saucepan. Add flour, stir until mixture begins to bubble. Lower heat and cook for an additional minute. Remove pan from heat and add milk and other liquid[1]

Stir until well blended and mixture comes to a boil and thickens. Add mushrooms and liquid to the mixture and blend.

[1]If you use wine, the milk will begin to curdle but will become smooth as you stir.

[2]Average sodium level for each ingredient. A good swap is Swanson Usalted Chicken Broth or Progresso's unsalted broth.

Mushroom Sauce Nutritional Data Per Tablespoon: Calories: 34.6, Protein: .585 g, Carbohydrate: 1.459 g, Dietary Fiber: .074 g, Total Sugars: .597 g, Total Fat: 2.993 g, Saturated Fat: 1.5 g, Monounsaturated Fat: .9 g, Polyunsaturated Fat: .303 g, Cholesterol: 6.424 mg, Trans Fatty Acids: 0 g, Total Omega-3 FA: .024 g, Total Omega-6 FA: .015 g, Calcium: 15.4 mg, Potassium: 49.7 mg, Sodium: 9.485 mg, Vitamin K: .381 mcg

MUSHROOM SOUP

LACTO OVO – 1 CARB CHOICES

Makes 3-cups

Sodium Per Recipe: 164.2 mg Sodium Per Cup: 54.7 mg

This soup also works well with our green bean casserole dish. When serving as a meal, you can double the recipe. You can also add more mushrooms if you like or lower the amount listed, but I wouldn't go below 8-ounces of mushrooms.

12 ounces fresh (your) favorite mushrooms, chopped (17.5 mg)
2 tablespoons Spanish or white onions, chopped (.4 mg)
2 garlic cloves, minced (1.02 mg)
1 tablespoon unsalted butter (1.562 mg)[1]
3 tablespoons all-purpose flour (separated)[2] (.417 mg)
2 cups Maureen's Chicken Broth (43.4 mg)[3]
1 cup half and half or light cream (99.2 mg)
¼ teaspoon granulated onion powder (.324 mg)
¼ teaspoon white pepper (.03 mg)
⅓ teaspoon ground nutmeg (.088 mg)
½ teaspoon ground coriander seed (.315 mg)
1 tablespoon chives, chopped (.09 mg)

Chop or slice mushrooms into your favorite size or shape. Chop onions, mince garlic.

In a large nonstick 2 or 4-quart skillet, add olive oil, the onions, garlic and mushrooms. Stir over medium heat until onions are translucent or soft.

Keep stirring and slowly add the two tablespoons of the flour.

Add in Maureen's Chicken Broth and while stirring heat until the soup thickens slightly Stir in the milk or half and half with the last tablespoon of flour. Season with pepper, nutmeg and the dash of mace.

Continue stirring until its warm to serve or use in another recipe. May store in fridge for a day or so, covered. Reheat to serve or use. Garnish with the chives.

[1] If using a skillet that is not nonstick, then add one more tablespoon of unsalted butter for the sautéing.

[2] To help make the soup "thicker," you can replace one tablespoon of flour with one-tablespoon of cornstarch.

[3] You may want to add another ½ cup of broth before stirring down over heat. Or use Swanson or Progresso unsalted chicken broth. Add 12 mg sodium per serving.

Cream of Mushroom Soup Nutritional Data Per Serving: Calories: 224.5, Protein: 8.792 g, Carbohydrate: 16.3 g, Dietary Fiber: 2.146 g, Total Sugars: 3.218 g, Total Fat: 15 g, Saturated Fat: 8.691 g, Monounsaturated Fat: 4.213 g, Polyunsaturated Fat: .981 g, Cholesterol: 47.6 mg, Trans Fatty Acids: 0 g, Total Omega-3 FA: .185 g, Total Omega-6 FA: .103 g, Calcium: 108 mg, Potassium: 568.6 mg, Sodium: 54.7 mg, Vitamin K: 3.275 mcg

CROCKPOT CHICKEN
with Mushroom Sauce

FLEXITARIAN – 0 CARB CHOICES

Serves 4 to 6

Sodium Per Recipe: 541.6 mg Sodium Per Serving (6): 90.3 mg

Use the Mushroom Sauce on the previous page to make this delicious dinner entree. Add a vegetable or salad and Voila! A day at a work with dinner waiting.

8 chicken thighs, boneless, skinless (282.1 mg)
1¾ cups Mushroom Sauce (Previous page) 227.6 mg)
4 cups, cooked yolk less Fettucini noodles[1] (31.9 mg)

Place meat in crockpot and cover with sauce. Cook on low for 7 hrs.or high for 4 hrs.

Mix the sour cream and 2-tablespoons flour together.

Remove meat, keeping it warm.

Stir the sour cream mixture into the sauce in the crockpot. Turn the crock-pot on high, cover and cook for another 30-45 minutes until sauce thickens.

Serve sauce over the chicken or the pork with half cup of rice or noodles.

[1]Egg noodles may be all you can find. They work well. Yolkless noodles lower cholesterol levels in noodles.

Crockpot Chicken with Mushroom Sauce Nutritonal Data: Calories: 300.5, Protein: 16.7 g, Carbohydrate: 23.9 g, Dietary Fiber: 1.133 g, Total Sugars: 2.864 g, Total Fat: 15.2 g, Saturated Fat: 6.846 g, Monounsaturated Fat: 4.578 g, Polyunsaturated Fat: 2.078 g, Cholesterol: 92.3 mg, Trans Fatty Acids: .073 g, Total Omega-3 FA: .182 g, Total Omega-6 FA: .06 g, Calcium: 75.8 mg, Potassium: 387 mg, Sodium: 90.3 mg, Vitamin K: 3.237 mcg

PASTA RECIPE

VEGAN – 1 CARB CHOICES

Makes 13.25 ounces[1]

Sodium Per Recipe: 166.8 mg   Sodium Per Ounce: 12.6 mg

There are various ways to make your own pasta. Some are complicated while some are not so difficult. Using a pasta maker is a good idea if you have the equipment to do so. But for a lasgna or even some noodles that taste exceptionally fresh and delightful, you can do it with a rolling pin and a sharp knife. This is a rolling-pin recipe. Pasta by the way, does not "need" salt. So, we are ahead of the game right from the kick off. You can also make pasta with just eggs and flour. However, we are excluding the cholesteral heavy yolks in this recipe. Yolks generally offer a "softer" pasta, but adding olive oil works well to replace the yolks.

1½ cups semolina flour[2] 2.505 mg)
3 egg whites, beaten (164.3 mg)
2 tablespoons filtered water (trace)
2 tablespoons extra virgin olive oil (trace)

Semolina makes a "grain texture" pasta. For a silkier pasta, use all-purpose flour as written in the footnotes.[2]

Combine ingredients in a medium bowl or use your processor with a bread paddle. If in a bowl, mix together and then ball with your hands. With a processor pulse it a few times until dough is combined. Remove and ball with your hands. Cover with a light towel for about 25 minutes and then roll it out on a lightly floured board to the thickness (or thinness) you want. It will get thicker as it boils. Press hard on the rolling pin.

If using for lasagna, you do not have to boil it. Otherwise boil for about 12 to 15 minutes or until tender. Serve hot. A nice quick sauce is a combination of fresh lemon juice, mincded garlic and olive oil

Pasta usually measures one cup of cooked noodles per each 2-ounces. Double recipe to make one 9" x 13" lasgna with triple layers.

[2]You can use 1 1/2 cups all-purpose unbleached flour or white pastry flour instead. Use two egg whites and one yolk, 2 teaspoons olive oil and begin with a 1/4 cup of filtered water. Knead by hand or in a processor.

Calories: 90.3, Protein: 3.212 g, Carbohydrate: 13.8 g, Dietary Fiber: .737 g, Total Sugars: .053 g, Total Fat: 2.324 g, Saturated Fat: .332 g, Monounsaturated Fat: 1.038 g, Polyunsaturated Fat: .779 g, Cholesterol: 0 mg, Trans Fatty Acids: 0 g, Total Omega-3 FA: .016 g, Total Omega-6 FA: 0 g, Calcium: 3.737 mg, Potassium: 47.3 mg, Sodium: 12.6 mg, Vitamin K: .444 mcg

HALF & HALF BREAD

Bread Machine Recipe

VEGAN – 1 CARB CHOICES

Makes One Loaf

Sodium Per Recipe: 25.3 mg   Sodium Per Slice (16): 1.58 mg

When a visitor to Megaheart wanted a whole wheat bread she could make in her bread machine, but also said some white flour was okay, we came up with this one. And it's a beauty. Try it out, we think you'll like it. P. S. You can add a tablespoon of flaxseed if you want a bit more fiber.

1 cup, less 1-tablespoon filter, warmed water (trace)
2 tablespoons red wine vinegar (2.384 mg)
2 tablespoons extra virgin olive oil (trace)
1½ cups best for bread flour (3.75 mg)
1½ cups white whole wheat flour[1] (9 mg)
2 tablespoons vital wheat gluten (4.5 mg)
2 crushed 500 mg Vit. C tablet,
or 1/8 teaspoon ascorbic acid (trace)
1 tablespoon sugar (trace)
¼ teaspoon granulated onion powder (.324 mg)
2½ teaspoons bread machine yeast (5 mg)

Place ingredients in your bread pan in order listed or the order your bread machine manufactures lists. Keep sugar and yeast apart from each other. Set machine on whole wheat, 1.5 pounds light or medium crust. (Medium crust will be a bit crunchier.)

Enjoy!

[1]Vegans may exchange transfat free shortening for butter (in crust) and water for the milk in the pie. If using the butter, then recipe is classifed Lacto Vegetarian.

Half & Half Bread Nutritional Data Per Slice:Calories: 105.5, Protein: 3.718 g, Carbohydrate: 18.4 g, Dietary Fiber: 1.824 g, Total Sugars: .891 g, Total Fat: 2.12 g, Saturated Fat: .31 g, Monounsaturated Fat: .893 g, Polyunsaturated Fat: .715 g, Cholesterol: 0 mg, Trans Fatty Acids: 0 g, Total Omega-3 FA: .014 g, Total Omega-6 FA: 0 g, Calcium: 6.375 mg, Potassium: 72.1 mg, Sodium: 1.58 mg, Vitamin K: .619 mcg

SMOKED FOWL

FLEXITARIAN – 1½ CARB CHOICES
Serves 2

Sodium Per Recipe: 288.3 mg   Sodium Per Serving (6): 144.2 mg

When I asked my absolutely favorite chef, Scott Leysath if we could smoke or brine fowl (ducks, chicken, turkey and other game birds) he replied with how and why. Below are his instructions for brining and then smoking a bird. Scott has a TV show and his sense of humor shows through here as well.

The No-Salt Brining Process:

You can smoke anything without a brine and it'll taste just fine. I use brine more often with poultry and game birds, as much to get the blood out as to add some flavor. It will pass through a chicken, turkey, duck, etc. and exchange blood with brine. For a good no-salt brine, submerge your birds in a bucket of filtered water seasoned with garlic powder, onion powder, Italian seasonings, in a refrigerator overnight. It won't have the same cook-time effect as brining with salt, but it will add flavor and moisture.

The No-Salt Smoker Process

Once your bird is "brined" pat dry and rub with extra virgin olive oil and your favorite seasonings. Smoke at 225 degrees until internal temperature is 165 -175 degrees. Meat won't be "cured," so you'll have to refrigerate or freeze it as you would any other cooked meat. It will taste great.

See Smoked Salmon, next page.

SMOKED SALMON

FLEXITARIAN – **0** CARB CHOICES

Fish Size: 3 pounds

Sodium Per Recipe: 20 mg Sodum Added Per Ounce: .417 mg

This recipe is from Scott Leysath, *The Sporting Chef*

The Rub

1/2 cup extra virgin olive oil (trace)
2 tablespoons fresh lemon juice (.305 mg)
1/4 teaspoon (or more to taste) cracked black pepper (.231 mg)
1 teaspoon Trader Joe's 21 Seasoning Salute[1] (trace)
8 cloves garlic, minced (4.08 mg)
1/4 cup brown sugar, packed (15.4 mg)
Option: Cayenne Pepper if you want to balance the sugar for a sweet&hot flavor. (trace)

Combine olive oil, lemon juice, cracked black pepper, minced garlic, spice mix, and brown sugar.

You can also add something spicy (like chili powder or cayenne) to balance the sugar, if you like it sweet-hot. Let the olive oil mixture sit at room temp for at least an hour so that the flavors blend together. You could even heat it over low heat and then let it cool for a while.

For the salmon, remove the skin and any of the dark/gray funk on the skin side of the fillet. Place the fillet on a large piece of plastic wrap. Rub the olive oil mixture over both sides of the fish and wrap with the plastic wrap. Refrigerate for 6 - 12 hours.

Pat fish down to remove excess, season some more with the dry no-salt seasoning and smoke in a 160 degree smoker for 2 hours then increase heat to 250 degrees and smoke for 1 hour more or until just done, but not dry.

Oh yeah...and they still have to be frozen since they're not preserved, but frozen salmon is easy to work with and assuming that you don't refreeze it, you can do anything with it you do with "regular" smoked salmon. I freeze my smoked salmon all the time.

[1]Trader Joe's blend is similar to other multi-spice blends from Costco, McCormick and other spice makers. Make sure the one you buy does not have salt added.

Smoked Salmon Nutritional Data Per Ounce: Calories: Calories: 25.9, Protein: .037 g, Carbohydrate: 1.351 g, Dietary Fiber: .016 g, Total Sugars: 1.132 g, Total Fat: 2.336 g, Saturated Fat: .336 g, Monounsaturated Fat: 1.121 g, Polyunsaturated Fat: .772 g, Cholesterol: 0 mg, Trans Fatty Acids: 0 g, Total Omega-3 FA: .01 g, Total Omega-6 FA: 0 g, Calcium: 1.948 mg, Potassium: 4.455 mg, Sodium: .417 mg, Vitamin K: .516 mcg

APPLE GLAZED STUFFED CHICKEN

FLEXITARIAN – 2½ CARB CHOICES

Serves 4

Sodium Per Recipe: 404.9 mg Sodium Per Serving: *101.2* ***mg***

Many years ago when I traveled a great deal in my work I was able to take Maureen to Sun Valley, Idaho to a convention that included many famous people. There was a restaurant there that served Chicken Cordon Bleu. It was excellent but also put me on a path of developing more chicken dishes including this stuffed chicken. The marvel of the evening was that we were surrounded by many of those who made headline stories back then, yet we were more into the chicken than the glitter. That's how good it was. From that evening came this and other stuffed chicken recipes.

4 5-oz chicken breast halves, pounded[1] (383.5 mg)
1 teaspoon extra virgin olive oil (trace)
¼ cup chopped onion (1.6 mg)
1 cup dried no-salt homemade bread,cubed[2] (5.628 mg)
⅓ cup fresh[3] cranberries or golden raisins (5.794 mg)
1 large apple, processed into apple juice (1.84 mg)
⅓ cup filtered water (trace)
1 tablespoon of sugar or 2 packets of Splenda (trace)
⅛ teaspoon white or ground black pepper (trace)
1 tablespoons orange zest (grated peel) (.36 mg)
1½ cups orange juice with added calcium (3.735 mg)
½ cup filtered water (trace)
2 tablespoons cornstarch (1.44 mg)
1 tablespoon sugar or 2 packets Splenda (trace)
Pepper to taste

Preheat oven to 350° F

In a small nonstick saucepan cook onions in olive oil until tender (about 2 minutes).

In a small bowl combine bread cubes and cranberries or raisins, add in the cooked onions and stir.

In another pan bring the water and sliced or chopped apple to a boil. Stir that into the bread-cranberry-onion mix. Stir in sugar or Splenda and the pepper (to taste). Set aside.

Lay chicken breasts on stretch plastic wrap and fold wrap over chicken. Pound chicken until it's about ¼-inch thick. Remove plastic wrap and place the stuffing at the center lengthwise. Pull both sides up and tuck one under the other (should be a tight fit). Use toothpicks to hold the rolls together.

Place each roll into a shallow, oiled (spray oil works well) dish. Bake at 350° F for about 40 to 45 minutes or until your themometer reads about 160° F to 165° F.

While chicken is cooking, make the sauce. Combine the water and cornstarch in a small pan and stir until creamy smooth. Add in the orange juice, zest and sugar[1] and bring to a boil over medium heat. Stir often. Sauce will thicken. Add pepper to taste (but not too much). Spoon over finished chicken rolls. Serve with steamed asparagus or strong beans and a yellow vegetable like Acorn squash.

[1] Boneless and Skinless Chicken Breasts. Diabetics you can leave out the bread and and raisins to lower carbgs appreciably. Replace them with a few apple chunks and use ½ cup fresh cranberries. One-tablespoon sugar contains 12.6 grams of carbs. Carb Choices will drop to 1.5.

[2] May cut all in half to make a serving for two.

[3] Pounded to about a quarter inch thick. See instructions.

[4] Use any unsalted homemade bread except whole-wheat. Data based on one Don's Sandwich Bun.

[5] Fresh cranberries use ½ cup. Sodium (1 mg). Golden Raisins 1/3 cup sodium (5.794 mg) Recipe data uses the raisins.

[1] If using Splenda instead of sugar, add just before glaze is finished cooking.

Stuffed Chicken with Apple Glaze Nutritional Data: Calories: 350.8, Protein: 37 g, Carbohydrate: 40.6 g, Dietary Fiber: 3.213 g, Total Sugars: 13.6 g, Total Fat: 4.411 g, Saturated Fat: .859 g, Monounsaturated Fat: 1.699 g, Polyunsaturated Fat: 1.058 g, Cholesterol: 85.6 mg, Trans Fatty Acids: .037 g, Total Omega-3 FA: .097 g, Total Omega-6 FA: 0 g, Calcium: 223.6 mg, Potassium: 743.2 mg, Sodium: 101.2 mg, Vitamin K: 3.211 mcg

THAI STIR FRY

FLEXITARIAN – 1½ CARB CHOICES

Serves 2

Sodium Per Recipe: 288.3 mg Sodium Per Serving (6): 144.2 mg

We often make this dish with a variety of whatever vegetables we have on hand. I prefer the red wine vinegar but the cider vinegar works just as well. You can prepare the chicken for this your favorite cooking from baking, the BBQ, or stir-fry. Don't overcook it, however.

2 cups cooked fettuccini[1] (6 mg)
2 tablespoons cider or red wine vinegar) (2.384 mg)
½ cup orange juice (1.24 mg)
2 teaspoons brown sugar (2.576 mg)
1 teaspoon cornstarch (.749 mg)
1 tablespoon sesame oil (trace)
6 ounces cooked chicken, cut to bite size pieces[2] (153.4 mg)
2 cloves garlic, minced (1.02 mg)
1 tablespoon fresh ginger, minced (.78 mg)
½ teaspoon red pepper flakes (.27 mg)
2 celery stalks (64 mg)
2 medium carrots (42.1 mg)
2 broccoli florets (7.26 mg)
12 snow peas (1.632 mg)
6 asparagus stalks, cut bite size (1.92 mg)
3 medium mushrooms (about 3 tablespoons) (2.7 mg)
1 tablespoon toasted sliced unsalted almonds (.284 mg)

Mix first 4 ingredients in a small bowl and set aside.

Heat sesame oil in 12-inch fry pan over medium heat and add garlic, ginger and sprinkle with red pepper flakes. Stir-fry for a minute or until aromatic. Add celery, carrots, broccoli and asparagus. Stir-fry until vegetables turn bright but still crisp. Add mushrooms, snow peas, and stir-fry for another 2 minutes.

Remove all vegetables from heat and place in bowl. Then add chicken and rice to same pan and reheat.

When rice and chicken are warm, add vegetables to chicken and rice and reheat if necessary. You may use any fresh vegetables that you enjoy in place of those recommended.

[1]or 1 cup cooked brown rice (1.95 mg) (boil or steam)

[2]Equals about 8-ounces raw chicken (white breast meat)

Crockpot Chicken with Mushroom Sauce Nutritonal Data: Calories: 300.5, Protein: 16.7 g, Carbohydrate: 23.9 g, Dietary Fiber: 1.133 g, Total Sugars: 2.864 g, Total Fat: 15.2 g, Saturated Fat: 6.846 g, Monounsaturated Fat: 4.578 g, Polyunsaturated Fat: 2.078 g, Cholesterol: 92.3 mg, Trans Fatty Acids: .073 g, Total Omega-3 FA: .182 g, Total Omega-6 FA: .06 g, Calcium: 75.8 mg, Potassium: 387 mg, Sodium: 90.3 mg, Vitamin K: 3.237 mcg

ASPARAGUS SOUP

FLEXITARIAN – 1 CARB CHOICES

Makes: 4 cups

Sodium Per Recipe: 249.8 mg *Sodium Per Cup: 62.5 mg*

This soup is very good. Sometimes we add a dash of lemon or lime, but it really doesn't need it. Watch the vitamin K level if you're on blood thinner. Makes sure your daily intake of vitamin K isn't radically exceeded. Asparagus and spinach are considered high in vitamin K. See the nutrient panel at the bottom.

1½ pounds fresh asparagus[1] (12 mg)
2 cups raw spinach leaves (47.4 mg)
1 large potato, peeled and cut into bite size pieces (3.8 mg)
1 tablespoon onion flakes (1.05 mg)
2 teaspoons salt free seasoning[2] (1.296)
3 cups Maureen's Chicken Broth[3] (65 mg)
1 cup 2% fat milk with vitamin A added (100 mg)
white pepper to taste (trace)
Optional: Dollop of sour cream when served (19.2 mg)

Remove lower stems of asparagus and clean thoroughly. Cook in small amount of filtered water for 3 to 4-minutes or until they turn bright green. Chop into 1-inch pieces. Set aside.

In another pot, over medium flame, heat 3 cups of chicken broth and add potato and onion flakes. Cook until potato soft (about 15 minutes). Add spinach for another 2 minute and then add the asparagus pieces. Cook an additional five-minutes.

Remove from stove and process with a blender or hand-held mixer in two different batches. Add 1-cup milk and process until well blended.

Return to pot to reheat.

Serve hot.

* Can be made with water and low sodium Herbox (but remember Herbox leaves an after-taste of potassium chloride.

[1] After discarding lower stems you should have between 12 and 14 ounces.

[2] Such as Trader Joe's 21 Seasonings Salute and Costco's salt-free multi spice container. (many spice producers now have similar seasonings and without salt)

[3] Or use Swanson or Progresso Unsalted Chicken Broth. Add 15 mg sodium per cup.

Asparagus Soup Nutritional Data Per Cup: ***Calories: 118.8, Protein: 8.331 g, Carbohydrate: 14.7 g, Dietary Fiber: 4.467 g, Total Sugars: 7.822 g, Total Fat: 4.127 g, Saturated Fat: 1.95 g, Monounsaturated Fat: 1.239 g, Polyunsaturated Fat: .534 g, Cholesterol: 16.5 mg, Trans Fatty Acids: 0 g, Total Omega-3 FA: .079 g, Total Omega-6 FA: .035 g, Calcium: 149 mg, Potassium: 628.5 mg, Sodium: 62.5 mg, Vitamin K: 137.1 mcg***

BREAD MACHINE BAGELS

LACTO OVO – 2½ CARB CHOICES

Makes 8 to 10 Large Bagels

Sodium Per Recipe: 17.5 mg   Sodium Per Tablespoon: 8.435 mg

Make the dough in your bread machine, form and boil, then bake in your oven. It's not nearly as difficult as it may sound. Well worth the effort if you love bagels.

The Dough

1¼ cups warmed[1] filtered water (trace)
2 tablespoons Red Wine Vinegar (2.384 mg)
⅓ teaspoon ascorbic acid2 (trace)
¼ teaspoon granulated onion powder (.324 mg)
2 tablespoons white sugar (trace)
3¼ cups white unbleached bread flour (7.5 mg)
2¼ teaspoons bread machine dry yeast (3.5 mg)

For Boiling

3 quarts boiling filtered water (trace)
3 level tablespoons white sugar (trace)
1 tablespoon cornmeal (.567 mg)
1 egg white (54.8 mg)
3 tablespoons poppy seeds[2] (6.864 mg)

Place ingredients for dough into bread machine and set machine for dough.

When dough is ready, place on lightly floured bread board and after pressing down on it, let it rest for ten minutes.

After ten minutes, break into eight to ten balls rolling dough around in your hands until they are smooth. (9 makes a pretty good sized bagel, reducing that count downward makes larger bagels). Press down on each ball until ball is about 1-inch or slightly less thick. Punch a hole in the center with your thumb. Using your other hand, twirl the ball around your thumb to make the hole larger and even. Set dough on board again and let rise for about thirty or more minutes, covered with a light clothe or paper towel.

Bring a pot of water, three or four quarts, to a boil. Stir in the sugar after it boils. (This creates a light glaze on the bagels.)

While water is working up a boil, add a few drops of water to your egg white and whisk it briskly. Set aside with basting brush.

Prepare a cooling rack with paper towels on it. This will be used to drain the bagels after you lift them from the boiling water.

Place parchment paper on a baking sheet and sprinkle the paper with cornmeal.

Preheat Oven to 375o F (190 degrees C)

Using a large pancake turner or other flat tool, carefully place your bagels into the boiling water. You don't need to cook them all at the same time. If this is your first time, start with one at a time. Boil for 1 minute, flipping the bagel half way through. Drain briefly on paper towels set on the cooling rack.

Place drained bagels baking sheet. Glaze tops with egg white, and sprinkle with your choice of toppings.

Bake in oven for 20 to 25 minutes, or until well browned.

With another effort, you can easily convert these to your favorite bagels: Cinnamon Raisin, Onion, sesame seed, even some low sodium cheese (just shred and add to the dough mix).

[1]105°F to 110° F (40.5° C to 43.3° C). Very hot water kills the yeast, cold water hampers the dough development.

[2] May also convert to making raisin cinnamon, onion, sesame seed or add a 1/2 cup grated low sodium cheddar to the dough recipe.

Bagels, Based on 9 Bagels Made Nutritonal Data Per Bagel: Calories: 205.1, Protein: 5.693 g, Carbohydrate: 41.2 g, Dietary Fiber: 2.012 g, Total Sugars: 7.268 g, Total Fat: 1.763 g, Saturated Fat: .218 g, Monounsaturated Fat: .265 g, Polyunsaturated Fat: 1.048 g, Cholesterol: 0 mg, Trans Fatty Acids: 0 g, Total Omega-3 FA: .027 g, Total Omega-6 FA: 0 g, Calcium: 49.8 mg, Potassium: 94.3 mg, Sodium: 8.435 mg, Vitamin K: .131 mcg

MUSTARD SAUCE

VEGAN – 0 CARB CHOICES

Makes 4-Tablespoons

Sodium Per Recipe: 17.5 mg Sodium Per Tablespoon: 4.38 mg

Works well with white fish, barbecued steaks or burgers and light fowl, domestic and game.

2 tablespoons white balsamic vinegar (7.36 mg)
2 teaspoons Grey Poupon®, East Shore®, Hain® or Mendocino® honey mustard (10 mg)
1 teaspoon mustard powder (.165 mg)
1 tablespoon extra virgin olive oil (trace)

Combine all ingredients and whisk together until well blended. Whisk again, just before serving.

Mustard Sauce Nutritonal Data: Calories: 46.8, Protein: .245 g, Carbohydrate: 2.651 g, Dietary Fiber: .121 g, Total Sugars: 2.252 g, Total Fat: 3.737 g, Saturated Fat: .515 g, Monounsaturated Fat: 1.845 g, Polyunsaturated Fat: 1.201 g, Cholesterol: 0 mg, Trans Fatty Acids: 0 g, Total Omega-3 FA: .037 g, Total Omega-6 FA: 0 g, Calcium: 6.458 mg, Potassium: 14.6 mg, Sodium: 4.381 mg, Vitamin K: .78 mcg

CINNAMON BUN CLONES

LACTO OVO – 6+ CARB CHOICES[1]

Makes 12 Cinnamon Buns

Sodium Per Recipe: 317 mg   Sodium Per Tablespoon: 26.4 mg

This recipe is what I came up with in an effort to come close to duplicating a popular commercial bun. Follow the directions and you might be pleasantly surprised at the results. Get outside help to eat them all.

Step One

1 cup filtered water (110° F) (trace)
1 tablespoon red wine vinegar (1.192 mg)
2 large eggs, room temperature (140 mg)
⅓ cup extra virgin olive oil (trace)
4½ cups bread flour (11.2 mg)
1 tablespoon vital wheat gluten (2.25 mg)
1 level tablespoon grated orange peel (.18 mg)
¼ teaspoon onion powder (.324 mg)
⅓ teaspoon ascorbic acid[2] (trace)
½ cup white sugar (trace)
1 level tablespoon bread machine yeast (6 mg)

Step Two

1 cup brown sugar, packed (61.6 mg)
2½ tablespoons ground cinnamon (1.95 mg)
⅓ cup butter, softened (8.315 mg)
1 cup golden or black seedless raisins, packed (19.8 mg)
½ cup chopped unsalted walnuts (1.17 mg)

Step Three

1 large egg white (54.8 mg)
(Set egg in room temperature for about an hour before using)

Step Four

¼ cup butter, softened (6.242 mg)
1½ cups confectioners' sugar (1.8 mg)
½ teaspoon vanilla extract (.189 mg)

Here's How

Place Step One ingredients into your bread machine pan and select dough.

When dough has risen in machine roll it out onto a lightly floured surface covered with light clot, press down once and allow it to rest for about ten minutes.

While dough is resting, in a small bowl, stir together the brown sugar and cinnamon in Step Two.

Uncover dough and roll out gently to about 16 x 20 or 21-inches and about ¼" to a 1/3" thick. We want a rectangle. Baste dough with melted butter (from Step Two above) and then sprinkle sugar cinnamon mix evenly. Then spread the raisins and unsalted walnuts over that.

Whisk the egg in a small bowl with a dash of water. Set aside.

Roll into a log lengthwise and cut into 12 evenly measured rolls. Start by slicing in the middle, then the middle of the two logs, then into the middle of the four logs, etc. Place rolls (curl side up) in a lightly greased 9 x 13-inch baking dish or pan. Baste the egg-white over the top of the buns (the curls will be facing up). Cover with high lid or light cloth and let rise in warm spot until nearly doubled, about 30 to 45 minutes or possibly an hour (depending on temperature of your warming spot).

If your buns have been rising outside of your oven, then carefully place into your oven on the middle rack and close the door. Turn oven on to 400° F. Bake for about 20 minutes or until golden brown. Remove and let the pan or dish cool on a rack for about an hour before Spreading the topping on. (If using a convection oven, set temp to 375° F.)

We prefer to let bread and buns like these rise in the oven. You'll get an additional boost to the rise when you do. Heat the oven to about 100o F first. The best way to do this is to the turn the oven to 200o F and let it sit for 2 minutes. Then turn it off. If you're using your oven to let these rise, then you won't have to cover them. If rising in the oven, when they are ready, just turn the oven on to 400° F and bake for about 15 to 20 minutes (until golden brown).

[1] Diabetics you can lower the carbohydrates in this recipe by cutting the sugar in Step One to 1/4 cup, (Splenda does not work at all with yeast), replacing the brown sugar with Sugar Twin Brown (per their instructions) or cutting it in half. Leave out the raisins. The topping can be made with a Granulated Splenda and butter and a dash of orange zest and vanilla. This will produce a glaze instead of the white sugar coating. See nutritional data below for the results.

[2] Or 3 crushed 500 mg vitamin C tablets.

Cinnamon Bun Clone Nutritional Data Per Bun: Calories: 491.3, Protein: 8.455 g, Carbohydrate: 90.7 g, Dietary Fiber: 3.271 g, Total Sugars: 45.2 g, Total Fat: 13.6 g, Saturated Fat: 6.33 g, Monounsaturated Fat: 3.149 g, Polyunsaturated Fat: 2.97 g, Cholesterol: 59 mg, Trans Fatty Acids: 0 g, Total Omega-3 FA: .533 g, Total Omega-6 FA: .239 g, Calcium: 59.8 mg, Potassium: 246.6 mg, Sodium: 26.4 mg, Vitamin K: 2.06 mcg

Cinnamon Bun For Diabetics Nutritional Data Per Bun 3 Carb Choices: Calories: 321.8, rotein: 7.967 g, Carbohydrate: 42.7 g, Dietary Fiber: 2.721 g, Total Sugars: 4.582 g, Total Fat: 13.5 g, Saturated Fat: 6.306 g, Monounsaturated Fat: 3.142 g, Polyunsaturated Fat: 2.944 g, Cholesterol: 59 mg, Trans Fatty Acids: 0 g, Total Omega-3 FA: .529 g, Total Omega-6 FA: .239 g, Calcium: 37.1 mg, Potassium: 119.3 mg, Sodium: 19.5 mg, Vitamin K: 1.578 mcg

ANGEL HAIR PASTA
With Barbecued Chicken

FLEXITARIAN – 2 CARB CHOICES

Serves 6

Sodium Per Recipe: 419.6 mg Sodium Per Slice: 69.9 mg

Barbecue the chicken the day you make this or the day before. Store in fridge overnight if need to. Use your favorite mushroom for this recipe.

4-6 large barbecued chicken breasts, sliced diagonally into 4 inch thick strips (306.8 mg)
4 tablespoon olive oil (trace)
4 tablespoons usalted butter (6.248 mg)
1 shallot, finely diced (2.4 mg)
2 garlic cloves, minced (1.02 mg)
2 cups fresh mushrooms, hard part of stems removed and stems and caps sliced thick (7 mg)
1 cup Maureen's Chicken Broth[1] (21.6 mg)
¼ cup fresh parsley, minced (8.4 mg)
½ cup tomatoes, seeded and diced (4.5 mg)
¼ teaspoon granulated onion powder (.324 mg)
freshly ground black pepper to taste
5 cups hot, cooked angel hair pasta (40 mg)
5 ounces grated fresh mozzarella (no salt added)[1] (22.4 mg)

Heat olive oil and 2 tablespoons of butter in a large skillet over medium heat. Add shallot and garlic, sauté 2 to 3 minutes. Add mushrooms and sauté until they release juices. Add Maureen's chicken stock, increase heat to medium-high and cook, uncovered for 5 minutes. Add chicken, parsley and tomatoes. Stir to warm. Remove from heat and stir in remaining 2 tablespoons butter. Serve over pasta and garnish with cheese.

[1]Or use Swanson Unsalted Chicken Broth or other brand of choice. Add 4 mg sodium per serving.

Angel Hair Pasta w/Barbecued Chicken: Calories: 443.1, Protein: 32.2 g, Carbohydrate: 37 g, Dietary Fiber: 2.256 g, Total Sugars: 1.886 g, Total Fat: 18.2 g, Saturated Fat: 8.664 g, Monounsaturated Fat: 5.395 g, Polyunsaturated Fat: 2.259 g, Cholesterol: 119.1 mg, Trans Fatty Acids: .058 g, Total Omega-3 FA: .179 g, Total Omega-6 FA: .205 g, Calcium: 208.6 mg, Potassium: 426.9 mg, Sodium: 69.9 mg, Vitamin K: 44.4 mcg

PANFORTE

VEGAN – 2 CARB CHOICES
Serves 16

Sodium Per Recipe: 58.7 mg Sodium Per Slice: 3.669 mg

An Italian (Tuscany) Christmas dessert. Slice into thin servings and serve after dinner with tea or coffee. (Italians serve with a liqueur.)

7 ounces unsalted almonds, freshly ground (1.134 mg)
4 ounces unsalted almonds, whole (1.985 mg)
4 ounces unsalted walnuts, freshly ground (2.268 mg)
4 ounces unsalted hazelnuts, freshly ground (trace)
10 ounces candied orange & lemon peel, chopped (42.5 mg)
2 ounces dried figs, finely chopped (5.67 mg)
7 ounces white granulated sugar (trace)
4 ounces honey (not raw honey) (4.536 mg)
pinch of:
ground cinnamon (trace)
ground cloves (trace)
coriander (trace)
nutmeg (trace)
2 tablespoons all-purpose flour (.312 mg)

Preheat oven to 325° F.

Line 8" baking dish with parchment paper.

Stir honey and sugar together in double boiler (honey in sugar in the bowl above the boiling water). Stir constantly until sugar has dissolved.

Mix in the rest of ingredients except for the cinnamon flour mix.

When spread evenly across the pan, dust with the cinnamon flour mix.

Bake for forty (40) minutes. Cake will not rise.

When done, move to cooling rack and blow off or dust off any flour that didn't back into the panforte. Will store wrapped in aluminum foil for up to three weeks.

Dust with confectioner's sugar when serving.

Mustard Sauce Nutritonal Data: Calories: 301.2, Protein: 6.587 g, Carbohydrate: 31 g, Dietary Fiber: 4.165 g, Total Sugars: 23.2 g, Total Fat: 18.8 g, Saturated Fat: 1.507 g, Monounsaturated Fat: 10.1 g, Polyunsaturated Fat: 6.315 g, Cholesterol: 0 mg, Trans Fatty Acids: .002 g, Total Omega-3 FA: .651 g, Total Omega-6 FA: 1.496 g, Calcium: 74.7 mg, Potassium: 249.6 mg, Sodium: 3.669 mg, Vitamin K: 1.805 mcg

SUNDRIED TOMATO PESTO

VEGAN – 0 CARB CHOICES

Makes Approx. 16 Tablespoons

Sodium Per Recipe: 101.6 mg   Sodium Per Tablespoon: 6.352 mg

Use with chicken, pork, Don's Pesto Sandwich.

⅓ cup pine nuts, lightly browned in an oven at 350° F. (.891 mg)
1 cup basil leaves (1.696 mg)
2 garlic cloves (1.02 mg)
⅓ cup sundried tomatoes in oil (96.6 mg)
⅓ cup olive oil (trace)
white or black pepper to taste (trace)
Optional: Dash of granulated onion powder (trace)

Place all ingredients in a food processor and blend to make a coarse paste. Season with pepper and a dash of granulated onion powder. To store, cover paste with a little additional olive oil, cover and refrigerate.

Sundried Tomato Pesto Nutritional Data Per Tablespoon: Calories: 64.1, Protein: .604 g, Carbohydrate: 1.092 g, Dietary Fiber: .287 g, Total Sugars: .112 g, Total Fat: 6.697 g, Saturated Fat: .796 g, Monounsaturated Fat: 3.972 g, Polyunsaturated Fat: 1.476 g, Cholesterol: 0 mg, Trans Fatty Acids: 0 g, Total Omega-3 FA: .052 g, Total Omega-6 FA: .013 g, Calcium: 6.953 mg, Potassium: 61.6 mg, Sodium: 6.352 mg, Vitamin K: 15.2 mcg

BÉCHAMEL SAUCE

VEGAN – 0 CARB CHOICES

Makes Approx. 1 cup

Sodium Per Recipe: 106.3 mg   Sodium Per Tablespoon: 6.46 mg

Basic sauce used to make other sauces. Create your own sauces by adding assorted ingredients such as low-sodium cheeses, spices, herbs and citrus juices.

2 tablespoons unsalted butter (3.124 mg)
2 tablespoons unbleached all-purpose flour (.312 mg)
1 cup nonfat or low fat milk w/ Vitamin A&D (103 mg)
white pepper to taste (trace)

In a medium saucepan over medium heat, melt butter. Add flour while whisking until mixture is bubbly. Cook for 2 minutes, whisking frequently. Do not allow mixture to brown. Reduce heat, if necessary. Gradually blend in milk in a thin stream while whisking and cook until sauce boils and is smooth and thick. Season with salt and pepper.

Bechamel Sauce Nutritional Data Per Tablespoon: Calories: 21.5, Protein: .632 g, Carbohydrate: 1.506 g, Dietary Fiber: .026 g, Total Sugars: .783 g, Total Fat: 1.462 g, Saturated Fat: .921 g, Monounsaturated Fat: .377 g, Polyunsaturated Fat: .059 g, Cholesterol: 4.122 mg, Trans Fatty Acids: 0 g, Total Omega-3 FA: .012 g, Total Omega-6 FA: .038 g, Calcium: 19.7 mg, Potassium: 25.4 mg, Sodium: 6.646 mg, Vitamin K: .127 mcg

SWEET-HOT BARBECUE SAUCE

VEGAN – 0 CARB CHOICES

Makes Approx. 3.5 cups

Sodium Per Recipe: 153.7 mg Sodium Per Tablespoon: 9.609 mg

This recipe is based on a Scott Leysath barbecue sauce. It works with all meats including game meat.

- **1 tablespoon unsalted butter (1.562 mg)**
- **1 medium onion, finely diced (4.4 mg)**
- **2 garlic cloves, minced (1.02 mg)**
- **2 tablespoons lemon peel, shredded (.72 mg)**
- **1 cup packed brown sugar (61.6 mg)**
- **½ teaspoon chili flakes (13.1 mg)**
- **½ teaspoon cayenne pepper (.27 mg)**
- **½ teaspoon granulated onion powder (.648 mg)**
- **¼ teaspoon freshly ground black pepper (.231 mg)**
- **¼ cup no salt added or Contadina tomato paste (**
- **2 8-ounce cans no salt added tomato sauce (64.2 mg)**
- **½ cup apple cider vinegar (5.975 mg)**

In a medium sauce pan over medium heat, heat butter and sauté onions, garlic and lemon peel until onions become translucent, but not brown. Add sugar and cook for 3 more minutes, stirring often. Add remaining ingredients, bring to boil, reduce heat to low and cook for 30 minutes.

Sweet-Hot Barbecue Sauce Nutritional Data Per Tablespoons:Calories: 68, Protein: .34 g, Carbohydrate: 15.4 g, Dietary Fiber: .428 g, Total Sugars: 14.2 g, Total Fat: .775 g, Saturated Fat: .468 g, Monounsaturated Fat: .195 g, Polyunsaturated Fat: .048 g, Cholesterol: 1.908 mg, Trans Fatty Acids: 0 g, Total Omega-3 FA: .007 g, Total Omega-6 FA: .019 g, Calcium: 17.6 mg, Potassium: 82 mg, Sodium: 9.609 mg, Vitamin K: .751 mcg

CRANBERRY-APPLE CRISP

LACTO OVO – 3 CARB CHOICES

Serves 9

Sodium Per Recipe: 76.4 mg   Sodium Per Tablespoon: 8.492 mg

We make this for guests or special events. It's usually set out buffet style. It's a tad high in carbs and calories, so when I embibe, it's with just a auarter-cup serving. That pretty much cuts all the nutritional data numbers in half.

The Fruit

4 medium to large Granny Smith or other cooking apples, cored, sliced (7.28 mg)
1 cup frozen or fresh cranberries (11.7 mg)
½ teaspoon ground cinnamon (.13 mg

The Crisp

¾ cup packed brown sugar (46.2 mg)
½ cup white, unbleached all-purpose flour (1.25 mg)
½ cup unsalted walnuts, chopped finely (1.17 mg)
⅓ cup unsalted butter, softened (8.24 mg)
¾ teaspoon ground cinnamon (.195 mg)
¾ teaspoon ground nutmeg (.264 mg)

Preheat oven to 350° F. Grease an 8" x 8" square baking dish or pan with trans-fat free shortening or unsalted butter.

In a small bowl mix the apples and cranberries together with the ½ teaspoon ground cinnamon. Place this mix into the baking dish.

In a small bowl combine The Crisp ingredients until evenly mixed and crumbly. Spread evenly over the top of the apples and cranberries.

Bake for about 35 minutes or until apples puncture with a fork. (Don't overcook.)

Serve warm or hot with a dollop of nonfat whipped cream or a spoonful of vanilla ice cream.

Cranberry Apple Crisp Nutritional Data Per Serving:Calories: 313.6, Protein: 7.025 g, Carbohydrate: 48.7 g, Dietary Fiber: 8.146 g, Total Sugars: 26.4 g, Total Fat: 11.5 g, Saturated Fat: 4.824 g, Monounsaturated Fat: 2.372 g, Polyunsaturated Fat: 3.505 g, Cholesterol: 17.9 mg, Trans Fatty Acids: 0 g, Total Omega-3 FA: .704 g, Total Omega-6 FA: .18 g, Calcium: 61 mg, Potassium: 439.8 mg, Sodium: 8.492 mg, Vitamin K: 2.671 mcg

PUMPKIN PUDDING

LACTO OVO – 1/2 CARB CHOICES

Serves 6 to 8

Sodium Per Recipe: 455.8 mg

Sodium Per Serving (8): 57 mg Sodium Per Serving (10): 45.6 mg

I like to make the filling for a pumpkin pie, but instead of laying it over piecrust I put the pudding into 6-ounce custard dishes or when serving to guests, into Ramekins. (See www.megaheart.com/kit_cabitnet.html) The ramekins we use are shown there, as are Pyrex custard cups. The Pyrex holds 6-ounces while the Ramekins hold 8-ounces. This almost-a-pie recipe lowers carbohydrates to a level most diabetics can accept. Calories are way down, too.

1 cup canned pumpkin (12.2 mg)
¾ can evaporated milk (300.5 mg)
2 large eggs (140 mg)
1 cup Splenda granulated (trace)
½ teaspoon vanilla extract (.189 mg)
1 teaspoon ground cinnamon (.26 mg)
¼ teaspoon ground cloves (1.276 mg)
½ tsp ground allspice (.731 mg)
½ teaspoon ground ginger (.288 mg)

Preheat oven to 350° F (175 degrees C).

Beat canned pumpkin, evaporated milk and eggs in a large bowl until evenly combined. Add Splenda, vanilla extract and ground cinnamon, cloves and nutmeg; continue to beat well until mixture is well combined.

Ladle mixture into custard cups, fill only ¾. After cooking and when cooling starts, the pumpkin will fall a bit. Fill cup with whipped cream topping when serving. (I use the nonfat whipped cream in a pressure can – fewer calories and lower sodium and carb content.)

Bake 35 minutes, or until a toothpick inserted in the center comes out clean. Cool for at least an hour before serving.

Pumpkin Pudding Nutrition Data Per Serving (8): Calories: 91, Protein: 4.37 g, Carbohydrate: 9.894 g, Dietary Fiber: 1.295 g, Total Sugars: 1.16 g, Total Fat: 4.046 g, Saturated Fat: 2.07 g, Monounsaturated Fat: 1.32 g, Polyunsaturated Fat: .271 g, Cholesterol: 63.2 mg, Trans Fatty Acids: 0 g, Total Omega-3 FA: .043 g, Total Omega-6 FA: 0 g, Calcium: 115 mg, Potassium: 193.9 mg, Sodium: 57 mg, Vitamin K: 5.234 mcg

Pumpkin Pudding Nutrition Data Per Serving (10): Calories: 72.8, Protein: 3.496 g, Carbohydrate: 7.915 g, Dietary Fiber: 1.036 g, Total Sugars: .928 g, Total Fat: 3.237 g, Saturated Fat: 1.656 g, Monounsaturated Fat: 1.056 g, Polyunsaturated Fat: .217 g, Cholesterol: 50.5 mg, Trans Fatty Acids: 0 g, Total Omega-3 FA: .034 g, Total Omega-6 FA: 0 g, Calcium: 92 mg, Potassium: 155.1 mg, Sodium: 45.6 mg, Vitamin K: 4.187 mcg

RED POTATOES & RED PEPPERS

VEGAN – 1/2 CARB CHOICES

Makes 4 Servings

Sodium Per Recipe 56 mg *Sodium Per Serving: 14 mg*

4 medium red potatoes, cut into 1/2-inch pieces (51.1 mg)
1 small red bell pepper, finely chopped (2.96 mg)
1 tablespoon extra virgin olive oil (trace)
2 teaspoons dried rosemary or thyme (1.2 mg)
½ teaspoon garlic powder (.364 mg)
¼ teaspoon granulated onion powder (.324 mg)

Place all ingredients into a small bowl. Stir until potatoes are oiled and the spices and red pepper pieces are evenly distributed on the potatoes.

Place in oiled baking pan.

Bake in preheated oven for about 45 minutes or with a roast in the roast pan for the last 45 minutes of the roast's cooking time.

Red Potatoes meet Red Peppers Nutritional Data Per Serving:
Calories: 189.4. Protein: 4.312 g, Carbohydrate: 35.7 g, Dietary Fiber: 4.308 g, Total Sugars: 3.045 g, Total Fat: 3.949 g, Saturated Fat: .625 g, Monounsaturated Fat: 1.706 g, Polyunsaturated Fat: 1.307 g, Cholesterol: 0 mg, Trans Fatty Acids: 0 g, Total Omega-3 FA: .056 g, Total Omega-6 FA: 0 g, Calcium: 31.1 mg, Potassium: 1019 mg, Sodium: 14 mg, Vitamin K: 7.825 mcg

TOMATO-BASIL BISQUE

VEGAN - ½ CARB CHOICES

Serves 4

Sodium Per Recipe: 119.2 mg Sodium Per Serving: 29.8 mg

This side dish is an old family recipe converted to a salt free dish. It's easy to make, and you can add more flavors to it with your own choice of spices or herbs. Chill for a few hours before serving.

3 cups peeled, seeded and chopped tomatoes (27 mg)
1 cup Maureen's Chicken Broth[1] (21.7 mg)
1 8-ounce can no-salt-added tomato sauce (70 mg)
¼ teaspoon granulated onion powder (.324 mg)
2 tablespoons fresh basil, chopped[2] (.212 mg)

Blanch the tomatoes to help with peeling.

Cut tomatoes into quarters and remove seeds (don't worry if a few are left behind).

Blend together the fresh tomatoes, broth, no salt added tomato sauce until smooth. Add in the basil and chill in refrigerator for a few hours before serving. combine tomatoes, vegetable or chicken broth, and tomato sauce. Cover and blend until smooth.

Stir in basil.

Cover and refrigerate before serving.

[1]Or use Swanson Unsalted Chicken Broth or other brand of choice. Add 4 mg sodium per serving.

[2]or 1 teaspoon dried basil. Crush the basil using a mortar and pestle or use a countertop coffee bean grinder.

Tomato-Basil Bisque Nutritional Data Per Serving: Calories: 53.1, Protein: 1.928 g, Carbohydrate: 9.805 g, Dietary Fiber: 1.85 g, Total Sugars: 3.928 g, Total Fat: .774 g, Saturated Fat: .178 g, Monounsaturated Fat: .24 g, Polyunsaturated Fat: .228 g, Cholesterol: 2.824 mg, Trans Fatty Acids: 0 g, Total Omega-3 FA: .015 g, Total Omega-6 FA: 0 g, Calcium: 20.4 mg, Potassium: 350.8 mg, Sodium: 29.8 mg, Vitamin K: 16.8 mcg

TWICE-BAKED POTATOES

A Microwave Recipe

LACTO OVO – 1 CARB CHOICES[1]

Serves 4 to 8[2]

*Sodium Per Recipe: 140.6 mg**

Sodium Per Serving (4): 35.1 mg *Sodium Per Serving (8): 17.6 mg*

A rare treat, twice-baked potato recipes abound. This is ours. We serve it only when guests join us since Maureen and I will split one,. Check the Nutrient Data at the end of the recipe to see if this fits into your dietary plan. This recipe may be halved.

4 medium russet potatoes, scrubbed clean, skin on (10.7 mg)
1 cup broccoli florets, well chopped (30 mg)
1 cup water (trace)
1 cup shredded low sodium Cheddar cheese, divided* (from 60 mg to 125 mg)
½ cup reduced-fat sour cream (73.2 mg)
3 garlic cloves, minced (1.53 mg)
¼ teaspoon white pepper (.03 mg)
3 scallions (green onions), thinly sliced the white part only (1.44 mg)

Scrub potatoes clean. Poke holes into potatoes with skewer or fork throughout. Cook in microwave on potato setting if you have one, but only until soft. Don't overcook.

With the cooked potato lying on the counter naturally, slice off the top third and set aside. We'll use the tops later. Using a large dinnerware soup spoon, scoop the insides (the meat of the potato) into a small to medium size bowl. Place the potato shells into individual serving dishes or all of them into an 8" x 8" baking dish (or larger if necessary).

In a medium to large bowl, mash the potatoes with a hand masher and then add 4-ounces of the shredded low sodium Cheddar, reduced or low fat sour cream, garlic and pepper to the potato. Mash these together making sure all is evenly distributed. Add this mix along with the to the broccoli and stir until well combined. (If you are going to add meat, then see footnote number 3 below before mashing potatoes.)

Fill the potato shells equally and top with the remaining 4 ounces of Cheddar. Microwave on High until the filling is hot and the cheese is melted, 2 to 4 minutes.

Serve hot.

* The USDA rates no salt, low sodium Cheddar at 23.6 mg sodium per cup, shredded. Heluvagood now has some salt in it and they rate that cheese at 25 mg per ounce. One cup shredded (not packed) nationally available Heluvagood equals about 5 ounces or 125 mg for this recipe's total amount. We are listing the higher amount. Should you be able to find no salt Cheddar cheese in your area, then you can subject about 25 mg of sodium per potato. The rest of the nutrient data would remain the same.

[1] This is a Lacto Ovo Vegetarian recipe if not using ground turkey. It is a Flexitarian recipe if using the mat. If using whole potato Carb Choices is one. If cutting in half, Carb Choices is one-half.

[2] We cut the servings in half when making this recipe. Potatoes will store in refrigerator covered or sealed up to two days. Microwave to heat when serving.

[3] Optional:

8-ounces lean ground turkey or chicken

If you add meat follow the below instructions.

While potatoes bake, brown the meat in a medium to large nonstick fry pan (skillet) over medium to high heat. Stir every few minutes. Transfer the meat to a medium to large bowl. Add in broccoli once it is cooked.

Twice Baked Potatoes Nutritional Data Per Serving (4): Calories: 215.4, Protein: 10.4 g, Carbohydrate: 15 g, Dietary Fiber: 1.716 g, Total Sugars: 3.051 g, Total Fat: 13.1 g, Saturated Fat: 8.247 g, Monounsaturated Fat: 2.602 g, Polyunsaturated Fat: .312 g, Cholesterol: 43.8 mg, Trans Fatty Acids: 0 g, Total Omega-3 FA: .117 g, Total Omega-6 FA: 0 g, Calcium: 276.1 mg, Potassium: 423.2 mg, Sodium: 35.1 mg, Vitamin K: 39.9 mcg

Twice Baked Potatoes Nutritional Data Per Serving (8): Calories: 107.7, Protein: 5.188 g, Carbohydrate: 7.521 g, Dietary Fiber: .858 g, Total Sugars: 1.525 g, Total Fat: 6.543 g, Saturated Fat: 4.123 g, Monounsaturated Fat: 1.301 g, Polyunsaturated Fat: .156 g, Cholesterol: 21.9 mg, Trans Fatty Acids: 0 g, Total Omega-3 FA: .058 g, Total Omega-6 FA: 0 g, Calcium: 138 mg, Potassium: 211.6 mg, Sodium: 17.6 mg, Vitamin K: 19.9 mcg

PLUM PUDDING

LACTO OVO – 3 CARB CHOICES[5]

Serves 12

Sodium Per Recipe: 479.5 mg
Sodium Per Serving Without Sauce: 40 mg
Sodium Per Serving With Sauce

This pudding comes straight out of the past and tastes just like the plum pudding of old, which was, as many might remember, the "flavor of Christmas." It's a bit high in calories and requires some changes to fit into a diabetic meal.

1½ cups white unbleached all-purpose flour (3.75 mg)
1 tablespoon Ener-G Baking Soda (trace)
1½ teaspoons Ener-G Baking Powder* (6.75 mg)
¼ teaspoon granulated onion powder (.324 mg)
1 teaspoon nutmeg (.352 mg)
½ teaspoon ground cloves (2.552 mg)
2 teaspoons ground cinnamon (.52 mg)
1 cup brown sugar, packed (61.6 mg)
3 cup white sugar[1] (trace)
½ cup expeller pressed canola oil (trace)
3 large eggs (210 mg)
2 cups grated carrots (151.8 mg)
2 cups grated potatoes[2] (18 mg)
1 tablespoon cocoa (1.026 mg)
2 cups unsalted walnuts, chopped (4.68 mg)
1 cup black seedless raisins, packed (or currants) (18.1 mg)

Requires a 2-quart size Steam Pudding Mold

Mix all ingredients together in a large bowl. together.

Put ineo greased steamer moldt[3]

Cut a circular piece of aluminum foil one-inch larger than the mold top. Grease one side and place it, grease side down, over the top of the mold. Press the overhand into the pot. Place the lid over this and lock the lid into place. (Some molds come with locking lids, others come with lids that "snap" into place.)

Place pudding mold into a large pot, run cold water into the larger pot about half way up the pudding mold pot. Place lid on larger pot and steam for two-hours.

When done, remove pudding mold from water pot, let cool for about a half hour to an hour. Remove pudding from mold and wrap with cheesecloth. Add brandy to taste[4]. Wrap with stretchable plastic wrap such as Saran Wrap.

TO SERVE: Remove wrap and cheesecloth, place back into the steamer mold, place back into large water pot and steam for another 1 and a half hours.

TO FLAME. If you want to present your pudding "flaming," then pour one cup hot brandy (heat in microwave) over the top and ignite. (**Caution:** Flaming the pudding can be dangerous.)

Hot Sauce

Combine in small pan, cook over medium heat, stir constantly until thick.

1 tablespoon cornstarch (.749 mg)
½ cup sugar (trace)
1 grated lemon peel (3.24 mg)
1 cup filtered water (trace)

Removed and then add:

2 tablespoons lemon juice (.305 mg)
1 tablespoon unsalted butter (1.562 mg)

* If making for salt-eaters, then replace Ener-G with 2 teaspoons baking soda. Replace Onion powder with 1 teaspoon salt. This adds 3,350 mg of sodium to the recipe.

[1] Or Splenda Granulated. [2] Russet, White, Red, Yukon

[3] If you don't have a steamer pudding pot, then use a baking pot and built a "lid" for it with aluminum foil. The pudding will rise. You can find the steam mold at Amazon at this link: http://www.amazon.com/gp/product/B00004S1CF/ref=as_li_tf_tl?ie=UTF8&tag=megahearcomsbook&linkCode=as2&camp=1789&creative=9325&creativeASIN=B00004S1CF

[4] For non alcoholic pudding, drizzle some fresh orange juice on the cheesecloth.

[5] Using Splenda reduces carbohydrates in recipe not using sauces by 200 g. or 16 g per serving, which would make it 49 grams or 3 Carb Choices Leaving Raisins out would reduce the recipe total another 13 grams making each serving 2 Carb Choices. Adding sauce to a serving would raise the carbohydrates by approximately

Plum Pudding Nutritional Data Per Serving (No Sauce): Calories: 487, Protein: 7.364 g, Carbohydrate: 67 g, Dietary Fiber: 3.624 g, Total Sugars: 44.4 g, Total Fat: 23.5 g, Saturated Fat: 2.388 g, Monounsaturated Fat: 8.018 g, Polyunsaturated Fat: 12 g, Cholesterol: 52.9 mg, Trans Fatty Acids: .036 g, Total Omega-3 FA: 3.452 g, Total Omega-6 FA: 1.693 g, Calcium: 91.9 mg, Potassium: 497.9 mg, Sodium: 40 mg, Vitamin K: 11 mcg

Plum Pudding Nutritional Data Per Serving with Sauce: Calories: 534.9, Protein: 7.491 g, Carbohydrate: 77.2 g, Dietary Fiber: 4.061 g, Total Sugars: 52.8 g, Total Fat: 24.7 g, Saturated Fat: 3.079 g, Monounsaturated Fat: 7.984 g, Polyunsaturated Fat: 12.2 g, Cholesterol: 55.4 mg, Trans Fatty Acids: .031 g, Total Omega-3 FA: 2.884 g, Total Omega-6 FA: 2.171 g, Calcium: 97.9 mg, Potassium: 513.9 mg, Sodium: 40.4 mg, Vitamin K: 8.526 mcg

PULL-APART TACOS

Crockpot Recipe

FLEXITARIAN - ½ CARB CHOICES

Serves 4

Sodium Per Recipe: 375.6 mg   Sodium Per Serving: 93.9 mg

Let the crockpot do the cooking for you. Six to eight hours later, you'll enjoy a really tasty treat with our enchilada sauce and the fresh veggies. Make our homemade flour tortillas beforehand, store in fridge or freezer and then enjoy. Or buy commercially produced corn tortillas that list sodium levels at 5 mg or lower. These usually don't have salt in them.

1 pound lean boneless pork shoulder roast (222.3 mg)[1]
1 cup Maureen's Chicken Broth[2] (21.7 mg)
½ cup Quick Enchilada sauce[3] (30.1 mg)
4 8-inch soft homemade no-salt flour tortillas or commer cially produced no-salt corn tortillas[4] (5.617 mg)
2 cups shredded Romaine or Iceberg lettuce (7.52 mg)
1 cup low sodium cheddar, shredded[5] (23.7mg)
1 medium size red tomato, chopped (about 1-large tomato)
1 medium avocado, thinly sliced (10.9 mg)
1 cup onion, chopped (6.4 mg)
4 tablespoons sour cream (38.4 mg)

Trim fat from pork roast and set into your crockpot. (Crockpot should be more than a 3-quart size, preferably a 4-quart crockpot. If yours is smaller, then cut the meat to help it fit into the pot.

Add broth. Cover; cook on low-heat setting for 8-hours or on the high setting for up to 5-hours.

Remove roast from crockpot and discard the broth.

Using two forks, shred meat, discarding fat.

Set aside two (2) cups of the meat. (Put any additional meat into a zipper lock (airtight) bag or container and refrigerate for another meal. You may also freeze this meat for up to two or three months.

Making the Meat Sauce

In a medium saucepan, over medium-low heat, cook the two cups of meat and the enchilada sauce for about ten minutes, covered. Stir occasionally.

While sauce is heating, warm your tortillas or shells either in an oven or a nonstick fry pay. If using corn tortillas, then fry in a nonstick pan with a touch of extra virgin olive oil added for flavor.

When ready to serve, place meat/sauce mixture in center of warm tortillas. Top as desired with lettuce, cheese, tomatoes, onions, avocado and a dollop of sour cream.

Serve immediately.

[1] Nutrient Data based on 2 cups of cooked pork roast. You can use more meat like a 2 ½ to 3 or more pound roast. Just set the extra meat aside for a leftovers recipe the following day.

[2] Prepare Maureen's Chicken Broth and store in fridge or freezer in Mason jar. Recipe can be found on page:

[3] PrepareEnchilada Sauce early and store in fridge. Recipe can be found on next page.

[4] Super Tortilla Recipe on following page.

[5] It's getting more and more difficult to find low sodium cheddar cheese. If you can find it locally, then Heluvagood has a lower sodium cheese that does use some salt. The rating for that cheese is 25 mg per ounce. If you use this cheese, then add the difference to each Taco.

Pull-Apart Tacos Nutritional Data Per Serving: Calories: 667, Protein: 40.6 g, Carbohydrate: 49.6 g, Dietary Fiber: 5.85 g, Total Sugars: 4.44 g, Total Fat: 34.2 g, Saturated Fat: 11.8 g, Monounsaturated Fat: 16.3 g, Polyunsaturated Fat: 2.817 g, Cholesterol: 115.4 mg, Trans Fatty Acids: .024 g, Total Omega-3 FA: .37 g, Total Omega-6 FA: .403 g, Calcium: 296.6 mg, Potassium: 1062 mg, Sodium: 93.9 mg, Vitamin K: 42.1 mcg

SUPER TORTILLA

VEGAN - 2 CARB CHOICES

Makes 12 8" Tortillas

Sodium Per Recipe: 20.5 mg *Sodium Per Serving: 1.706 mg*

These tortillas will match any you might otherwise buy I the market. Easy to make, they can be frozen for up to three or four months. Place a piece of wax or parchment paper between each one when freezing.

4 cups unbleached all purpose flour (10 mg)
1 tablespoon white wine vinegar (.15 mg)
½ cup extra virgin olive oil (trace)
1½ cups filtered water (trace)
2 teaspoons fresh squeezed lime juice (.19 mg)
2 teaspoons Ener-G Baking Powder (9 mg)

Combine flour and onion powder in a medium sized bowl. Bring in the olive oil and vinegar stirring with a wooden spoon. Add the lime juice. Add the water slowly. Mix together while doing so and when the dough cleans the side of the bowl stop adding the liquid. Too much water can make a tortilla tough.

Add in the Featherweight and knead using your hands with your fingers working the dough for about 8 turns (to get the Featherweight into the dough).

Form the dough into a ball and cover with plastic or cloth.

Let sit for about 30 minutes to two hours in a room temperature location.

Heat your nonstick flat surface griddle or a large nonstick fry pay over medium to medium high heat. You won't need oil or butter to "fry" these if you use the nonstick.

Cut or with your hands form 12 even sized balls. If using a Tortilla press, follow their instructions. But after forming the shell, place on lightly floured board and placing a piece of wax paper over the tortilla, roll out to an even thinner disc.

If not using a press, lightly flour the board. Press a ball of dough over your forefinger to create a hole. Set the ball on the bread board, hole side down, and roll out the dough with a pin (and wax paper as described above). To make a circle, roll it once, then turn the dough ninety degrees, then roll again and continue doing that until you've rolled it out thinly. These balls should make an 8 to 12" disc.

When a splash of water bounces on the griddle or fry pan, you are ready to cook the discs. You can prepare all the discs and then cook them, or prepare and cook, prepare and cook and so on. Each disc should cook in about 20 to 30 seconds. Turn disc when it bubbles and cook other side for about 5 to 10 seconds.

You can store in refrigerator overnight in zip lock bags or stack with wax paper between each disc, put into zip lock bag and freeze for future use.

***Flour Tortilla Nutritional Data Per Tortilla:** Calories: 233.2 Protein: 4.33 g, Carbohydrate: 32.5 g, Dietary Fiber: 1.16 g, Total Sugars: 0 g, Total Fat: 9.415 g, Saturated Fat: 1.281 g, Monounsaturated Fat: 6.67 g, Polyunsaturated Fat: .93 g, Cholesterol: 0 mg, Calcium: 43.2 mg, Iron: 2.048 mg, Potassium: 133.4 mg, Sodium: 1.706 mg, Vitamin K: 4.41 mcg, Folate: 64.6 mcg*

ENCHILADA SAUCE

VEGAN – 0 CARB CHOICES

Makes 3 Cups

Sodium Per Recipe: 11.9 mg Sodium Per Tablespoon: .248 mg

This sauce workes great with enchiladas and tacos, especially our Pork PullApart Tacos.

1 dozen dried New Mexican or California chilies (5.46 mg)
1 large onion quartered (6 mg)
3 cloves garlic (1.53 mg)
6 cups filtered water (trace)

Place the chilies and the other ingredients into a 2-3 qt. sauce pan and simmer for 30 minutes.

Working with half the cooked chili mixture, transfer it and ¾ c. cooking liquid (use tongs to remove chilies) into a bowl and use your Braun mixer to puree mixture. You also may use a blender. When mixture is pureed, pour it into a sieve and stir the mixture with a spoon so all sauce except the very coarse parts seep through the sieve into another bowl. Repeat this procedure with the other half.

This sauce is easy to make and excellent to use for enchiladas as well as the Pull Apart Tacos featured in this cookbook. Add no-salt-added tomato sauce if making enchiladas. May be stored in the refrigerator or frozen in smaller containers for convenient use.

*These chilies are the large dried chilies

***Enchilada Sauce Nutritoiinal Data Per Tablespoons:** Calories: 1.934, Protein: .06 g, Carbohydrate: .441 g, Dietary Fiber: .093 g, Total Sugars: .186 g, Total Fat: .011 g, Saturated Fat: .002 g, Monounsaturated Fat: .001 g, Polyunsaturated Fat: .005 g, Cholesterol: 0 mg, Trans Fatty Acids: 0 g, Total Omega-3 FA: 0 g, Total Omega-6 FA: 0 g, Calcium: 1.114 mg, Potassium: 7.652 mg, Sodium: .271 mg, Vitamin K: .151 mcg*

GREEN BEAN CASSEROLE

LACTO OVO – 1 CARB CHOICES

Serves 4

Sodium Per Recipe: 142.9 mg Sodium Per Serving: 35.7 mg

If you can find a no-salt cheddar in your area, I recommend you use it instead of Heluvagood.

½ pound fresh green beans, blanched (13.2 mg)
1 medium onion, sliced for rings, broiled lightly[1] (4.4 mg)
½ cup mushrooms, diced (large) (1.75 mg)
2 cloves garlic (
½ cups shredded fresh Mozzarella cheese (17.8 mg)
½ cup reduced fat or lower sodium sour cream (73.2 mg)
1 tablespoon unsalted butter (1.562 mg)
1 tablespoon all-purpose flour (.162 mg)
⅛ teaspoon granulated onion powder (.648 mg)
½ teaspoon white sugar (trace)
¼ cup Panko original[2] (30 mg)

Clean trim string beans, cut in half, place into pot with enough water to bring them to a boil. Let boil lightly for about 10 minutes. Drain in colander and splash with ice cold water. Set aside.

Slice onion and push out rings. Lay on cooking sheet covered with parchment paper. Broil for about 5 minutes on each side. Set aside.

Chop mushrooms, mince galric, set aside. Grate low sodium mozzarella or low sodium Swiss, set aside.

Melt unsalted butter in a medium to large skillet over medium heat. Stir in flour until smooth, and cook for one minute. Stir in the granulated onion powder, sugar, chopped onion, mushrooms, and sour cream. Add blanched and trimmed green beans, and stir to coat. (May slice beans into bite size pieces.)

Transfer the mixture to a 8" x 8" casserole dish. Spread shredded cheese over the top. Sprinkle Panko over that.

Bake for 30 minutes in the preheated oven at 350° F, or until hot. Cheese will bubble slightly.

[1] Spray with light coat of oil. Broil carefully, they can burn up in a hurry.

[2]Check Panko package for sodium level. Most should state 25 to 35 mg sodium per 1/4 cup.

Green Bean Casserole Nutritional Data Per Serving: Calories: 209.9, Protein: 8.64 g, Carbohydrate: 13.4 g, Dietary Fiber: 2.83 g, Total Sugars: 4.738 g, Total Fat: 14.2 g, Saturated Fat: 8.714 g, Monounsaturated Fat: 2.878 g, Polyunsaturated Fat: .57 g, Cholesterol: 44.3 mg, Trans Fatty Acids: 0 g, Total Omega-3 FA: .135 g, Total Omega-6 FA: .077 g, Calcium: 228.7 mg, Potassium: 284.4 mg, Sodium: 35.7 mg, Vitamin K: 9.109 mcg

How to Blanch Your Greenbeans
& Other Vegetables

Blanching is when we partially cook vegetables and with a swift use of icy water cool them so they remain crunchy. The Green Bean Casserole asks for blanched green beans when using fresh beans. You may also use blanching for vegetables in salads and some pasta dishes. If you set out a plate of veggies for dips or as appetizers, try blanching them first. They will be easier to eat, not so hard on the digestive tract and they'll burst with natural flavors when eaten.

First, wash your green beans and cut the ends off. While doing this, bring a medium to large pot of water to a boil. Set aside a large bowl with ice water for shocking the beans after they boil.

Place the beans (a handful at a time) into the boiling water. Don't get the pot crowded – you want the beans floating freely if possible. We put them in slowly to help keep the water boiling at a consistent rate. Test the beans for doneness after a minute or so. The beans should remain crisp, but cooked.[1]

When cooked, remove the beans and put them into the ice-water quickly, pushing them down under water. This halts the cooking process. Like meats, vegetables will continue to cook until cooled.

When beans are "ice" cold, drain them well. Make sure they are cold. Any warmth at all will continue the cooking process.

[1] This process works for all vegetables. Some like broccoli can be tested using a knife into the thick stem. If the knife holds and lifts the broccoli, then it's not cooked. Same with carrots, celery and other stalk veggies. If the knife slide in and out, the vegetable is cooked.

DON'S MUSHROOM BURGER

FLEXITARIAN – 3+ CARB CHOICES

Makes 1 Burger

Sodium Per Burger: 63.7 mg

I love hamburgers. So, even though I had to lower my fat content and sodium to "below the line," I figured out how to make one I could enjoy anytime I wanted. Try it, you'll like it. The fat has also been reduced here.

1 sesame sandwich bun (12.3 mg)
1 inner leaf Romaine lettuce (.48 mg)
2 -ounces lean ground beef* (37 mg)
4 medium to large mushrooms, diced (3.68 mg)
1 thin or medium slice red onion, diced (.42 mg)
1 teaspoon honey mustard (5 mg) (3.3mg)
1 slice medium tomato (1.8mg)
1 ounce (slice) low sodium Swiss or Cheddar cheese (3.92 mg)**

Mix mushrooms and diced onion into meat. Cook meat mixture in nonstick pan, pressing down hard to make it bun size. Toast the buns inner side only, let cheese melt on top bun. Layer mustard on lower bun. Add no-salt-added ketchup if you like. Place meat against the melted cheese when the meat is done. Close sandwich. Delicious.

*May use turkey or chicken burger instead.

**Low sodium no-salt-added cheeses may list on their FDA labels from 5 mg to 10 mg per ounce.

Mushroom Burger Nutritional Data Per Burger: Calories: 475.2 . Protein: 29.8 g, Carbohydrate: 51.9 g, Dietary Fiber: 3.46 g, Total Sugars: 11 g, Total Fat: 16.6 g, Saturated Fat: 7.187 g, Monounsaturated Fat: 6.61 g, Polyunsaturated Fat: 1.63 g, Cholesterol: 76 mg, Trans Fatty Acids: .191 g, Total Omega-3, FA: .193 g, Total Omega-6 FA: .004 g, Potassium: 763.1 mg, Sodium: 63.7 mg, Vitamin K: 11.2 mcg

MUSHROOMS WITH SOY SAUCE

VEGAN – 1 CARB CHOICES

Serves 2

Sodium Per Recipe: 17.8   *Sodium Per Serving: 8.905 mg*

Mushrooms are loaded with vitamin D and that's just one of the good things about them. One of the others is that they make great side dishes for many entrees including omelets pork, beef, fish and fowl! Serve over the meat of your choice.

1 tablespoon extra virgin olive oil[1] (trace)
8 ounces sliced mushrooms (crimini, white, portabella)(11.2 mg)
3 cloves garlic, minced (3.06 mg)
2 teaspoons Don's Soy Sauce (3.55 mg)
white pepper to taste (trace)

In a nonstick skillet[1] stir mushrooms in olive oil until mushrooms have softened – about five minutes. Stir in the garlic and continue to cook and stir for a minute. Add the soy sauce and continue to cook the mushrooms until the liquid has evaporated – about three to five more minutes.

[1] If using other than nonstick, add one more tablespoon of extra virgin olive oil.

Mushrooms with Soy Sauce Nutritional Data Per Serving: Calories: 114.2 , Protein: 4.091 g, Carbohydrate: 10.5 g, Dietary Fiber: 1.34 g, Total Sugars: 4.844 g, Total Fat: 7.435 g, Saturated Fat: 1.064 g, Monounsaturated Fat: 3.365 g, Polyunsaturated Fat: 2.495 g, Cholesterol: 0 mg, Trans Fatty Acids: 0 g, Total Omega-3 FA: .032 g, Total Omega-6 FA: 0 g, Calcium: 30 mg, Potassium: 463.4 mg, Sodium: 8.905 mg, Vitamin K: 1.644 mcg

FRENCH DIP SANDWICH

Crockpot Recipe

FLEXITARIAN – 2 1/2 CARB CHOICES

Servings: 6 servings

Sodium Per Recipe: 767 mg   Sodium Per Sandwich: 117.5 mg

We had some leftover roast beef last week and I mentioned that we hadn't yet tried a French dip sandwich. Maureen's eyes brightened. She couldn't believe it. So we experimented and after some pleasant but not quite perfect tries with the leftovers we started from scratch with a fresh brisket and turned it into a Crockpot (slow cooker) recipe. With her chicken broth and some of our own sauces we succeeded with a very tasty French dip sandwich. We hope you like it as well. Our Worcestershire sauce worked a touch better than our soy sauce, but both were excellent.*

1 cup sweet onion[1] (1.5 mg)
1 2½-pound fresh beef round roast[2] (612.4 mg)
2 cloves garlic, minced (1.02 mg)
1 teaspoon ground dried thyme[3] (.77 mg)
½ teaspoon white pepper (.06 mg)
1 cup Maureen's Chicken Broth or Beef Broth[4] (21.7 mg)
¾ cup filtered water (trace)
1 tablespoon Don's Soy (1.77 mg) or Worcestershire sauce[5] (24.7 mg)
1 medium red or green sweet pepper, seeded, julienned (4.76 mg)
6 French Dip Buns[6] (15.5 mg)

Bake bread ahead of time or while crockpot is cooking.

Place onions in a 4-quart or larger crockpot. Cut fat from raw beef. Place meat on top of onions. Mix garlic, thyme, pepper together and rub on meat. Pour broth, and soy or Worcestershire sauce over meat and make sure it's covered with the broth.

Cover and cook on low or slow-heat setting. If using brisket you'll have to cook it longer than a round or a bottom. Possibly as long as ten hours. For the other beef 8 hours will do the trick. If cooking on high or fast cook setting, about four hours is all that's needed for the round or bottom with another hour tacked on if cooking the brisket.

Add red pepper slices to the slow cooker after about two or three hours at high setting or after about 4-hours on low setting.

When ready, move meat to a cutting board; cut thin slices cross-grain. Remove visible fat. Remove onions and red pepper from cooker with a slotted ladle or spoon.

Divide sliced meat into 6 portions (you may have more meat than needed.

Just seal it and save for another meal or freeze for a meal later on). Evenly layer the bun bottoms with the onions and pepper slices, leaving the sauce behind for dipping.

Skim fat off the sauce.

You can dip one of two ways. Either dip the tops and then place them on the sandwich, or set a plate or small bowl out for each person served a sandwich, with sauce on it to dip as they eat. .

[*]Also excellent with our beef broth. (See Index)

[1] Vidalia or Walla Walla work well. One large onion should fill a cup with the rings. Slice onion into ½ inch rings, push out all rings before placing into crockpot.

[2] Your choice of boneless, round, or bottom. If you prefer brisket add about 160 mg sodium per recipe or 25 mg per sandwich).

[3] You can exchange the thyme for a favorite compatible spice like marjoram, sage, or give it a different flavor with oregano or savory.

[4] Either works well. See Index for beef broth recipe. [1]Or use Swanson Unsalted Chicken Broth or other brand of choice. Add 4 mg sodium per serving.

[5] Soy Sauce data was used for the totals for this recipe. If using Worcestershire, add 4 mg sodium per sandwich.

[6] (See index for Baguette Buns) or make Ciabatta Buns. Either one should be halved lengthwise to make the dip. (*See No Salt, Lowest Sodium International Cookbook*), If you want to lower the sodium and carbohydrates, then

French Dip Nutritional Data Per Sandwich (Rosemary Baguette Buns): Calories: 604.3, Protein: 45.1 g, Carbohydrate: 39.9 g, Dietary Fiber: 2.004 g, Total Sugars: 6.16 g, Total Fat: 28 g, Saturated Fat: 9.596 g, Monounsaturated Fat: 12.1 g, Polyunsaturated Fat: 2.679 g, Cholesterol: 119.1 mg, Trans Fatty Acids: 0 g, Total Omega-3 FA: .268 g, Total Omega-6 FA: 0 g, Calcium: 29.4 mg, Potassium: 787.9 mg, Sodium: 117.5 mg, Vitamin K: 9.408 mcg

FRENCH DIP BUNS

LACTO OVO – 2 1/2 CARB CHOICES

Makes 12 4" long buns.

Sodium Per Recipe: 122.6 mg *Sodium Per Bun: 10.2 mg*

Baguettes are distinctive in flavor and with ingredients. A standard baguette might call for flour, water, yeast, salt and poolish. Poolish is basically sourdough. For our French Dip Recipe, we come close to a baguette but we leave out the poolish and add in lemon or orange zest, a bit of gluten and olive oil and egg whites (a good binder). We get the same results except for the sourdough flavor. If you want to make this with sourdough, then judge your sourdough liquidity when exchanging amounts of flour and water. For buns, designed for sandwiches like our French Dip Sandwich, it's best to stick to the recipe below.

The Dough

1 cup warmed (100° F to 105° F) filtered water (trace)
¼ cup white granulated sugar trace)
¼ cup extra virgin olive oil (trace)
2 egg whites, large eggs (109.6 mg)
¼ teaspoon ascorbic (trace)
1 tablespoon orange or lemon peel grated (.15 mg)
¼ teaspoon ascorbic acid (trace)
1 tablespoon vital wheat gluten (2.25 mg)
4 cups best for bread white flour (10 mg)
1 tablespoon bread machine yeast (6 mg)

After Machine Rise and Before Baking

½ egg white, whisked with a ¼ teaspoon filtered water (trace)
2 tablespoons Albers, Quaker or other cornmeal for dusting (1.134 mg)

Directions

Place dough ingredients in bread pan in order listed or in your manufacturer's order.

Just before dough is ready, set baking rack in oven in middle or one rack height below middle. Turn oven on for two minutes to 200° F. Then turn off. leave door closed. Separate the remaining egg saving the white in a small bowl. Add the water and whisk briskly. Have a basting brush handy.

When dough is ready to remove, roll out on lightly floured breadboard cut in half. Work with the first ball by pressing down on it forming a rectangle about 4" wide and about 12" long. Your dough will be about ½" thick. Make sure the sides are even. Using a sharp knife, begin sliced in the middle (the width that is) and then evenly to the right and left to form 6 buns.

Brush egg white over entire bun, then place these on the parchment paper sideways to the ends of the jelly roll pan. (The ends of each bun facing the sides of the pan.) Do the same with the second ball of dough. You should have two rows of six buns reaching down the length of the pan.

With a very sharp knife, make two slashes about a quarter inch deep about two-inches apart diagonally across the top of the buns. Set on middle rack of oven and close door to allow buns to rise.

After 45 to 60 minutes, turn oven on to 375° F. Buns should be fully baked in 15 to 20 minutes. They'll turn to a moderately dark golden brown.

Remove, cool on racks. Use with our French Dip Sandwiches or with hamburgers, chicken salad sandwiches, or serve with your favorite salad. (This recipe also may be converted into a Parker House Roll recipe producing about 30 rolls.

May store in zipper lock bags for a few days or freeze.

To reheat, place in microwave and reheat for about 10 to 20 seconds.

[1] or 3- 500 mg vitamin C tablets, crushed

French Dip Buns Nutritional Data Per Bun: Calories: 215, Protein: 5.4 g, Carbohydrate: 36.3 g, Dietary Fiber: 1.184 g, Total Sugars: 4.35 g, Total Fat: 5.097 g, Saturated Fat: .735 g, Monounsaturated Fat: 2.278 g, Polyunsaturated Fat: 1.714 g, Cholesterol: 0 mg, Trans Fatty Acids: 0 g, Total Omega-3 FA: .029 g, Total Omega-6 FA: 0 g, Calcium: 7.845 mg, Potassium: 55.6 mg, Sodium: 10.2 mg, Vitamin K: 1.109 mcg

BANANA PUDDING

LACTO OVO VEGETARIAN – 2.5 CARB CHOICES

8 servings

Sodium Per Recipe: 317.2 *mg* *Sodium Per Serving:* 43.3 *mg*

3 egg yolks (24.5 mg)
½ cup sugar or half sugar half Granulated Splenda (trace)
¼ cup cornstarch (2.88 mg)
2 cups nonfat milk with vitamin A added (205.8 mg)
1 tablespoon butter (1.562 mg)
1 teaspoon vanilla (.378 mg)
3 large firm but ripe bananas (about 1- pound peeled, meat only) (4.08 mg)
1 cup (total) pressurized whipped cream (78 mg)

Beat egg yolks slightly in small bowl and set aside.

Combine sugar or Splenda mix, and cornstarch in a medium-size saucepan over medium heat until well blended. Stir in nonfat milk until smooth. Cook slowly while stirring until mixture thickens and boils for 1-minute. Remove from heat and pur half the milk mixture into a small or medium size bowl.

Whisk beaten egg yolks into the half of the milk mixture in the new pan. Stir back into milk mixture in the saucepan. Over medium heat, cook while stirring constantly for 1 minute or until mixture thickens slightly. Stir in butter and vanilla. Stir until butter melts.

Transfer mixture to a bowl. Place over ice water. Let stand, stirring frequently, until cold. When chilled, spoon half the pudding mix into shall pudding bowls or ramekins.

Peel and slice two bananas. Set slices over the top of the cream filling. Cover with remaining cream filling, spreading evenly with a flat spoon or spatula. Place a slice from the third banana in the center of each bowl and push down to meet level of pudding leaving the top of the banana exposed. Place a piece of waxed paper directly on top of each pudding. Refrigerate 2 to 3 hours or until chilled and firm. Add dollops of whipped cream when serving. Serve cold.

[1] It is possible to get 10 servings from this recipe.

Greeen Beans with Almonds Nutritional Data: Calories: 105.2, Protein: 1.635 g, Carbohydrate: 6.459 g, Dietary Fiber: 2.207 g, Total Sugars: 2.344 g, Total Fat: 8.764 g, Saturated Fat: 1.181 g, Monounsaturated Fat: 4.467 g, Polyunsaturated Fat: 2.702 g, Cholesterol: 0 mg, Trans Fatty Acids: 0 g, Total Omega-3 FA: .062 g, Total Omega-6 FA: 0 g, Calcium: 27.1 mg, Potassium: 144.1 mg, Sodium: 3.96 mg, Vitamin K: 9.39 mcg

GREEN BEANS WITH ALMONDS
& CARAMALIZED SHALLOTS

VEGAN – 1 CARB CHOICES

4 servings

Sodium Per Recipe: 15.8 mg   *Sodium Per Serving: 3.46 mg*

¼ cup unsalted, blanched slivered almonds (1.44 mg)
3 teaspoons extra virgin olive oil[1] (trace)
2 small shallots, thinly sliced (1.2 mg)
1½ teaspoons granulated white sugar[2] (trace)
white pepper to taste (lightly) (trace)
½ pound fresh green beans, ends cut off, sliced diagonally at the center[3] (13.2 mg)

Using a nonstick skillet over low heat, toast almonds by stirring constantly until lightly toasted. Careful, they can burn quickly. This should take no more than three to four minutes. Set aside.

Blanch green beans in boiling water for a few minutes until they turn bright green and can be pierced with a fork. Then stop the cooking process by plunging them in ice water. Drain and set aside.

In the same nonstick pan you used for the almonds, add the olive oil. Heat oil to medium and add shallots, cook until softened. Sprinkle the mixture with sugar and white pepper. Cook until the sugar dissolves and the shallots caramelize about 6 to 8 minutes.

Add the green beans and mix gently, reheat until ready to serve, and top with toasted almonds.

[1] May use canned precooked unsalted (no salt added) green beans or frozen beans. By weight, 1 no salt added can would equal ½ pound beans.

[2] Or half sugar half Splenda. Splenda by itself will not caramelize.

Greeen Beans with Almonds Nutritional Data: Calories: 105.2, Protein: 1.635 g, Carbohydrate: 6.459 g, Dietary Fiber: 2.207 g, Total Sugars: 2.344 g, Total Fat: 8.764 g, Saturated Fat: 1.181 g, Monounsaturated Fat: 4.467 g, Polyunsaturated Fat: 2.702 g, Cholesterol: 0 mg, Trans Fatty Acids: 0 g, Total Omega-3 FA: .062 g, Total Omega-6 FA: 0 g, Calcium: 27.1 mg, Potassium: 144.1 mg, Sodium: 3.96 mg, Vitamin K: 9.39 mcg

SLOW-COOKED BBQ RIBS

FLEXITARIAN – 1.5 CARB CHOICES[1]

I like these cooked over the grill or in the slow-cooker. Cook on low for 8 hours. Makes a very nice meal with leftovers to enjoy later.

Serves 6 to 8

Sodium Per Recipe: 666.1 mg

Sodium Per Serving (6): 111 mg *Sodium Per Serving (8): 83.3 mg*

3 pounds boneless pork center rib country-style ribs1 (571.5 mg)
¼ teaspoon ground cloves (1.276 mg)
½ teaspoon no-salt chili powder (trace)
¼ cup light brown sugar, packed (15.4 mg)
3 cloves garlic, minced (1.53 mg)
1 medium onion, thinly sliced (4.4 mg)
½ cup unsweetened not-from-concentrate apple juice2 (4.96 mg)
1½ cups Don's Barbecue Sauce (67 mg)

For a five or six quart crockpot.
1
Lightly grease the crockpot bowl. Clean ribs meat with water, trim fat and pat dry with paper towels.

Place onions on bottom of cooker.

In a small bowl toss the meat pieces with the ground cloves, chili powder, brown sugar, and minced garlic.

Pour apple juice into pot and then lay the pork in.

Cover and cook on **low** for 8 hours. Drain any liquid that remains and then with the meat still in the crockpot bowl, pour barbecue sauce over the pork. Stir to make sure sauce is evenly distributed. Cover pot and cook on low for another hour or longer if you like.

[1] 1 Carb Choices if serving 8.

[2] May use up to four pounds. Cut as much fat off meat as possible.

[3] Or filtered water.

Barbecued Ribs Nutritional Data Per Serving (8): Calories: 432.2, Protein: 34.5 g, Carbohydrate: 17 g, Dietary Fiber: .765 g, Total Sugars: 14.1 g, Total Fat: 24.5 g, Saturated Fat: 8.369 g, Monounsaturated Fat: 11.1 g, Polyunsaturated Fat: 2.642 g, Cholesterol: 102.1 mg, Trans Fatty Acids: 0 g, Total Omega-3 FA: .18 g, Total Omega-6 FA: 0 g, Calcium: 31 mg, Potassium: 794.9 mg, Sodium: 83.3 mg, Vitamin K: 1.709 mcg

Barbecued Ribs Nutritional Data Per Serving (6): Calories: 576.3 , Protein: 46 g, Carbohydrate: 22.7 g, Dietary Fiber: 1.02 g, Total Sugars: 18.7 g, Total Fat: 32.7 g, Saturated Fat: 11.2 g, Monounsaturated Fat: 14.7 g, Polyunsaturated Fat: 3.522 g, Cholesterol: 136.1 mg, Trans Fatty Acids: 0 g, Total Omega-3 FA: .24 g, Total Omega-6 FA: 0 g, Calcium: 41.3 mg, Potassium: 1060 mg, Sodium: 111 mg, Vitamin K: 2.278 mcg

SLOW-COOKED POT ROAST

FLEXITARIAN – 0 CARB CHOICES

This is a terrific way to cook a pot roast, especially if you set it up before leaving for the day. Leftovers are useable in sandwiches or other meals.

Yield 6 to 8 servings

Sodium Per Recipe: 939 mg

Sodium Per Serving (6): 156.5 mg Sodium Per Serving (8): 117.4 mg

1 medium to large onion, sliced, rings pushed out (4.4 mg)
¼ cup filtered water (trace)
1½ tablespoons Don's Italian Seasoning1 (.494 mg)
⅛ teaspoon ground cloves (.638 mg)
1 2½ pound boneless beef chuck roast (873.2 mg)
3 cloves garlic, minced (1.53 mg)
1 large carrot, peeled, sliced (49.7 mg)
½ cup mushrooms, halves (1.75 mg)
2 tablespoons aged balsamic vinegar (7.36 mg)

Spread the onion slices out into the bottom of the crockpot. Pour water in. You might need a few more tablespoons of water to ensure onions are wet.

Punch the meat with a four pronged fork throughout. Rub the spice mix and ground cloves into the meat on both sides. Use more spice mix if you like the flavor a lot.

Place the roast into the crockpot on top of the onions.

Place carrots around the meat. Add balsamic to the pot either on the meat or in the water.

Cover the pot, set to Low, and cook until the roast is tender. Check in four hours. If the roast hasn't contributed more liquid to the cooker, then add another ¼ cup filtered water. If you won't be there for the eight hours, then add it in the beginnig for insurance. If you want it to make gravy, then add ¼ cup of flour and stir that with a ½- cup of filtered water and place that into the pot instead of the ¼ cup of water listed in the ingredients. Flour adds calories and carbohydrates.

[1] Or a "hotter" spice mix like Trader Joe's 21 Seasonings or other commerical salt free spice mixes.

Crockpot Pot Roast Nutritional Data Per Serving (6): Calories: 302.7, Protein: 37 g, Carbohydrate: 4.593 g, Dietary Fiber: .821 g, Total Sugars: 2.256 g, Total Fat: 14.1 g, Saturated Fat: 5.278 g, Monounsaturated Fat: 6.225 g, Polyunsaturated Fat: .565 g, Cholesterol: 122.9 mg, Trans Fatty Acids: 0 g, Total Omega-3 FA: .044 g, Total Omega-6 FA: 0 g, Calcium: 34.8 mg, Potassium: 702.2 mg, Sodium: 156.5 mg, Vitamin K: 1.745 mcg

SPINACH CHICKEN WRAPS

FLEXITARIAN – 0 CARB CHOICES

Serves 4 to 8[1]

Sodium Per Recipe: 486.7mg Sodium Per Serving (4): 121.7 mg

4 medium skinless, boneless chicken breast halves (about 20-ounces) (360 mg)
2 ounces chopped fresh or frozen spinach, washed, well-drained[2] (44.9 mg)
2 ounces low-sodium Swiss Cheese[3] (
3 ounces sour cream (about 7 to 10 tablespoons) (67.2 mg)
1 small onion chopped finely (2.8 mg)
1 cup chopped mushrooms (3.5 mg)
½ lemon (or lime), juice only (.47 mg)
2 tablespoons olive oil (trace)

Oil an 8 x 10 casserole dish. Set aside.

Place chicken breast on cutting board between plastic wrap (Saran or other). Pound with flat side of meat mallet (not the checkered side) to about ¼ to 3/8 inch thick. (Thin but not over beaten.)

In a medium size bowl combine the sour cream, onions, garlic and mushrooms. (May exchange ricotta or Farmer's cheese for the sour cream.)

Slice each of the two slices of Sargento's in half. Place each half on a pounded breast. Spoon the sour cream and onion mix onto the chicken, leaving about a half-inch open area around the edges. Evenly spread the chopped spinach on top.

Roll up, overlapping one side over the other. Pin down with three toothpicks, ensuring the chicken won't split open while cooking.

Place evenly spaced into your baking dish.

Bake, covered by foil, for 15 minutes. Remove foil, drizzle a bit of the olive oil over the meat at the seal on top. Leave uncovered and continue baking for another 40 minutes or until chicken is done. Use a thermometer in the meat (170° F).

About five minutes before it's done, drizzle the rest of the olive oil over the meat and squeeze lemon juice over the same area.

Remove chicken from oven, serve hot.

We like to serve cranberries with this dish and if you don't have fresh cranberries, canned whole berries workk or a good cranberry chutney.

Recommended side dish: green beans cooked with a bit of oil and some sliced mushrooms with a dash of white pepper or an Italian spice mix (unsalted of course).

Serve hot.

[1] We often serve only half of each half-breast, which doubles our servings.

[2]Spinach contains vitamin K, but it shouldn't upset your blood thinner readings if spinach is included in your diet now and then. Protime (INR) readings are used to adjust your blood thinner levels. If your diet is predictable, then your medications were adjusted for the levels of vitamin K you consume through food.

[3] Other brands may also have low sodium per ounce or per slice but not be no salt added. Sargento's works for us at 25 mg sodium per slice (eight tenths of an ounce). Swiss is one of the cheeses that is lower in sodium than most others. Check FDA panels on packages. Fresh mozzarella packed in water also works well and has about the same amount of sodium.

Spinach Chicken Wraps Nutritional Data Per Serving (4): Calories: 327.1, Protein: 38.1 g, Carbohydrate: 4.819 g, Dietary Fiber: .832 g, Total Sugars: 2.291 g, Total Fat: 17.1 g, Saturated Fat: 6.43 g, Monounsaturated Fat: 5.446 g, Polyunsaturated Fat: 2.675 g, Cholesterol: 103.8 mg, Trans Fatty Acids: 0 g, Total Omega-3 FA: .138 g, Total Omega-6 FA: .004 g, Calcium: 177.1 mg, Potassium: 220.2 mg, Sodium: 121.7 mg, Vitamin K: 70.8 mcg

RANCH DRESSING MIX

VEGAN - 0 CARB CHOICES

Make and store with other spices in an airtight jar. (We use old spice jars this way. Use for salads, party mixes, some casseroles.

Makes: 17 Tablespoons

Sodium Per Recipe: 76.2 mg   Sodium Per Serving: 4.483 mg

- **4 tablespoons dried parsley, crushed (28.9 mg)**
- **4 teaspoons dried dill weed (25.8 mg)**
- **4 teaspoons granulated onion powder (14.9 mg)**
- **4 teaspoons dried onion flakes (4.2 mg)**
- **2 teaspoons garlic powder (1.456 mg)**
- **1 teaspoons ground pepper (.924 mg)**

Place all ingredients in a pint or quart size jar, seal the jar and shake well. Transfer to smaller spice jar. Shake each time before using. Store in airtight jar on shelf for up to two months or you may store in fridge.

Salad dressing: Mix in with sour cream and or plain yogurt, a bit of extra virgin olive oil and possibly a touch of buttermilk or half and half. Mix in spices to taste.

Dip: Mix into sour cream to taste.

Ranch Dressing Mix Nutritional Data Per Tablespoon: Calories: 14, Protein: .568 g, Carbohydrate: 3.211 g, Dietary Fiber: .48 g, Total Sugars: 1.124 g, Total Fat: .077 g, Saturated Fat: .008 g, Monounsaturated Fat: .017 g, Polyunsaturated Fat: .014 g, Cholesterol: 0 mg, Trans Fatty Acids: 0 g, Total Omega-3 FA: .001 g, Total Omega-6 FA: 0 g, Calcium: 28.3 mg, Potassium: 78 mg, Sodium: 4.483 mg, Vitamin K: 5.432 mcg

CHICKPEA SANDWICH FILLING

VEGAN – 0 CARB CHOICES

When using this recipe, I often load up a sandwich with freshly sliced tomato, onion, some good lettuce, aged balsamic vinegar and sometimes fresh basil. Although this mix is terrific all by itself, the added nutrients from the above ingredients are beneficial and of course, tasty. Note the 0 Fats in the nutrient data.

Makes Enough For: 4 Sandwiches

Sodium Per Recipe: 102.1 mg Sodium Per Sandwich (4): 17 mg

1 (14.5 ounce) can Eden Organic No Salt Added Garbanzo beans, drained (70 mg)
½ medium stalk celery, chopped (16 mg)
½ medium onion, chopped (2.2 mg)
1 tablespoon Yo Cheese or Greek Style Yogurt1 (11.6 mg)
1 tablespoon lemon juice (.153 mg)
1 teaspoon dried dill weed (2.08 mg)
white pepper to taste (trace)

Place drained and rinsed Eden Organic chickpeas into a medium size bowl. Either mash with a potato masher, a handheld processor or a sturdy fork. Mix in celery, Yo Cheese, onion, lemon juice, dill weed , and pepper to taste.

Serve on any of our homemade sandwich breads.

Chickpea Sandwich Filling Nutritional Data Per Serving (4): Calories: 115.9, Protein: 6.678 g, Carbohydrate: 19 g, Dietary Fiber: 4.748 g, Total Sugars: .766 g, Total Fat: 1.354 g, Saturated Fat: .012 g, Monounsaturated Fat: .006 g, Polyunsaturated Fat: .007 g, Cholesterol: .115 mg, Trans Fatty Acids: 0 g, Total Omega-3 FA: .001 g, Total Omega-6 FA: 0 g, Calcium: 17.6 mg, Potassium: 55.9 mg, Sodium: 16.8 mg, Vitamin K: 1.52 mcg

BUTTERNUT SQUASH SOUP

FLEXITARIAN* – 2 CARB CHOICES

Makes 8 cups

Sodium Per Recipe: 113.7 mg   Sodium Per Cup: 17 mg

Maureen does it again. A fabulous soup. Not the low calories, very low sodium and nearly 4 grams dietary fiber. Flavor is high and texture is wonderful.

1 medium butternut squash (39.2 mg)
2 medium onions (8.8 mg)
2 medium green apples (trace)
2 tablespoons extra virgin olive oil (trace)
4 cups Maureen's Chicken Broth[1] (87.7 mg)
2 teaspoons dried thyme (.77 mg)
1 teaspoon Chinese 5-spice (trace)
black peppercorns, ground, to taste (trace)

Preheat Oven to 400° F

Peel squash and apples. (We use a large OXO peeler for the squash.) Cube squash into bite size pieces, cut up apples and onions and add these ingredients to a large mixing bowl. Pour olive oil on veggies and mix thoroughly. Sprinkle with herbs and spices. Transfer to baking dish and bake 40 to 50 minutes at 400° F, stirring at least three times.

When veggies are soft remove them from the oven and beat them in small batches with a hand-held blender or mixer.

Using 1-cup of Maureen's Chicken broth at a time, return to pot to reheat. This will make 8-cups of soup.

Delicious with a dollop of crème fraiche or sour cream.

*Flexitarian (semi-vegetarian) because of the chicken broth.

[1]Prepare broth earlier. You can store our chicken broth in your fridge in sealed quart jars for up to a week. The broth also freezes well and will store that way up to three or four months. Thaw in fridge for a few days before using. You don't want to thaw it outside of the fridge since is chicken broth. Or use Swanson Unsalted Chicken Broth or your favorite brand. Add 12 mg per serving if using branded unsalted chicken broth.

Butternut Squash Soup Nutritional Data Per Cup: Calories: 136.7, Protein: 3.019 g, Carbohydrate: 23.9 g, Dietary Fiber: 3.909 g, Total Sugars: 8.571 g, Total Fat: 4.578 g, Saturated Fat: .796 g, Monounsaturated Fat: 2.871 g, Polyunsaturated Fat: .648 g, Cholesterol: 5.648 mg, Trans Fatty Acids: 0 g, Total Omega-3 FA: .077 g, Total Omega-6 FA: 0 g, Calcium: 78.5 mg, Potassium: 560.3 mg, Sodium: 17 mg, Vitamin K: 8.09 mcg

ROLLS / BUNS FOR ALL SEASONS

LACTO OVO — 2 CARB CHOICES
Makes: 18 Sandwich Buns or
Makes 36 Dinner Rolls
Sodium Per Recipe: 192.4 mg
Sodium Per Sandwich Bun (18): 10.7 mg
Sodium Per Dinner Roll (36): (5.345 mg

This recipe is brand new (2016). It's for white bread rolls, buns, sliced bread and could even be rolled out for thick pizza dough. The dough is elastic enough to even make pizza crust, cinnamon buns or baked cinnamon/raisin loaves. Measure exactly as instructed below, let it rise, remove and shape into servings that you want.

2 cups warmed filtered water (105° F to 110° F) (trace)
½ cup first pressed or expeller canola oil (trace)
2 tablespoons cider vinegar (1.49 mg)
2 large eggs (140 mg)
1 teaspoon vanilla extract or vanilla flavoring (.378 mg)
4 ¾ cups white, unbleached bread flour (11.9 mg)
2 tablespoons vital wheat gluten (5.916 mg)
¼ cup potato flour (22 mg)
1 tablespoon malted barley flour (.75 mg)
¼ teaspoon ascorbic acid (3 to 4 vitamin C tablets crushed) (trace)
1 tablespoon sugar (trace)
2 tablespoons Splenda (trace)
2 tablespoons granulated soy lecithin (trace)
1 tablespoon plus 2 teaspoons bread machine yeast (10 mg)

Glaze
1 egg white (64 mg)
1 tablespoon filtered water (trace)

Place ingredients in bread pan in order listed. Make sure yeast is in a pocket of the flour and not near the sugar or Splenda. Set machine for "dough" and after the rise[1] roll out onto lightly floured bread board.

While dough is being prepared in machine, prepare your pans, cookie sheets or muffing/dinner roll pans with parchment paper for bread pans or cookie sheets or flour dusted oil for muffin pans. Also set an egg out to come to room temp. When ready, whisk the egg white and water together using a basting brush.

When ready, roll dough out on to board and knead with hands for just a couple of times. Then ball up and slice in half with very sharp knife.

1. For burger buns I use English muffin rings to cut out a bun size piece. Place these on parchment paper on cookie sheets. Brush on egg white mix, sprinkle with toasted sesame seeds.

Let rise in warm place for 45 minutes to an hour. Bake in 375o F oven for 15 to 20 minutes or until done.

2. For dinner rolls, prepare pans an pull enough dough to roll into 1" balls. Set three to four of these into each muffin cup and when done, set aside to rise for about 40 minutes.

3. Bread Loaves: Slice the dough into three or four sections. Knead each until smooth, about a minute or less. Lay into parchement paper covered loaf pans. Let rise for 45 minutes to an hour in warm place. Bake in oven at 375o F for about 20 minutes or until golden brown. May bake all loaf pans on same rack in a convection oven.

Allow all breads to cool on rack for at least 20-minutes before "testing" or serving. The bread needs to "finish" cooking while cooling on the rack.

Remember: Don't open oven door to check bread while it's baking. If you have a window and an interior light, use that to check.

[1] Dough may push against lid before the timer ends. Remove dough if it gets that high and following instructions.

Nutrient Data Per Sandwich Bun (18): Calories: 202.8, Protein: 5.593 g, Carbohydrate: 28.8 g, Dietary Fiber: 1.304 g, Total Sugars: .987 g, Total Fat: 7.025 g, Saturated Fat: .681 g, Monounsaturated Fat: 4.103 g, Polyunsaturated Fat: 1.929 g, Cholesterol: 23.5 mg, Trans Fatty Acids: .024 g, Total Omega-3 FA: 1.119 g, Total Omega-6 FA: 1.129 g, Potassium: 89.9 mg, Sodium: 10.7 mg, Vitamin K: 4.433 mcg

Nutrient Data Per Dinner Roll (36): Calories: 101.4, Protein: 2.796 g, Carbohydrate: 14.4 g, Dietary Fiber: .652 g, Total Sugars: .494 g, Total Fat: 3.512 g, Saturated Fat: .341 g, Monounsaturated Fat: 2.051 g, Polyunsaturated Fat: .964 g, Cholesterol: 11.8 mg, Trans Fatty Acids: .012 g, Total Omega-3 FA: .56 g, Total Omega-6 FA: .564 g, Potassium: 45 mg, Sodium: 5.345 mg, Vitamin K: 2.217 mcg

100% WHOLE WHEAT BREAD[1]

LACTO OVO - 1 CARB CHOICES
Makes 56 Slices
Sodium Per Recipe: 202 mg Sodium Per Slice: 3.608 mg

This "fail-safe" whole wheat bread recipe is our very best effort to date. We think you'll love it. You can make it without sugar, but we do recommend a level tablespoon to help the yeast activate. One (1) level tablespoon of sugar contains 12.6 g of carbohydrates or in the case of this recipe .225 grams of carbs per slice. To help you compare that to "reality," one medium banana contains 27 grams of carbohydrates. In other words, one banana contains more carbs than two level tablespoons of sugar. If you want to make this bread without sugar, add 1 teaspoon of yeast to the recipe.

We used whole wheat from "Wheat Montana, Farms & Bakery." We use the whole wheat that is "Prairie Gold Premium 100% Whole Wheat Flour." It is unbleached and it's white whole wheat. White and Red Whole Wheat have the same nutrients, but white whole wheat bakes better for bread loaves. Visit this page at Amazon.com to find the Whole Wheat Flour we created and tested for this recipe.

2 cups warmed filtered water (105° F to 115° F) (trace)
2 large eggs (140 mg)
1 teaspoon vanilla extract (.378 mg)
2 tablespoons apple cider vinegar (1.49 mg)
½ cup expeller pressed canola oil (trace)
4½ cups whole wheat flour (27 mg)
1 tablespoon of white granulated sugar (trace)
2 tablespoons granulated Splenda or other sucralose (trace)
3 tablespoons vital wheat gluten (8.155 mg)
2 tablespoons granulated soy lecithin (trace)
2 tablespoon potato flour (11 mg)
2 tablespoons plus 1-teaspoon active dry bread machine yeast (14 mg)

Place ingredients into bread machine pan in order listed. Set for dough.

Prep while dough making is in process.: 4 bread loaf pans with parchment paper, or two loaf pans and a baking sheet to make bread "rounds." Cover sheet with parchment paper or silicon sheets.

After dough cycle is finished, or when dough reaches lid of your machine, roll out onto lightly floured board and with a very sharp knife, slice into four sections.

Roll each piece into a smooth log that will fit into a loaf pan.

Place into parchment paper lined loaf pans, baste with light coat of nonfat milk, let rise in a warm place for about an hour or until it's at least double. We have seen it rise more, but don't wait too long to place into oven.

Set rack to low middle area of oven(s). Set a small aluminum pan with a half inch to an inch of water into oven off to the side or at the back.

Preheat oven to 375° F. When ready, set two loaves on rack apart from each other and bake for about 15 to 25 minutes (Our oven takes approximately 25 minutes). If loaf sounds hollow when you snap it with your fingers, it's done.

Remove and set onto rack to cool. Best not to slice the bread for the first fifteen to twenty minutes.

Repeat above baking for next loaf or loaves unless you have two ovens and are able to bake both batches set at the same time. Enjoy.

[1]To make this bread without sugar, add 2 tablespoons malted barley wheat and one teaspoon of yeast for a total of 2 tablespoons plus 2 teaspoons. Reduce Splenda by 1 tablespoon. (Splenda is included simply for a sweeter bread. You may also exclude it entirely.)

Nutritional Data Per Slice (56): Calories: 62.2, Protein: 2.139 g, Carbohydrate: 7.862 g, Dietary Fiber: 1.306 g, Total Sugars: .302 g, Total Fat: 2.824 g, Saturated Fat: .307 g, Monounsaturated Fat: 1.389 g, Polyunsaturated Fat: .872 g, Cholesterol: 7.554 mg, Trans Fatty Acids: .008 g, Total Omega-3 FA: .386 g, Total Omega-6 FA: .363 g, Potassium: 56 mg, Sodium: 3.608 mg, Vitamin K: 2.47 mcg

RAPID WAFFLES

LACTO OVO — 2 CARB CHOICES
Makes 1 Waffle
Sodium Per Waffle: 87.5 mg

In a rush? Here's a great rapid waffle. You can double this waffle recipe or triple it, etc. Works for Belgian waffle makers or the standard round waffle-maker. The nutrient values are for one single waffle in either machine, using either two thick or four thinner slices of homemade, salt free bread. Now, don't inhale too deeply, we know that waffle batter contains a variety of high sodium ingredients from baking soda to baking powder and of course gobs of salt. A standard waffle can contain as many as 1,000 mg of sodium with commercial (restaurant) waffles being even higher. The calories in many waffles come from sugar, flour and what we put on top, such as syrup, powdered sugar or even sour cream.

2 standard size slices of homemade bread[1] (11.3 mg)
1 large egg, whisked with milk (70 mg)
1 tablespoon half and half or nonfat milk (6.15 mg)
Ground cinnamon to taste (.078 mg)

Preheat waffle iron. If iron is nonstick you will not need to oil it. If you must oil it, do so with a can of spray olive oil or canola oil.

Sprinkle cinnamon on sliced bread.[2]

Whisk egg with nonfat milk or half & half in a flat bowl where you can lay your sliced bread evenly.

When iron Is hot, lay bread onto whisked egg and milk mix and then turn over. When well over, place on half of the iron. So the same with the second slice.

Close waffle maker, sealing it as tightly as possible and wait for "green light."

When waffle is cooked remove and serve as you usually would. It will amaze you.

[1] Enough to cover most of the waffle iron but not fully. If using our 100% whole wheat bread, circa 2016, sodium levels per slice will be about 3.5 mg.

[2] We prefer our 100% whole wheat bread recipe or the sugar-free white bread recipe.

Nutrient Data Per Waffle:
Calories: 297.6, Protein: 15.6 g, Carbohydrate: 35.3 g, Dietary Fiber: 6.141 g, Total Sugars: .426 g, Total Fat: 11.8 g, Saturated Fat: 3.22 g, Monounsaturated Fat: 4.838 g, Polyunsaturated Fat: 2.218 g, Cholesterol: 243.6 mg, Trans Fatty Acids: 0 g, Total Omega-3 FA: .409 g, Total Omega-6 FA: 0 g, Potassium: 304.4 mg, Sodium: 87.5 mg, Vitamin K: 5.523 mcg

LENTIL & GARBANZO BEAN SOUP

VEGAN — 2.5 CARB CHOICES

Sodium Per Recipe: 279.5 mg Sodium Per 1-Cup serving: 46.6 mg

Garbanzo beans are pureed and stirred into the lentil soup to help flavor and thicken it. Before cooking always examine, sort, and rinse lentils well. Lentils require no soaking.

4 tablespoons extra virgin olive oil, divided (trace)
1 medium onion, chopped (4.4 mg)
1 carrot, finely chopped (42.1 mg)
3 cloves garlic, minced (1.53 mg)
3 to 6 teaspoons curry powder to taste1 (4.68 mg)
1 cup lentils, sorted and rinsed, see step one below (11.5 mg)
1 carton(32 oz.)unsalted Swanson or other unsalted broth/stock2 (180 mg)
1 can no-salt-added garbanzo beans, drained (35 mg)
2 tablespoons fresh lemon juice (.305 mg)

Step One

In a large pot, for each pound of lentils (about 2 cups)
add 6-8 cups hot filtered water.
Simmer gently with lid tilted until desired tenderness is reached, about 15-20 minutes. Make sure you don't overcook them.

Step Two

In a large pot or Dutch oven, heat 2 tablespoons extra virgin olive oil over medium high heat. Sauté onion and carrots until onion is tender, 5 minutes. Stir in garlic and curry powder; sauté 1-minute. Stir in lentils and stock. Bring to a boil, reduce heat and simmer, covered, until lentils are tender, 35 to 40 minutes. Meanwhile, puree garbanzo beans in a food processor with lemon juice, 4 tablespoons filtered water and the remaining 2 tablespoons extra virgin olive oil until smooth. When lentils are tender, stir in garbanzo bean mixture. Simmer for 10 to 15 minutes until temperature reaches 165° F, measured by a food thermometer. Season with white or black pepper and more curry powder, if desired.

[1] You can adjust the curry flavor to your taste; begin by adding 3 telaspoons and increase as you like.

[2] Use either chicken, beef or vegetable broth. Water works too, but then you'll need more curry or white or black pepper.

Nutrient Data Per Cup: Calories: 295.4, Protein: 13.7 g, Carbohydrate: 36.1 g, Dietary Fiber: 14.4 g, Total Sugars: 3.254 g, Total Fat: 11.1 g, Saturated Fat: 1.437 g, Monounsaturated Fat: 4.631 g, Polyunsaturated Fat: 3.305 g, Cholesterol: 0 mg, Trans Fatty Acids: 0 g, Total Omega-3 FA: .083 g, Total Omega-6 FA: 0 g, Potassium: 563.7 mg, Sodium: 46.6 mg, Vitamin K: 6.498 mcg

Recipe Suggests:	Vol.	May Exchange with:
1 (8-inch) round cake pan	4 cups	1 (8 x 4)-inch loaf pan, *or* 1 (9-inch) round cakepan, *or* 1 (9-inch) pie plate
2 (8-inch) round cake pans	8 cups	2 (8 x 4-inch) loaf pans 1 (9-inch) tube pan 2 (9-inch) round cake pans 1 (10-inch) Bundt pan 1 (11 x 7-inch) baking dish 1 (10-inch) springform pan
1 (9-inch) round cake pan	6 cups	1 (8-inch) round cake pan 1 (8 x 4-inch) loaf pan 1 (11 x 7-inch) baking dish
2 (9-inch) round cake pans	12 cups	2 (8 x 4-inch) loaf pans 1 (9-inch) tube pan 2 (8-inch) round cake pans 1 (10-inch) Bundt pan 2 (11 x 7-inch) baking dishes 1 (10-inch) springform pan
1 (10-inch) round cake pan	11 cups	2 (8-inch) round cake pans 1 (9-inch) tube pan 1 (10-inch) springform pan
2 (10-inch) round cake pans	22 cups	5 (8-inch) round cake pans 3 or 4 (9-inch) round cakepans 2 (10-inch) springform pans
9-inch tube pan	12 cups	2 (9-inch) round cake pans 2 (8-inch) round cake pans 1 (10-inch) Bundt pan
10-inch tube pan	16 cups	3 (9-inch) round cake pans 2 (10-inch) pie plates 2 (9-inch) deep dish pie plates 4 (8-inch) pie plates 2 (9x5-inch) loaf pans 2 (8-inch) sq. baking dishes
11 x 7 x 2-inch baking dish	6 cups	1 (8-inch) square baking dish 1 (9-inch) square baking dish 1 (9-inch) round cake pan

10-inch Bundt pan	12 cups	2 (9-inch) sq. baking dishes 1 (9x13-inch) baking dish 2 (9-inch) round cake pans 2 (8-inch) round cake pans 1 (9-inch) tube pan 2 (11x7-inch) baking dishes 1 (10-inch) springform pan
9 x 13 x 2-inch baking dish	15 cups	1 (10-inch) Bundt cake pan 2 (9-inch) round cake pans 3 (8-inch) round cake pans 1 (10 x 15-inch) jellyroll pan
10 x 15 x 1-inch jellyroll pan	15 cups	1 (10-inch) Bundt pan 2 (9-inch) round cake pans 2 (8-inch) round cake pans 1 (9 x 13-inch) baking dish
9 x 5-inch loaf pan	8 cups	1 (9 x 2-inch) deep dish pie plate 1 (10-inch) pie plate 1 (8-inch) square baking dish
8 x 4-inch loaf pan	6 cups	1 (9-inch) square baking dish 1 (8-inch) round cake pan
9-inch springform pan	10 cups	1 (11 x 7-inch) baking dish 1 (10-inch) round cake pan 1 (10-inch) springform pan 2 (8-inch) round cake pans
10-inch springform pan	12 cups	2 (9-inch) round cake pans 2 (8 x 4-inch) loaf pans 1 (9-inch) tube pan 2 (9-inch) round cake pans 1 (10-inch) Bundt pan 2 (11 x 7-inch) baking dishes 2 (8-inch) round cake pans
8-inch square baking dish	8 cups	1 (9 x 2-inch) deep dish pie plate 1 (9 x 5-inch) loaf pan 2 (8-inch) pie plates
9-inch square baking dish	8 cups	1 (11 x 7-inch) baking dish 1 (9 x 2-inch) deep dish pie plate 1 (9 x 5-inch) loaf pan 2 (8-inch) pie plates

Glossary

The following are general definitions. No recommendations for use or non use are made by the authors. Data and suggested levels of consumption are based on USDA or NIH recommendations. The authors recommend sodium levels prescribed by your doctor, however encourage you to discuss the successes we've had with very low sodium intake. The authors also recommend that if you want to try for lower levels of sodium than suggested herein, that you speak with your doctor so that he/she knows you are going to consume lower levels of sodium. The American Medical Association recommends between 1300 mg and 1800 mg a day for healthy people. Chef Don has held his level at 500 mg and below per day since 1997.

Ablation, Cardiac – A noninvasive procedure generally performed on patients with abnormal heart rhythms. Used to treat rapid heart beats. These heart beats usually involve the upper chambers of the heart (atria). Known as SVTs or super ventricular tachycardias. Known generally as atrial fibrillation (A-Fib), atrial flutter, atrial tachycardia, AV nodal reentrant tachycardia and AV reentrant tachycardia. When successful, cardiac ablations reduce or relieve any need for the patient to take lifelong antiarrhythmic medications. Some ablations treat heart rhythm disorders that occur or begin in the lower chambers, but these are infrequent. Ablations of the lower chambers carry more danger than of the upper chambers since they can cause sudden cardiac death. The risk of sudden cardiac death might also be a reason for a cardiac ablation, however, in this case you may also receive an implantable cardioverter device (ICD). The ablation may prove worth it since it decreases the frequency of abnormal heart rhythms in the ventricles. The reduction of ICD shocks after the ablation makes the procedure well worth it.

New to the ablation arena is a device known as a stereotaxis system. See: Stereotaxis and visit *www.stereotaxis.com.*

Accent Flavor Enhancer – See MSG and Flavor Enhancers.

Ala Carte – À la carte or a la carte is a French phrase meaning "from the card," or menu. More literally translated it means "by the bill of fare." It can mean one of two things in a restaurant – either each individual item you order is priced separately, or there are options to the courses listed.

Almonds (nuts) – Whole almonds with skins on provide the human heart many benefits. Nearly a score of flavonoids are found in the almond seed skin alone. Those combined with the vitamin E in the meat of the nut make almonds a serious fighter against heart disease and other maladies. They are in other words, loaded with high octane antioxidants. Unsalted almonds contain magnesium, phosphorus, potassium, tryptophan and smaller amounts of vitamin A, a whopping 8.97 mg of vitamin E, zinc, riboflavin, manganese, and folate. Other nutrients per quarter-cup include protein (7.62 g), dietary fiber (4.07 g), Monounsaturated fat (11.6 g), polyunsaturated fat (4.364 g) and only .345 mg of sodium. Almonds are available year round. Almonds are really the seed of the almond fruit tree. That is why you will hear the seed often referred to as the almond nut. Almonds are credited with lowering LDL (the bad cholesterol), protection against diabetes and cardiovascular disease, and the ability to help us lose body weight. A quarter cup of almonds has about 206 calories, but studies have shown that if you eat nuts two times a week you are more likely to lose or not gain weight as opposed to those who do not eat nuts. Remember, peanuts are not part of this equation. Peanuts are legumes, not nuts.

Alpha-carotene – Alpha carotene is the second most common form of carotene. Carrots have both alpha and beta-carotenes at high levels. These provide health benefits when they neutralize free radicals that may cause damage to cells. Carotenes are the reason yams, carrots, butter, and other fruits and vegetables are orange. Carotenes are also responsible for the orange colors in dry foliage. Additional orange colored foods that contain carotene include cantaloupe, mango, apricots, winter squash and pumpkin. Carotene is also found in non orange colored foods like kale, spinach, beet greens, mustard greens, cilantro, fresh thyme and broccoli. (See: Free radicals)

Amino acids – Amino acids are known as the building blocks of proteins. An amino acid is classified as *essential* when our body synthesis is inadequate to meet metabolic need. When that happens, we must be supplied with amino acids as part of our diet. These acids can affect everything from growth to the body's natural treatment of injury and disease. Amino acid deficiency can result in poor health. One of the essential amino acids we ingest in many foods is tryptophan. It is one of the necessary essential amino acids. Other important amino acids include leucine, isoleucine, valine, phenylalanine, methionine, threonine, lysine, and histidine.

Anthocyanins – A flavonoid found in different fruits. It neutralizes free radicals, offering a possible reduction in the risk of cancer.

Anti-inflammatory (food) – See Anti-inflammatory Section in this book.

Antioxidants – Substances that prevent oxidation. Neutralizes the damaging effects of free radicals in certain cell components. Oxidation has been linked to cancer, aging, atherosclerosis, ischemic injury, inflammation and neurodegenerative diseases (Parkinson's and Alzheimer's). Antioxidants include carotene, vitamins C and E and selenium.

Artisanal Salt – These are "marketing" salts or heavily promoted table and sea salts. They are "flavored," and boast added minerals. Problem is that sodium is sodium and the added minerals are inconsequential when it comes to health matters or added nutrients. There are a variety of them on the market today. If you are on a low sodium diet, do not use.

Ascorbic acid – Also known as vitamin C. Fortunately many fruits and vegetables have vitamin C, which is essential for the development and maintenance of connective tissue. It's the vitamin C that intensifies production of new cells in the healing of wounds. It is also an antioxidant that keeps free radicals from linking with other molecules, which in turn would form damaging compounds that might attack tissue. Vitamin C plays a big roll in protecting our immune system as it helps to ward off infections. It can also reduce serious allergic reactions. Another benefit is its role in the synthesis of hormones and other body chemicals. We use ascorbic acid in no-salt bread recipes since it helps as a bread leavening agent when added with gluten, vinegar and sugar.

Atherosclerosis – A condition that can bring about a stroke or heart attack. When too much cholesterol builds up in our blood vessels, blood accumulates along the walls and begins the blocking process. (See: Cholesterol)

Atrial fibrillation (A-fib) – A cardiac arrhythmia often characterized by rapid out-of-sync beating of the atria (upper heart chambers). More infrequently this can occur as well in the lower chambers. This results in poor or ineffective atrial contractions. A-fib causes poor blood flow, shortness of breath, and weakness that can often bring the victim to his/her knees or cause them to pass out. A-fib patients are nearly always prescribed a blood thinner to prevent possible clotting. A-fib without protective medications can cause a stroke. An alternative to antiarrhythmic medications for A-fib is a surgical cardiac ablation. This procedure might be needed more than once. (See: Ablation)

Au Gratin – With potatoes (on a restaurant menu) it means the potatoes are covered with bread crumbs or crumbs mixed with butter and grated cheese, and then cooked or browned in an oven. Other foods can be prepared au gratin as well.

Baking Powder (double acting) – Having 320 mg to 480 mg per teaspoon, baking powder is used mostly to leaven quick breads and cakes. A baking powder replacement brand called Featherweight has only 13.2 mg of sodium per tablespoon (USDA). Ener-g Foods, Seattle, WA, has a double-acting baking powder with 0 mg sodium.. Both can be found in health food stores, some grocery stores, or online from *Healthy Heart Market.* The primary ingredient for Featherweight is Potassium Chloride. This is not salt and neither is it "potassium salt." However, if you are monitoring your potassium then you may want to evaluate Featherweight more closely before using it. To use in converting one of your own recipes, the general rule is to exchange three times the amount of Featherweight for the standard baking powder. However, you may not like the biting taste Featherweight gives if you use too much of it. So, I usually try just doubling the amount when first making a recipe. Often it works, but sometimes it doesn't. Mix it into the batter immediately prior to placing into oven. Stir in thoroughly. Make sure oven is preheated and ready for you to place the batter in. Ener-g baking powder has no flavor and is mostly calcium carbonate.

Baking Soda – Baking soda has approximately 821 mg to 1,000 mg of sodium per teaspoon. Generally used to leaven breads and cakes, baking soda is often added by commercial food servers (restaurants) and some processors to vegetables in cooking, and is often included in antacids and toothpaste. We should try to avoid using baking soda and ask in restaurants whether it was used on our food even as a freshener. Fortunately for home chefs, a good baking soda replacement is available from Ener-G Foods in Seattle, Washington. You can buy it online at *Healthy Heart Market.* It's called Ener-G Baking Soda. It works best when using two to three times the standard amount (from any given recipe). Ener-G does a good job.

Bangers – British for sausages. During WWII a shortage of meat caused sausage processors to put more water into the popular British sausage. When British citizens fried them the water would burst making a "banging" sound. They were thereafter referred to as bangers.

Basic Metabolic Panel (BMP) – A basic metabolic panel is a blood test that measures your glucose level, electrolyte and fluid balance, and kidney function. Your BMP may also produce any or all of the following: blood levels of sodium, potassium, chloride, carbon dioxide, calcium total protein, albumin, bilirubin, alkaline phosphates, AST and ALT (formerly called "serum") blood urea nitrogen, and creatinine. ALT is a test for your liver and also kidneys, heart, muscles and pancreas. AST (aspartate aminotransferase) measures the amount of this enzyme in the blood.

Baseline – In medicine (pertaining to us personally) a baseline is basically the information collected at the beginning of our medical visits or the beginning of a new diagnosis from which variations found later in fresh tests are measured.

Beta Carotene – The most common carotenoid found in many fruits and vegetables. It neutralizes free radicals. (See: Alpha-carotene)

Bioflavonoids – See Flavonoids.

Blanching – Scalding vegetables in boiling water or steam for a short time. Usually done before freezing or peeling. (See: Braising)

Blood Glucose – Primary (simple or monosaccharide) sugar made by the body from carbohydrates, protein and fat in our diet. Glucose moves through the bloodstream to provide energy to all our cells. In order for glucose to function, it needs help from insulin. Also known as dextrose.

Blood Pressure (bp) – An important vital sign. Blood pressure (bp or BP) is the force (or pressure) per unit area where pressure is exerted on the blood vessels. To cut to the meaning of this for us lay readers, body fluids can put lots of pressure on blood vessels thereby causing our bp to rise. Ergo, cut sodium, which causes the retention of body fluids, and you'll lower your bp. Blood moves away from the heart through arteries and capillaries and toward the heart through veins.

Most of us are unaware that blood pressure risks are higher with us than we realize. If your blood pressure is over 120/80 then you are at risk and should, according to many researchers and doctors, cut your salt and start a medication program. Any level higher than 120/80 can be considered dangerous. The National Heart, Lung, and Blood Institute refer to the area between "normal" and "hypertension" as "pre-hypertension." Visit the NHLBI online to obtain more information. It is definitely worth a visit. (http://www.nhlbi.nih.gov/)

Blood Sodium (Also: Serum Sodium) – Sodium levels in our blood are tested with a standard blood test. The normal range for blood sodium levels is 135 to 145 milliequivalents per liter (mEq/L). Normal value ranges may vary slightly among different laboratories. Mine has not changed in 13 years of a very low sodium diet, but then I don't take diuretics, which are often the leading cause of lowered blood sodium. Other factors can also cause low or high blood sodium. These include recent trauma, surgery, or shock. Also lower blood sodium causes include anabolic steroids, birth control pills, certain antibiotics, clonidine, corticosteroids, cough medications, laxatives, methyldopa, nonsteroidal anti-inflammatory drugs (NSAIDs).

Consuming large or small amounts of salt or fluid may affect a few points but mostly only when these events happen in "bursts." Other causes could be intravenous (IV) fluids containing sodium or certain other medications, including the hormone aldosterone, which tells the kidneys when to hold sodium in the body instead of passing it in the urine.

Your health care provider will instruct you, if necessary, to discontinue drugs that may interfere with the blood test. Do not stop or change your medications without your doctor's knowledge.

Drugs that can increase blood sodium levels include: anabolic steroids, birth control pills, certain antibiotics, clonidine, corticosteroids, cough medications, laxatives, methyldopa, nonsteroidal anti-inflammatory drugs (NSAIDs), drugs that can reduce blood sodium levels include: carbamazepine, diuretics, sulfonylureas, triamterene and asopressin. Data provided by NIH. (See: Hyponatremia)

Blood Thinners – Also known as an anticoagulants. Blood thinners are used to prevent or stop platelets present in blood plasma from developing into clots. Generally prescribed for heart patients, and patients with stroke, or aneurysms. The most common blood thinner often used before stroke or heart attacks or other heart problems is aspirin in doses of 81 mg per day (aspirin is known as a member of the salicylate family). Most prescribed blood thinners for heart and stroke patients is Warfarin, which is also known by its brand name of Coumadin. Frequent blood tests are needed to ensure that blood thinner levels remain within safe levels. These tests are known as ProTime or prothrombin time. (Also see: INR) There is a chance that we eat natural blood thinners everyday. If we change or alter or dietary intake of these substantially, we can affect our blood thinner level. Salicylate blocks vitamin K, a blood coagulator. Some spices, herbs, fruit and other foods have enough salicylate to perform as natural blood thinners. These include cinnamon, cayenne, curry, dill, ginger, licorice, oregano, paprika, thyme, turmeric, and peppermint. Fruits include blueberries, cherries, cranberries, grapes, oranges, prunes, raisins, strawberries, tangerines. Vinegar, wine and honey also contain measurable levels of salicylate. It is a myth that eating foods with vitamin K will impact your blood thinner medications enough to alter your health. If you maintain a balanced diet then your blood thinner will work efficiently. You won't have to adjust your diet at all, but once in a while you may have to adjust your medication. This can happen if you radically change your diet by either adding huge amounts of vitamin K food like kale or spinach, or if you change your normal pattern of eating them. It is far better to eat these foods for all the added nutrients they offer than to cut them out of your life. For a clear explanation of this, visit www.clotcare.com/clotcare/vitaminkandwarfarin.aspx

Blood work – The drawing of blood and lab evaluation to determine levels of body chemicals, or infections, or signs of diseases.

Braising – Generally to slow cook with liquid.

BMR – Basal Metabolic Rate refers to the number of calories your body burns at rest to maintain normal body functions. BMR is the total number of Kcalories per day your body burns even while sleeping. Note: BMR changes with age, as well as with weight, height, gender, diet and exercise habits. See: Calorie(s).

Brine or Brined (Commercially processed) – It's no longer safe for low-sodium eaters to trust any of the meat or fish that has been commercially processed "fresh" or otherwise. Today, many are brining chicken, pork, turkey, shrimp and other shell fish. Some do it to extend shelf life, others might claim it "adds flavor." Another unfortunate but big reason is that it adds the taste of salt, which our damaged palates have become accustomed to. Shrimp processors are salting nearly all shrimp, even the shrimp that may be displayed as fresh in your local market. (New federal USDA rulings state that all meats and fish and produce must now be displayed with a notice of where each product was produced. You'll find that much of your shrimp comes from countries you'd never even thought about as a food source.) Before purchasing shrimp, ask the counter–help to show you the package it was in before they displayed it. You'll see the FDA label on the package and probably find that the sodium level is high due to added salt; if not, then you've found a winner. Finding natural chicken, turkey and pork is becoming more and more difficult as well.

Brining red and white meats is a process that soaks salt through all the meat cells and cannot be washed off. The labels that processors place on packaging might state, "Natural," "No Additives," "Fresh," etc. Processors are raising the sodium levels of meat from around 72 mg per 4-ounce serving to over 500 mg per 4-ounce serving. FDA labels should show about 80 mg to 100 mg per 4-ounce serving and nothing higher for these "fresh" cuts of meat. If the meat you are buying does not have a label, the odds are that it may have been brined. Ask your butcher for the official FDA and USDA information. He must give it to you. Be especially careful when eating in a friend's home or a restaurant. If they serve either of the above meats, you can almost always expect they purchased the higher sodium variety, which is usually the cheaper cut as well.

BUN – See Creatinine.

Buttermilk, Low Sodium – *Known brands with low sodium include, Knudsen (130 mg), A&P(125 mg), Borden (130 mg), Borden Skim-Line (150 mg), Crowley (130 mg), Drigold Trim (130 mg) and Weight Watchers (140 mg)*

Calcium – Calcium is a mineral that builds and strengthens bones;

it's also important for helping muscle contraction, especially our heartbeat. Recent research has shown that calcium and vitamin D might prevent colon cancer. Calcium also helps control the function of nerves and with blood clotting. Young people up to about age eighteen, should consume at least 1,300 milligrams of calcium per day. After age eighteen the range of calcium ingestion suggested is between 1,000 mg and 1,200 mg a day. Calcium sources include milk, yogurt, cheese and dark green leafy vegetables like collard greens and kale. Calcium fortified foods supply significant levels as do fish. Each of *The No Salt, Lowest Sodium Cookbooks* lists calcium levels for every recipe as well recipes posted at megaheart.com

Calorie(s) – Scientifically referred to as Kcalorie. In science calories refer to the amount of energy needed to increase the temperature of one milliliter (ml) of water one-degree centigrade. However, in our personal lives it's referred to as "energy." Our metabolic rate is the *energy* that is measured in calories or Kcalories. A Kcalorie is one-thousand calories or referred to as "kilogram calorie," thusly the K. These Kcalories are expended by our body to maintain "normal" functions while at rest. This "effort" consumes about 70% of our usable calories. Our basal metabolic rate, (See: BMR), is influenced by other factors including gender, age, weight, height, temperature, food, exercise and many other habits.

Carbohydrate(s) – Often maligned in the media, carbohydrates are needed by our bodies. Carbohydrates are organic compounds that consist of carbon, such as sugar, which also has complex polymers that play important roles in nutrition. Carbohydrates in food provide four-calories per gram. The chief source of energy for plants are its carbohydrates. Cutting through the science, we need only to know that carbohydrates relate to their structural core of simple sugars. These range from simple sugars and saccharides to monosaccharides, glucose, fructose, sucrose, maltose and lactose. Also included are starch, dextrin, glycogen and cellulose. (Did you know you were eating such sweetness?) Today, it is the carbohydrate intake that is measured by most diabetics, as opposed to sugar intake, although sugar itself has a high level of carbohydrates. The best sources of carbohydrates are whole grains, vegetables, fruits and beans, especially black beans. These promote good health by delivering vitamins, minerals, fiber, and a host of important phytonutrients. Highly processed foods contain high levels of carbohydrates. These include white bread, white rice, pastries, sugared sodas, and other highly processed foods. These "easily digested" carbohydrates may contribute to weight gain, interfere with weight loss, and promote diabetes and heart disease.

Carb Choices – Basically, a Carb Choice is a single serving of any food containing 15 grams of carbohydrate. Although the number 15 is really an average it's a basic guideline. Zero to five grams for instance is known as "0 Carb Choice," but 6 to 10 is one-half. From 11 to 20 is referred to as 1 carb choice. The full table is available at various sites and in many diabetic cookbooks. We have based our recipes in this book on the standard table. Diabetics also practice a food exchange based on this table. It's a challenging balancing act but it can be done and once accustomed to it, dietary needs are met efficiently.

Carcinogens – There are two types of carcinogens. Natural and synthetic. Both are known to cause cancer in humans at varying levels. *The following comment is printed directly from the American Cancer Society's Web site at cancer.org.* "Cancer is caused by changes (mutations) in a cell's DNA—its genetic "blueprint." Some of these changes may be inherited from our parents, while others may be caused by outside exposures, which are often referred to as environmental factors. Environmental factors can include a wide range of exposures, such as lifestyle factors (nutrition, tobacco use, physical activity, etc.), naturally occurring exposures (ultraviolet light, radon, infectious agents, etc.), medical treatments (chemotherapy, radiation, and immune system-suppressing drugs used after organ transplants, etc.), workplace and household exposures, and pollution.

"Substances and exposures that can lead to cancer are called *carcinogens*. Some carcinogens do not act on DNA directly, but lead to cancer in other ways. For example, they may cause cells to divide at a faster than normal rate, which could increase the chances that DNA changes will occur.

"Carcinogens do not cause cancer in every case. Substances labeled as carcinogens may have different levels of cancer-causing potential. Some may cause cancer only after prolonged, high levels of exposure. And for any particular person, the risk of developing cancer depends on many factors, including how they are exposed to a carcinogen, the length and intensity of the exposure, and the person's genetic makeup."

Carotenoids (See also: Phytonutrients) – Of all the phytonutrients, we probably know the most about carotenoids, the red, orange and yellow pigments in fruits and vegetables. The carotenoids most commonly found in vegetables (and in plasma) are listed below along with common sources of these compounds. Fruits and vegetables that are high in carotenoids appear to protect humans against certain cancers, heart disease and age related macular degeneration. Some foods have high amounts of beta-carotene and alpha-carotene. Food Sources: Apricots, carrots, mangoes, squash, yams/sweet potatoes.

Chestnuts (nuts) – Contain beta-carotene, magnesium, phosphorus, potassium, vitamins A, B1, B2, B3, B6, E, and K, and iron. One-quarter cup has 87.6 Kcal and only .715 mg of sodium. Low in fat with about 1.8 g of fiber and 10.4 mg of calcium. These also help prevent heart disease and the common cold.

Chili Powder – The powder from grinding a red chili. Mild, medium and hot versions are available for flavoring foods, but usually used with meats, beans and in many spice mixes. Contains vitamins A, C and dietary fiber as well as potassium and iron. Containing capsaicin, which makes chili powder an excellent anti-inflammatory food. Also known to relieve pain. Some research has proved chili peppers value in reducing blood cholesterol and triglyceride levels. Cayenne and chili peppers have a high level of beta carotene. Chili also kills bacteria that may cause ulcers. See Wayzata Chili Powder for unsalted version. The familiar product of Grandma's Chili Powder was discontinued in 2009, but replaced by the company with "Williams Seasoning," which is the same product.

Chinese Restaurant Syndrome – In 1968 the New England Journal of Medicine first reported "Chinese restaurant syndrome." The article explained how many people felt sick after eating at Chinese restaurants. The culprit was thought to be MSG. Examples of high blood sodium levels were suggested, and caused by MSG, although even to this day true allergy to MSG has never been identified. According to Dr. Trevor Beard[1], "Allergy is the correct word when an antigen such as pollen reacts with an antibody in the human tissues or blood stream. The reaction to MSG is not like that. It takes the form of intolerance to large doses (the same principle seen with drug intolerance). No harm has ever been linked with the small doses of MSG that occur naturally in breast milk, tomatoes and mushrooms; every case of MSG sensitivity identified so far has been a standard example of food intolerance, with symptoms only at doses above the individual's threshold of tolerance."

The culprit for feeling unwell or flushed after eating in a Chinese restaurant is probably caused mostly by the excessive salt used. A Chinese restaurant meal can have as few as 5,474 mg of sodium.

Cholesterol – Cholesterol is classified as a lipid. It is not a fat. Instead, cholesterol can be thought of as a waxy substance that occurs naturally in all parts of the body. Conflicting with some media reports, some cholesterol is essential for us and is found in all cell membranes. It is necessary for the production of bile acids and steroid hormones. That's the cholesterol your doctor might mention that our bodies manufacture. To learn more find a legitimate medical book in your local library or visit webmd.com on-line. Other sites that explain this and other health challenges include well-known clinics like Mayo Clinic (mayoclinic.

com/), Cleveland Clinic (clevelandclinic.org), Harvard Medical School (Harvard.edu/), and The National Institutes of Health (nih.org).

Dietary cholesterol on the other hand, is found only in animal foods and it can raise the "bad" cholesterol in our bodies, causing harm to our coronary system and ultimately to our heart. It is more than plentiful in organ meats and in egg yolks. It is not found in extra virgin olive oil. It is basically absent in fresh fruits and vegetables.

When we are tested for cholesterol the lab is searching for our HDL–LDL –Triglyceride levels. If we have too much LDL cholesterol in our blood, it can adhere to the walls of our arteries. This is known as plaque. Plaque can narrow our arteries, or deadlier yet, block them. (Yes, I want you to think about that the next time you don't purchase "lean" meat.) High levels of cholesterol in the blood can increase our risk of heart disease or stroke. Unfortunately for many of us, our cholesterol levels rise when we get older. Outward signs or symptoms of this are usually absent. That's why we need the blood tests. If your family has a history of high cholesterol, you'll want to manage yours carefully and adjust your diet accordingly. If you are overweight or eat a lot of fatty foods, then we suggest strongly that you adjust your lifestyle soon. Remember to avoid partially hydrogenated products as well, whether it's in your margarine or a packaged baked good.

We can lower our cholesterol with increased exercise and by eating more fruits and vegetables. We may have to take a medication to help lower cholesterol as well.

For specific graphs and numbers of cholesterol, visit:

http://www.webmd.com/cholesterol-management/guide/understanding-numbers

An additional note about LDL – Lipoprotein(a) is a type of LDL generally linked more to genetic makeup than to lifestyle. A high level could contribute to atherosclerosis and heart disease, but it's best to get the standard or regular LDL levels tested first. If your doctor suspects you have or are at risk of atherocslcerosis, then he/she may test for lipoprotein(a).

Chronic fatigue syndrome (CFS) – According to the Center for Disease Control (CDC), between 1 and 4 million Americans suffer from Chronic Fatigue Syndrome. At least a quarter are unemployed or on disability because of CFS. Yet, only about half have consulted a physician for their illness. The earlier a person with CFS receives medical treatment the greater the likelihood that the illness will resolve. Equally important, about 40% of people in the general population who report symptoms of CFS have a serious, treatable, previously unrecognized medical or psychiatric condition (such as diabetes, thyroid disease, substance abuse). CFS is a serious illness and poses a dilemma for patients, their families, and health care providers.

Cinnamon, ground – Lots of manganese, but also contains dietary fiber, calcium and iron. Anti inflammatory qualities are impressive. Has a history of being used medicinally for everything from boosting brain function, protecting against heart disease, to protecting colons and works well as an anti-clogging agent. A popular spice for everything from cookies to sauces. It is the bark of a cinnamon tree.

Citric Acid – Isolated for the first time in 1784 from lemon juice it is an essential component of the Krebs cycle. In layman's terms, it is the primary energy source in cells. Citric acid occurs abundantly in citrus fruits, although commercial synthesis is by fermentation of molasses. It is used in food as an antioxidant as well as enhancing the effect of other antioxidants, and also as an acidity regulator (used in canning and bread). Present in virtually all plants, it has been used as a food additive for over 100 years.

Clarified Butter – Clarified butter is unsalted butter that has been produced by separating the milk solids and water from the butter fat. (Clarified lard works the same way.)

CoEnzyme Q-10 – Plays a role in the body's production of adenosine triphosphate (ATP), the basic energy component of the human cell. Coenzyme Q-10 also plays a role in neutralizing harmful free radicals in cells. It's good for our heart and helps our body to convert food to energy. It is naturally manufactured by the body but begins to slow down production to nearly a stop at the age of 40 or so. Supplements are available. I take them, but check with your doctor first. You can find the best deal I've found at megaheart.com/supplements.html, possibly your pharmacy, but also at Costco. They are fairly expensive over the counter. I take 100 mg once a day. Let your doctor help figure that part out for you. Many cardiologists today recommend them. (See: Krebs cycle)

Collagen – Strengthens various parts of our body, including our muscles and blood vessels. It plays a necessary role in healing and it works as an antihistamine.

Convection or Conventional Oven – Heat distribution defines these two types of ovens. For the convection oven the heat is evenly distributed by a fan, usually at the back of the oven. The conventional oven provides heat generally from the bottom. Heat rises even in our small ovens. That is why some baked items might come out darker on one side than the other or if placed on a rack that's higher than the recipe suggests. In a convection oven you can bake two racks of cookies at the same time and with less heat. Both ovens can be powered by either gas or electricity

Cramp(s) – The research for cramp, or cramps, has been sporadic but convincing. Whether or not lowering our salt/sodium intake or sweating heavily while exercising has anything to do with it has been the question. The answers come up the same with all tests. Look for salt/sodium loading, or bouncing as it is often referred to. This means for instance, that you are going along fine with 500 mg a day and then one day you load up on 2,000 mg or more. That's called a bounce or loading. It may cause cramp. But a steady low-sodium diet does not in itself cause one. And sweating on a low-sodium diet doesn't off-load sodium or salt, either. Actually, it works the other way. The more salt / sodium you ingest, the saltier your sweat that drips to your lips tastes, but when not eating a high-–sodium diet, you won't taste the salt because it's not there. You will sweat the same amount, and the only way to replace it is with water. Drinks with high "shock" sodium levels are really more dangerous than helpful. Research done in Australia has shown that with less sodium, athletes performed much better than with the "shock" of too much sodium. A muscle cramp can be caused by a variety of things including alcohol, pregnancy, treated varicose veins, rigorous exercise or the first exercise of the year like your first tennis game when weather permits, and a cold bed may precipitate a muscle cramp. Swimming too, can cause cramps, which means that anyone learning how to swim should also learn how to handle cramps when in the water.

Cream of Tartar – A leavening agent used for stabilizing egg whites for meringue pie or other uses. Adds volume to the egg whites when beating. Lemon juice and vinegar also work with meringue, but cream of tartar doesn't create "another" flavor. It is produced from the processing of aging wine and is found on the insides of wine barrels. Also known as tartaric acid, cream of tartar is potassium hydrogen tartrate and is the leavening agent in baking powder. When used together with baking soda it produces double-acting baking powder.

Creatinine – Creatinine is chiefly filtered by the kidney. It is produced in our bodies from muscle metabolism or creatinine, an important molecule for energy production in muscles. Creatinine is cleared or excreted in our urine. Creatinine is a reliable indicator of kidney function. Levels are determined via blood test. (Related tests are known as: BUN, creatinine clearance, CMP, BMP or eGFR or efgr.) Normal levels of creatinine in the blood are approximately 0.6 to 1.2 mg per deciliter (dl) in adult males and 0.5 to 1.1 milligrams per deciliter in adult females.

Cruciferous – Certain variety of edible vegetables that show petals resembling a cross. These include broccoli, Brussels sprouts, cabbage, cauliflower, kale, bok choy, komatsuna, turnip root (greens), broccoflower, kohlrabi, horseradish, watercress, mustard seeds and collard greens. They contain phytochemicals, which have been shown to fight cancer. High in vitamin C and soluble fiber with multiple nutrients.

Curly Fries – Unique French fries characterized by their coil-like shape. They also look like springs. Made from whole potatoes that are cut using a special spiral slicer.

Dextrose – Simple carbohydrate, also known as glucose. Dextrose or sugar, is the primary source of energy for the body. It is chemically considered a simple sugar. Glucose is the main sugar our body produces and it does so from protein, fat and carbohydrates. Important to us is that the in largest portion comes from carbohydrates. This sugar is delivered to each cell via the bloodstream. Diabetics have learned that the cells cannot use the glucose without the help of insulin. Also found in Splenda. The amounts in Splenda will not cause a spike in blood glucose levels.

Diabetes – Congestive heart patients often develop diabetes. There are two types, Type 1 and Type 2. Type 2 diabetes, often called non-insulin dependent diabetes, is the most common form of diabetes; it affects nearly 95% of the 21 million patients who have diabetes. There is a great deal of misinformation about how to deal with diabetes. For on-line direction and help visit *www.diabetes.org*.

Dietary Fiber – Dietary fiber is an indigestible complex carbohydrate. Basically, dietary fiber is the thick cell wall of a plant. Fiber is categorized as: water-soluble or water-insoluble.

Water Soluble fiber has been shown to modestly lower cholesterol. Mysteriously even for science, human trials have demonstrated that diets higher in *water insoluble* fiber, which is generally not related to cholesterol, have an ability to protect against heart disease. We also know that water soluble fibers can lower blood-sugar levels. Some in the medical field believe that increasing fiber *decreases* the body's need for insulin, which is a bonus for diabetics.

It is the *water insoluble* fiber that acts as a stool softener. This helps our digestion and bowel movement by moving waste through our intestines at a quicker of more even pace. In other words, if you tend toward constipation or have diverticulosis, you may want to increase your water insoluble fiber intake. A regular movement is also thought to help prevent cancer.

Dietary Guidelines for Americans – The *Dietary Guidelines for Americans* has been published jointly every 5 years since 1980 by the Department of Health and Human Services (HHS) and the Department of Agriculture (USDA). The Guidelines provide authoritative advice for people two years and older about how good dietary habits can promote health and reduce risk for major chronic diseases. They serve as the basis for Federal food and nutrition education programs. For more information visit: *http://www.cnpp.usda.gov/*

Disodium Citrate – The sodium of citric acid. Used as an antioxidant in food and enhances other antioxidants. Also present as an acidity regulator and sequestrant. Look for it in gelatin products, sweets, ice cream, jam, colas, wine and processed cheeses.

Disodium Phosphate (or Sodium Phosphate) – Used in processed cheeses as an emulsifier and in some quick cooking cereals as an antioxidant synergist, stabilizer and buffering agent. It is also added to powdered milk to prevent gelation.

E. coli – *From USA Center for Disease Control (CDC) – "Escherichia coli* (abbreviated as *E. coli*) are a large and diverse group of bacteria. Although most strains of *E. coli* are harmless, others can make you sick. Some kinds of *E. coli* can cause diarrhea, while others cause urinary tract infections, respiratory illness and pneumonia, and other illnesses. Still other kinds of *E. coli* are used as markers for water contamination—so you might hear about *E. coli* being found in drinking water, which are not themselves harmful, but indicate the water is contaminated. It does get a bit confusing—even to microbiologists." A strain of E. coli associated with human illness from eating food with the bacteria can be transferred from animal to animal, and from animal to human. Also, the important one for us to watch out for, is that it can be transferred from animal to human via food. Transmission from person to person through close contact is a potential problem, especially among young children in school or other group settings."

Eggs & Cholesterol – A large egg has about 211.5 mg of cholesterol – all of it in the yolk. It is recommended that healthy people not consume more than 300 mg of cholesterol per day. There has been some confusion perpetrated in the media about eggs and cholesterol. Here's the bottom line. If you have heart disease or diabetes and you want to eat an egg (no more than one a day), then you will want to cut down on other foods that have cholesterol in them. If you like eggs you can always replace a single egg with the whites from two eggs. This works for omelets, baked goods, or salads including potato salads. If hard boiling the egg for salads or snacks, just remove the yolk. Sodium level for one egg white is 54.8 mg. *By the way, you can use eggs for up to five weeks after the "use by" date on the carton, as long as you have kept them refrigerated.*

Ejection Fraction (EF) – (EF) is one of the measurements of your heart needed to assess how well it is functioning. "Ejection" refers to the amount of blood that is pumped out of the heart's main pumping chamber with each heartbeat. "Fraction" refers to the amount of blood remaining in the chamber after each heartbeat. The EF then is a percentage of the blood within the chamber that is pumped *out* with each heartbeat. If you are diagnosed with an EF of 16 for instance, then only sixteen percent of your blood is leaving the chamber. That sets you up for clots, a reason you may be taking a blood thinner. An EF of 55 to 75 percent is considered normal. You can learn more about EF at various medical sites from Mayo, to Cleveland Clinic and WebMD.

Ener-G Baking Soda/Baking Powder Substitutes – (*www.ener-g.com*) Baking soda and baking powder are leavening agents in baked goods. They create the necessary gas for cookies, pancakes, etc. for a rise. Ener-G Calcium Carbonate works just like baking soda, but it's completely sodium free. On average the sodium in baking soda is about 150-250 mg per ¼ teaspoon, whereas Ener-G's baking soda substitute contains 0 mg per serving. Great for those looking to cut salt from their diets without having to sacrifice on taste or texture. For best results double or triple the amount of Ener-G Baking Soda in recipes when converting from standard baking soda. Ener-g's Baking Powder is double-acting, but still requires us to double an original recipes requirement for baking powder. Since you will also be removing salt from the recipe, you'll want to add some cream of tartar, vinegar, and possibly ascorbic acid. Free of gluten, wheat, casein, dairy, egg, corn, soy, yeast, nut, rice, potato, sodium, low protein, aluminum. Obtainable also from *healthyheartmarket.com* and at Whole Foods stores.

Enzyme – Enzymes are complex proteins that enable or help chemical reactions to occur. For example, digestive enzymes might assist our body to break down food into compounds that are more easily absorbed. Thousands of different enzymes are produced by our body. (See: CoEnzyme Q-10)

Essential Amino Acids – Essential Amino Acids are amino acids that your body does not have the ability to synthesize. Although hundreds of amino acids exist in nature, only nine are generally regarded as essential for humans (some say eight): histidine, isoleucine, leucine, lysine, methionine, phenylalanine, threonine, tryptophan, and valine, are considered essential, since they must be supplied by your diet. In other words, you've got to eat these to get them. The facts are that arginine, cysteine, glycine, glutamine, histidine, praline, serine and tyrosine are considered *conditionally essential* meaning they are not normally required in our diet, yet they may be required in diets of specific populations that do not synthesize these in adequate amounts. Again, another "confusing" food listing for us to "digest." Even scientists who specialize in this area have problems figuring this one out. For instance, "daily requirements" are only estimated and those vary from country to country and person to person.

Essential fatty acids (Eras) – A type of fatty acid that the body needs but cannot produce and which must be obtained from food.

Fatty acids – Fatty acids are generally classified as saturated, monounsaturated, or polyunsaturated. Fats that contain a majority of saturated fatty acids are solid at room temperature, although some solid vegetable shortening is up to 75 percent unsaturated. Fats containing mostly unsaturated fatty acids are usually liquid at room temperature and are called oils. Dietary fat is needed to carry fat-soluble vitamins A, D, E and K and to aid in their absorption from the intestine.

FDA Nutrition Panels (Labels) – On all processed food packages. Select nutrition values are posted per serving size, not per package contents. Check colas or fruit drinks for instance. You may see sodium level of 50 mg per serving, but the container may have two servings or more. Food manufacturers are allowed to label packages stating no salt added or unsalted, but they must also add "this is not a sodium free food." Most all food has some sodium in it. All stores should provide some access to information concerning nutrient levels of other foods like fresh produce or meats, or other foods locally packaged without FDA labels. Foods that are to be consumed on property are not at this time required to provide these labels. FDA is currently urging food processors to use realistic serving sizes on food packages so that consumers can better understand just how many calories and other nutrients they are really consuming.

Featherweight Baking Powder – A substitute Baking Powder. Ingredients include monocalcium phosphate, potato starch and potassium bicarbonate. Dietary content of potassium weighs in at 63.1 mg of potassium per 1/8 teaspoon and .5 mg of sodium.

Fiber – See Dietary Fiber

Flavonoids – Flavonoids are a class of water-soluble pigments that are found in many plants and provide a great antioxidant effect. More than four-thousand different flavonoids have been identified. These have been found in fruits, vegetables, tea, coffee, fruit drinks and even beer and wine. Some researchers believe they have antiviral, antiplatelet, anti-inflammatory, antitumor, anti allergy and antioxidant benefits. Flavonoids also contribute vitamins and enzymes. Flavonoids have helped with coronary heart disease and the preventions of heart attacks. Best bet? Eat the white coating on the inside of an orange peel.

Flavanones – A type of flavonoid found in citrus fruits which provides the health benefits of neutralizing free radicals and possibly reducing the risk of cancer.

Flavor Enhancers – Typically a product that is basically salt or MSG mixed with a few other ingredients, which are often lycopene or a few mild spices. *Don's Flavor Enhancer*, found in *The No–Salt, Lowest–Sodium International Cookbook* is a mix of many spices and works well with soups, stews and other dishes when attempting to reach for that "salt" flavor.

Foie Gras (pronounced fwa:'gra) – Liver of a duck or goose that has been fattened, often through forced feeding of corn. Foie Gras is French for "fat liver."

Folic acid (Folate, Folacin) (Vitamin B9) – Folic acid, also known as Vitamin B9, is referred to as folacin or folate. This vitamin can be manufactured by the body and be stored in the liver. Particularly needed for a developing fetus. According to the U.S. Centers for Disease Control and Prevention (CDC), if all women of childbearing age consumed sufficient folic acid (either through diet or supplements), 50 to 70 percent of birth defects of the brain and spinal cord could be prevented. Folic acid is critical from conception through the first four to six weeks of pregnancy when the neural tube is formed. This means adequate diet or supplement use should begin before pregnancy occurs. Recent research findings also show low blood folate levels can be associated with elevated plasma homocysteine and increased risk of coronary heart disease. Best dietary sources of folate include green vegetables, such as spinach and broccoli. It is also found in fruit, starchy vegetables, beans, whole grains, fortified cereal, and liver.

Food and Drug Administration (FDA) – The FDA is the US government agency that enforces laws on the manufacturing, testing, and use of drugs and medical devices. The Food and Drug Administration is part of the Public Health Service of the U.S. Department of Health and Human Services. It is the regulatory agency responsible for ensuring the safety and wholesomeness of all foods sold in interstate commerce except meat, poultry, and eggs (which are under the jurisdiction of the U.S. Department of Agriculture). FDA develops standards for the composition, quality, nutrition, safety and labeling of foods including food and color additives. (Visit *www.fda.gov/* for more information.)

Food Guide Pyramid – The Food Guide Pyramid is a graphic design used to communicate the recommended daily food choices contained in the Dietary Guidelines for Americans. Created by the U.S. Department of Agriculture and the U.S. Department of Health and Human Services. Visit: http://www.myfoodapedia.gov/Default.aspx. To calculate your five fruits and vegetables a day visit www.5aday.gov.

Free radicals – Substances created from exposure to oxygen, or background radiation (UVs), and other environmental factors. These unstable particles can and do cause cellular damage to the body, contributing to aging and disease. There is some belief that this damage may be repaired or prevented by antioxidants.

Fructose (monosaccharide or simple sugar) – Used by our bodies for energy. Has a low glycemic index. Look out for and avoid if possible high corn fructose in fruit drinks and other beverages. Natural fructose found in vegetables and fruits is about all each of us needs. A small bit of fructose helps our bodies to process glucose. A sudden shock of fructose however, seems to overpower our body's ability to process it. A steady diet of this overload of fructose can result in an appreciable gain of body weight. Fructose is processed in the liver. If too much fructose is ingested, the liver is overwhelmed and sends the unprocessed fructose into the bloodstream as triglycerides. Commercial food sources for this fructose include sodas, fruit drinks, nearly all packaged foods have it in one form or another (added by the processor). For *diabetics*, trying to find the high carbohydrates, often hidden in various sugars in most products, life has gotten tougher. Finding no-sugar or low-carbohydrate products in the grocery store is just as difficult as finding no-salt-added products. Fructose and sugars are hidden by various industry "code" words like corn sweetener, cane juice, dextrin, dextrose, fructose, fruit juice concentrate (which is fructose), glucose, high-fructose corn syrup, honey (high carbohydrates), invert sugar, lactose, maltodextrin, malt syrup, maltose, maple syrup, molasses, raw sugar, rice syrup, saccharose, sorghum or sorghum syrup, sucrose, syrup, treade, turbinado sugar, xylose, and just plain sugar. "Sugar Free" on many packages really doesn't mean "free of sugar." Make sure the package or container doesn't state that it's using sugar alcohol, which is a carbohydrate also known as polyols. Common code names for this high carbohydrate are maltitol, sorbitol, isomalt, mannitol, erythritol, lactitol, and xylitol.

Fungi – Any fungus of the kingdom of saprophytic and parasitic spore-producing eukaryotic (taxonomic group) typically filamentous organisms formerly classified as plants that lack chlorophyll and include molds, mushrooms, and yeasts.

Ginger – Spice. Research has shown that adding a teaspoon of ginger to food consumed for a few days before, during and after chemo can reduce nausea and vomiting. Ginger is used in recipes for lamb, seafood and vegetarian recipes and is also used in candies. Add crystallized ginger to cookies like biscotti and you'll get a truly enjoyable flavor. May interact with Coumadin/Warfarin. Should not be consumed by those with gallstone problems. Sometimes recommended to heart patients for blood thinning and cholesterol control.

Glucose – A sugar that occurs naturally. It has about half the sweetening power of regular sugar. It does not crystallize easily. Glucose comes from grape juice, honey, and certain vegetables, among other foods. Glucose is usually found in the form of dextroglucose.

Glutamine – Glutamine is an amino acid synthesized by the body from another amino acid, called glutamic acid or glutamate. It is the most abundant amino acid (building block of protein) in our blood. It is known as a *conditionally essential* amino acid. Our body can manufacture it, but under extensive physical stress our bodies cannot meet the demands with enough production of glutamine. Glutamine is stored in our muscles or in our lungs, where most of the glutamine is produced. Glutamine is needed to remove excess ammonia (a normal waste product in our bodies), but while doing this the extracted waste helps make other amino acids including the antioxidant glutathione. The importance of glutamine cannot be understated. It helps with the function of the brain and our digestion and immune cells rely on it for energy. Under normal healthy conditions we get enough glutamine from our diet and from what our body makes. However, some medical conditions might call for additional glutamine. These include injuries, surgery, infections, inflammatory bowel disease (IBD), HIV/AIDS, obesity, peritonitis, cancer, stress and osteoporosis. Supplements can be taken and may be helpful. Check with your doctor before taking any supplements of this or other minerals or vitamins. Dietary sources include animal proteins, plant proteins, milk, yogurt, ricotta cheese, raw parsley, spinach and cabbage.

Gluten – See Vital Wheat Gluten

Glycemic Index (GI) – is a measure of how carbohydrate-containing foods affect blood glucose levels. Not all carbohydrate foods are created equal, in fact, they behave quite differently in our bodies. The glycemic index or GI describes this difference by ranking carbohydrates according to their effect on our blood glucose levels. Choosing low GI carbs, the ones that produce only small fluctuations in our blood glucose and insulin level is the secret to long-term health reducing your risk of heart disease and diabetes and is the key to sustainable weight loss. (See: www.glycemicindex.com)

Grain(s) – Grains are the seeds or fruits of various food plants including cereal grasses. A few examples include wheat, corn, oats, barley, rye, and rice. Grain based foods include bread, cereals, rice, and pasta.

Grandma's Chili Powder – Once recommended by us in our cookbooks and at Megaheart.com. The manufacturer, Williams Foods, in Lenexa, Kansas discontinued this product in late 2009 but retintroduced it as Williams Original Chili Seasoning. Williams and another no salt added chili powder, Wayzata Bay Chili Powder, are available from Healthy Heart Market. Wayzata medium is at http://healthyheartmarket.com/wbchilipowder-med.aspx, and the hot is at http://healthy heart market .com/wbchilipowder-hot.aspx.

Grapefruit – Grapefruit and grapefruit juice can be dangerous when interacting with some medications, although it's perfectly safe with others. Unfortunately grapefruit juice interferes mostly with medications prescribed for heart disease, neurological or psychiatric challenges. Most studies have demonstrated that grapefruit juice is safe to consume when using over the counter drugs. You should consult with your doctor or pharmacist before consuming grapefruit juice or to learn if there's an alternative medication on the market that will allow you to drink grapefruit juice.

Drugs known to interact with grapefruit[2]:

Antibiotics: clarithromycin, erythromycin, troleandomycin
Anxiolytics: alprazolam, buspirone, midazolam, triazolam
Antiarrhythmics: amiodarone, quinidine
Anticoagulant: warfarin
Antiepileptic: carbamazepine
Antifungal: itraconazole
Anthelmintic: albendazole
Antihistamine: fexofenadine
Antineoplastics: cyclophosphamide, etoposide, ifosfamide, tamoxifen, vinblastine, vincristine
Antitussive: dextromethorphan
Antivirals: amprenavir, indinavir, nelfinavir, ritonavir, saquinavir
Benign prostatic hyperplasia treatment: finasteride;- Proscar, Propecia and others
Beta blockers: carvedilol
Calcium channel blockers: diltiazem, felodipine, nicardipine, nifedipine, nimodipine, nisoldipine, verapamil
Erectile dysfunction drugs: sildenafil, tadalafil
Hormone replacement: cortisol, estradiol, methylprednisolone, progesterone, testosterone
Immunosuppressants: cyclosporine, sirolimus, tacrolimus
HMG-CoA reductase inhibitors: atorvastatin, fluvastatin, lovastatin, simvastatin
Opioids: alfentanil, fentanyl, sufentanil
Selective serotonin reuptake inhibitors: fluvoxamine, sertraline
Xanthine: theophylline

Guar Gum – A natural food thickener similar to cornstarch, tapioca flour and locust bean gum. It is made from the seeds of the guar plant and works well as a stabilizer in food systems. It is used in ice cream to help prevent ice crystals from forming, and in sauces and salad dressings. It is sometimes used to give your mouth the feeling it has eaten "satisfying" fat. Also used in cosmetics. It's available for home cooking, and used in fresh gluten-free bread as a binder. (If you make gluten-free bread, you must use guar or Xanthan Gum or you'll get nothing but crumbs.) The guar plant is mostly grown in northern India and in Pakistan.

Haggis – Scottish dish made of minced sheep's heart, liver and lungs with onions, oatmeal, spices, suet, stock, and salt. Once boiled in the sheep's stomach it is now prepared in commercially produced casings. Appears like sausage. If presented to you without explanation you'd believe it was one of the tastiest sausages you'd ever eaten. High in sodium and saturated fats.

(HDL) (High Density Lipoprotein) – See: Cholesterol

Healthy Heart Market – Founded by heart transplant patient Pete Eiden, *www.healthyheartmarket.com* offers all the low-sodium products they can locate in the U.S. They are not affiliated with Megaheart.com nor any other site. They are located in Rogers, MN and offer quick shipping. It is now owned and operated by Lisa McComas and her husband. For updated sources for other low sodium foods visit *www.megaheart.com/wheretobuy.html.*

Herbs – We address only culinary herbs here. Herbs have been used since the beginning of mankind as "healers," and for other purposes but we know them for adding flavor, even though they may also help medicinally. Garlic, thyme, lavender, parsley, basil are recognizable herbs. Herbs come from the leafy green parts of a plant, while spices come from other parts including bark, root, fruit, seeds and berries. Some crossovers happen between spices and herbs like dill seed or dill weed and coriander seed and leaves.

Hooch – Sourdough starter separates in a refrigerator. The liquid that forms is known as hooch. It contains about 12 to 14% alcohol. If it is brown and starter is dry stir it back in. If sponge is too wet, throw out the liquid. It turns pink or orange, throw it out. It has spoiled.

Homocysteine (amino acid) – An excess of homocysteine has been linked to an increased risk of coronary disease, stroke, and other diseases such as osteoporosis and Alzheimer's. B vitamins and folic acid can help break down homocysteine in the body, but most doctors and researchers don't and will not recommend that you take supplements to ward off homocysteine. Instead, eat a healthy diet of fruits and vegetables. No studies are available to prove otherwise.

Hydrogenation – Hydrogenation is the process that converts unsaturated fats into saturated fats, which in turn allows processors to convert liquid oil into solid "shortening." It all started with "Oleo," now known as margarine. The word "oleo" comes from *oleic* fatty acid. In other words, processors take an unsaturated fat and turn it into a saturated fat. Just what we don't need. (See: Cholesterol)

Hypernatremia (also spelled hypernatraemia) – High blood sodium. Can also be referred to as dehydration. Water is excreted or lost from our bodies via different ways. These include perspiration, urine (sometimes brought about by diuretics), too much or too little blood sodium. If the fluids you take in consistently falls below the fluids that leave your body, the serum sodium level in your blood will begin to rise, leading to hypernatremia. Fortunately, our bodies are built to control this, however we have to keep an eye on this challenge if we are susceptible to excess loss of body fluids. Found more commonly in elderly or disabled patients who either don't or can't take in enough fluids. Can also be due to a medical condition called diabetes insipidus. Primary causes: severe vomiting or diarrhea, excessive exercise or sweating, burns, diuretics, kidney failure or malfunction, high fever or infections, excessive water/fluid consumption, CHF.

Symptoms include: lethargy, weakness, irritability, confusion or agitation, changes in blood pressure or heart rate/beat, swelling of tissue, nausea and edema. With more severe elevations of the sodium level, seizures and coma may occur.

Treatment includes: Your doctor might treat each case differently since so many variables can be involved. Treatments will range from medicines to adding or restricting fluids.

(Also see hyponatremia.)

Hypertension – Hypertension is basically an elevated arterial blood pressure that becomes persistent. It is the most common public health problem in developed countries and one where symptoms are simply not understood. I can attest to that. I must have had it for twenty years before "collapsing" with CHF. I had been treated for being "Type A," for having "Adult Onset Asthma," for being "High Strung," etc. All the while, it was hypertension and it could have been stopped in its tracks with a no-salt lifestyle. Since those days, a much stronger emphasis on lifestyle modifications has given our total diet a prominent role for both the primary prevention and management of hypertension. See our 28-day meal-planning guide in *The No Salt, Lowest Sodium Cookbook*. It's still the very best to use as a guide to make up your own plan. As to symptoms of hypertension, if your blood pressure gets extremely high, you might notice severe headaches or fatigue and confusion. Vision problems are also a sign as well as difficulty in breathing or an irregular heart beat. Chest pain can also indicate very high blood pressure as well as blood in the urine and for men, an unexplained impotence (ED) is yet another sign of possible hypertension. This is nothing to fool around with. Any one of these symptoms or multiples of them, demand that you see a cardiologist immediately.

Hyponatremia – Hyponatremia is a metabolic condition wherein there is not enough sodium in the body fluids outside the cells. This is the most common electrolyte disorder in the United States. Causes can be serious burns, CHF (congestive heart failure), medications that increase urine output (diuretics), kidney diseases (kidney failure), vomiting and diarrhea and liver cirrhosis syndrome of inappropriate antidiuretic hormone secretion (SIADH). Hyponatremia is something to be aware of and to remain cautious about if you have heart disease and take diuretics. Your doctor will ask for blood tests (BMP) a few times a year to make sure your blood sodium levels remain at healthy levels.

Treatment may include changing medication that affects blood sodium, increasing or decreasing how much water (fluids) you take in every day and sometimes saline solution.

Hypotension (below normal or low blood pressure) – Low blood pressure can cause dizziness and fainting. It may indicate endocrine, heart or neurological problems. Too low a blood pressure can starve the brain and other vital organs of oxygen and nutrients. This can lead to shock.

Immune System – Basically the immune system consists of cells and organs (or tissues) that work together to defend against diseases from the common cold to the flu, and even heart disease.

Inflammatory – See: Anti-inflammatory.

INR – International Normalized Ratio. See Prothrombin Time (ProTime).

Insulin – A naturally occurring hormone produced by the pancreas. It controls sugar glucose levels and allows our cells to use the glucose for energy. See: Blood glucose and Dextrose. When our body fails to function with insulin and glucose, we are then diagnosed with diabetes mellitus.

Inulin – A type of dietary fiber used to improve the "taste," stability, and acceptability of low-fat foods. A known water soluble fiber. Added to some foods, even a few brands of yogurt. It stimulates the growth of intestinal bifidobacteria. This puts it in a class known as probiotics. See: Probiotics.

Iodine – Essential to human life. Iodine is component of our two essential thyroid hormones, T4 (thyroxin) and T3 (triodothyronine.) In the USA, it's generally not necessary to use salt to get iodine. Iodine was never added to the salt in processed foods. Research shows that iodized salt is not needed in the USA since our diet includes many foods with iodine.

Sources: (Iodine content or levels in most foods that have iodine vary.) Seafood is generally rich in iodine. Cod, sea bass, haddock, and perch are all good sources. Kelp (seaweed) is the most common vegetable seafood that is a rich source of iodine and is added to many processed foods. Unsalted cheddar cheese also contains iodine. Some spinach contains healthy micro levels of iodine. Dairy products such as cow's milk, whole (boiled) eggs, mozzarella and yogurt also contain iodine. Strawberries are a good source as well. Other good sources are plants grown in iodine-rich soil. Daily requirements according to the NIH are:

Infants – 40 - 50 micrograms.
Children 1 - 3 years – 70 micrograms
4 - 6 years – 90 micrograms
7 - 10 years – 120 micrograms
11+ years – 150 micrograms
Pregnant women – 175 micrograms
Breast-feeding women – 200 micrograms
150 mcg of iodine is also available in some multivitamins.

We don't want to over consume iodine. Too much iodine can disrupt the thyroid and possibly cause either hypothyroidism, and with some of us it may increase the risk of thyroid cancer.

Jacket Potato – Baked potato.

KASL Flour – A special flour designed mostly for pizzas. Pizza crusts cook at high temperatures. KASL is known as Sir Lancelot flour at King Arthur's Flour Company and is generally sold in bulk to commercial establishments. Not presently sold in retail stores, but some pizza restaurants have been known to sell and even bag it for customers who ask.

Kneading – Process of combining bread ingredients especially flour and water and working them until the gluten (and gluten proteins) in the flour expand. Technically it runs gluten in strands throughout the dough, which constructs its elasticity and small carbon dioxide bubbles. If not kneaded enough, the loaf will probably collapse instead of rising. Kneading is often required twice. Never "punch" down as some recipes call for after the first kneading. If using a breadmaker, these two requirements are fulfilled smoothly and most all bread machine recipes will work well. Kneading bread dough was introduced by commercial bakers. For fun, why not try our no-knead bread recipe? (See: Index)

Krebs Cycle – Plays a major role in how living cells convert food into energy. It is a series of chemical reactions that generate a molecule called ATP (adenosine triphosphate), which almost all living things need to power themselves. Produced mostly from the proteins we consume. Some researchers believe Co-Enzyme Q-10 helps with this cycle as do apples.

Lactic Acid – A naturally occurring compound. Found in milk, molasses and fruit. Lactic acid occurs naturally in our blood when glycogen is broken down in the muscles. Also found in beer, canned vegetables and fruit and in fresh vegetables and fruit as well as a few other foods.

Sodium Lactate – Found in margarine, cheese, candy, ice cream and cakes as well as jams. It is the sodium of lactic acid and is used as a substance that promotes retention of moisture and as an antioxidant in food. It is capable of increasing the antioxidant effects of other substances as well. It has the ability to take up and retain moisture under some humidity and temperature conditions. Sometimes used as a substitute for glycerol.

Lactose – A sugar found in milk. It's also known as "milk sugar." It is the least sweet of all natural sugars. It is used in commercially produced candy and in baby formulas. Some who consume it find they cannot tolerate it.

Lactose Intolerance – (From Lactose.com) People who do not have enough lactase to digest the amount of lactose they consume may feel very uncomfortable when they digest milk products. Common symptoms, which range from mild to severe, include nausea, cramps, bloating, gas, and diarrhea. Symptoms begin about 30 minutes to 2 hours after eating or drinking foods containing lactose. The severity of symptoms depends on many factors, including the amount of lactose a person can tolerate and a person's age, ethnicity, and digestion rate.

Lard – Pig/hog fat. Mostly hydrogenated, which creates trans-fat in cooking fat/oil. Once used instead of butter because it was cheaper. But lard is clarified pork fat that is very high in cholesterol and trans fatty acids.

LDL – (See cholesterol)

Leavening Agent – An ingredient used mostly in baked goods (dough, batter) that creates a gaseous foaming action that creates "bubbles" needed for softness and extended freshness (shelf life). Leaveners react with acidity and other triggers including moisture and heat. Best known leavener is yeast. Other leaveners used by us and other chefs include buttermilk, sourdough starter, yogurt, sour cream, ginger beer and non-pasteurized beer, which contains live yeast.

Lecithin – A by-product of the refining of soybean oil. Contains healthy amount of choline, which is also found in egg yolks. Choline is known to help brain development and prevent heart disease. Lecithin is also found in red meats, spinach and nuts. Granulated soy lecithin produces a nutty flavor when added to homemade bread and helps keep the bread fresh longer.

L-lysine – Essential amino acid needed for healthy bodies. Our body does not produce L-lysine. Foods we eat to get L-lysine include red meat, pork, and poultry, cheese (particularly parmesan, which is too high in sodium for us to generally use), cod (and sardines, which are too high in sodium for us), nuts, eggs, soybeans especially tofu, isolated soy protein, and defatted soybean flour, which we recommend in our bread recipes for exchanges for diabetics, spirulina, and fenugreek seed (found in many spice mixes and rubs). Beans, diary products and other legumes, as well as other legumes also contain lysine.

Low-Sodium – The Food and Drug Administration (FDA) has set "official" levels of sodium for specific terminology to be used by food processors.

They are:

• Sodium-free – less than 5 milligrams of sodium per serving

• Very low-sodium – 35 milligrams or fewer per serving

• Low-sodium – 140 milligrams or fewer per serving

• Reduced sodium – usual sodium level is reduced by 25 percent

• Unsalted, no salt added (NSA) or without added salt – made without the salt that's normally used with food processing, but still contains the sodium that's a natural part of the food itself.

All of the above would be great if it meant anything to food processors. The terminology is per serving size, of course. And processors can pick whatever serving size they want. We can recognize a bottle of soda pop best. Mini-marts and other fast food suppliers sell 20 ounce bottles of colas with an FDA label that might state Sodium: 35 mg. As we've learned this means per serving size. Next we read near the top of the label that the serving size is 8 ounces. So this bottle has two and a half servings or 87.5 mg of sodium (caution, some sodas, like 7-Up are much higher). Although presented as a *very low sodium* item, it actually falls into the 140 mg or fewer *low sodium* category.

On my successful dietary plan, that bottle would fulfill one fifth of a day's supply of sodium.

Since 1997 we have lost many unsalted and no-salt-added products. However, many food brands have discovered the marketing tool of lowering salt in products, and the reason revolves around the baby-boomers. They are older now and in need of cutting their sodium intake.

The large food producers stepping into this low sodium arena include Campbell, Conagra, Heinz, Del Monte, among others. Just in 2007 alone over 660 products claimed they had reduced sodium. More than that jumped aboard in 2008 and 2009. For 2010 they have announced that a majority of products will have lowered sodium..

But so far, they haven't lowered their *salt* levels enough to make them much healthier. Lowering a can of soup from 1400 mg to 800 mg sodium per serving, is still unhealthy. On-line food tracking service *Productscan.com* (Now known as Datamonitor's Product Launch Analytics), provides data concerning new packaged goods. Productscan's on-line director Tom Vierhile, was quoted in an issue of USA TODAY as saying, "A little less salt makes consumers think they're doing the right thing."

For food processors, I'm afraid the motivation has more to do with marketing than our health. Otherwise they'd be cutting a lot more of the salt and high-fructose corn syrup.

Remember too, that processors are allowed to claim that anything between 35 mg and 140 mg of sodium per serving may be classified *Low Sodium.*

Reduced sodium levels refer to a 25% reduction of existing salt in the serving size of a product. Look out. It's a great ad, but the food my still be way over our daily limit.

So which foods changed?

Campbell's owns Pepperidge Farm, the bakery goods company. The indication from them is that they lowered salt a little bit and exchanged table salt with sea salt because it was a better tasting salt.

My problem with this promotion is that sea salt tastes exactly like table salt and more important, they are the very same chemical compound. They have the very same level of sodium. But some sea salt processors add other flavors to their salt claim better health and a "different" flavor. Salt is salt and table, kosher and sea salt have 2,350 mg of sodium per teaspoon. (USDA)

Many potato chip companies have introduced unsalted chips. The big surprise is that they taste much better than salted chips. When we serve chips at our house, those go first.

My hat's off to *Healthy Heart Market* who has an unsalted popcorn that seems superior to top brand names.

We do not recommend Morton Salt's new "Salt Balance" product. It is a blend of salt and potassium chloride, which makes up about 25% of the mix. That's like mixing table salt with Featherweight baking powder or one of the "soup" enhancers now offered. Those are mostly pure potassium chloride. Herbox Low–Sodium bouillon cubes are also nearly pure potassium.

Lupus – An autoimmune disorder that affects organ systems, skin, joints, and internal organs. Lupus can affect both men and women, but it is eight times as likely in women. It is not rare. Learn more about Lupus at *www.lupus.org.*

Lutein (Carotenoid) – One of the most abundant carotenoids at least in the North American diet. A phytonutrient found in leafy greens such as spinach, turnip greens and kale. Helps enhance or protect eyesight, and prevent cataracts and macular degeneration. Food sources include green vegetables, spinach, zucchini, Brussels sprouts, broccoli, romaine lettuce, kale and collard greens. A few of these also contain beta-carotene.

Lycopene (Carotenoid) – Natural pigment responsible for the deep colors in fruits, especially tomatoes. We need lycopene right from birth. However, an overdose or an underdose can lead to heart disease or cancer. It's best to get it in a balanced diet. Lycopene helps prevent oxidation of cholesterol, which slows down any development of atherosclerosis. It also protects our cells from damaging effects of free radicals. Food sources include tomatoes, watermelon, apricots, papaya, guava, salmon, shellfish (unsalted), cow's milk and egg yolks. Pink grapefruit contains lycopene as well, but grapefruit and grapefruit juice may interfere with some medications. Check your medications for interactions[3]. (See: Grapefruit)

Magnesium – Magnesium is an essential mineral for the human body. Many of the foods you now eat contain magnesium. If you aren't eating any of the foods listed here, you better get with it. Magnesium's job is too big. It helps with the contraction and relaxation of muscles, the promotion of certain enzymes in the body, production and the transportation of energy and the production of protein. If you're a "meat and potatoes" eater, you're in trouble. Magnesium is found in fruits and vegetables, especially avocados, apricots and bananas. It's in nuts (unsalted of course – like almonds, walnuts and pecans) Even though peanuts and cashews are arguably dietary "nuts," they are generally classified as legumes. No matter, each has high levels of magnesium. Magnesium is also found in well-known legumes like black beans, peas, seeds and other beans. Brown rice contains magnesium as do soy products like tofu, lecithin, and soy flour. Don't worry about overdoing it. Our bodies remove the magnesium we don't need. However, that's not usually the problem. Signs of too little magnesium can be muscle weakness, sleepiness or hyperexcitability.

Magnesium is also needed for bone, and fatty acid formation, activating B vitamins, blood clotting, and making new cells. The production and use of insulin also requires magnesium. Under certain circumstances magnesium has been found to improve vision in people with glaucoma. Similarly, magnesium has demonstrated an ability to lower blood pressure.

Maltodextrin – A complex carbohydrate. Maltodextrin is corn syrup solids composed primarily from fructose and glucose in a starch form. Complex means that the bonds that compose maltodextrin are very weak, and readily broken apart when ingested. The weak bonds and fragile composition of maltodextrin cause it to be easily digested a fraction slower than dextrose. Low amounts will not cause a spike in blood sugar. Found in Splenda packets and Granular Splenda. Store brands of "Sucralose" are the exact same mix as Splenda brand.

Manganese – A cup or two of tea a day can supply you with half of your daily needs for manganese. Manganese is an essential trace mineral required in small amounts to manufacture enzymes that are necessary for the metabolism of proteins and fat. Other than tea, it is found in spinach, split peas, unsalted nuts, oatmeal, pineapple, green leafy vegetables and a few other foods. It is essential for brain function and it supports the immune system and blood-sugar balance. Manganese is also involved in the production of cellular energy, reproduction, and bone growth. Works hand in hand with Vitamin K, B-complex and helps us to handle anxiety and stress.

Meat Alternatives for Vegans – Many of us wonder how vegans can enjoy a meal without a burger or steak or good barbecued chicken leg. The vegan answer is, "Easy!" Just use meatless foods like tofu meat substitutes (without added salt) or soy burgers. Vegans eat nuts so they visit health food grocery or food stores and purchase products that simulate what the rest of us eat – many of them made from soybeans. The big problem now, is finding some of these products without salt. They also use egg substitutes (made mostly from potato starch) and other dairy alternatives, which include fortified soy, rice or almond milk instead of cow's milk. Vegans use olive oil, water, homemade unsalted vegetable broth. For cheese, vegans use a product known as soy cheese, available in many health food stores. You can also try egg substitutes in baking. Just make sure the products are salt free or at least very low in sodium.

Meniere's Syndrome – a disorder of the inner ear that usually affects hearing and balance. Symptoms include episodes of dizziness, tinnitus and progressive hearing loss, although generally in one ear. It is thought to be caused by the drainage of fluids to the middle ear. More information is available from *www.menieres.org.* A no-salt, low-sodium liftestyle definitely helps those with Meniere's syndrome. See also nephrotic syndrome, Lupus, and diabetes.

Milligram (mg) – A milligram is a unit of measure equal to one one-thousandth of a gram (g).

Moderation – As in "eat everything in moderation." Lacks definition without knowing amounts and what each individual defines as moderation. It's much better to establish a good eating plan and sticking with it.

Monosodium Citrates – a sodium of citric acid. It is used as an antioxidant in food as well as to improve the effects of other antioxidants. It is also used as an acidity regulator and combiner. Found in jam, ice cream, coals and other carbonated beverages, milk powder, wine, processed cheeses and gelatin.

Mono Unsaturated Fats – While saturated fats increase the blood level of the "bad" LDL cholesterol, monounsaturated (one double bond) and polyunsaturated fats (two or more double bonds) generally found in vegetable oils work to lower "bad" or LDL cholesterol. An elevated LDL increases the risk of developing coronary heart disease. (See: Olive Oil section in this book)

MSG (Monosodium Glutamate) *(a free non essential amino acid glutamate known as additive 621)* – MSG is a big subject concerning a potentially big problem for some consumers[4] but not for all. Although a controversy concerning MSG remains alive, the FDA has calmed many with their research and research from Europe.

MSG is usually seen or used in a white crystalline form. It is also known as sodium glutamate and is a nonessential amino acid known as glutamic acid. Found in most processed foods, but not always labeled for it since some MSG is naturally present.

MSG additive #621 is commonly added to Asian cuisine, canned vegetables, soups, and processed meats. Made by a fermentation process using starch, beet sugar, cane sugar, or molasses, MSG is also sold as a white crystal substance that resembles salt and sugar. The product Accent is 100% monosodium glutamate.

Many consumers often equate all "free glutamate" products with MSG, but it is only one of several forms of glutamate – a major building block of proteins. Free glutamate, which results when glutamate is released during the breakdown of a protein molecule, occurs naturally in many foods, such as meat, milk, mushrooms, Parmesan cheese, and tomatoes. Glutamate is commonly found in food, primarily from protein sources. Foods and ingredients that contain glutamate as an inherent component are not required to list glutamate on the label. Examples include tomatoes, cheeses, meats, hydrolyzed protein products such as soy sauce, and autotyped yeast extracts. These ingredients are declared on the label by their common or usual names.

It's when MSG is added to food that the FDA requires "monosodium glutamate" to be listed on the label. Other salts of glutamic acid –such as monopotassium glutamate and monoammonium glutamate –also have to be declared on labels and can't be lumped together under "spices," "natural flavoring" or other general terms.[5]

Nationwide Food Consumption Survey (NFCS) – A national survey conducted by the USDA every ten years. It monitors the nutrient intake of a cross-section of the U.S. public.

Nephrotic Syndrome – Consists of a group of symptoms including protein in the urine (more than 3.5 grams per day), low blood protein levels, high cholesterol levels, and swelling or inflammation. The urine may also contain fat, which can be seen under the microscope. Symptoms include edema (swelling), swollen abdomen, swelling of the face, foamy urine, unintentional weight gain, poor appetite and high blood pressure. A no-salt diet is often prescribed.

Nitrite (Nitrate) – (Sodium) Nitrite is a food additive that has been used for centuries to preserve meats, fish and poultry. It also contributes to the characteristic flavor, color, and texture of processed meats such as hot dogs. Nitrite became a preservative of favor when processors discovered that it preserved the color of meat as well as the meat itself. Nitrite cured meats are protected against the deadly food bacterium, Clostridium (C.) botulinum.

About ninety to one-hundred-percent of the nitrates in our digestive tracts comes from vegetables and other sources. Those who eat cured meats probably have about ten-percent total in their tracts., Nitrates consumed in foods such as carrots and green vegetables are converted to nitrite during digestion. Nitrite in the body is instrumental in promoting blood clotting, healing wounds and burns, and boosting immune function to kill tumor cells.

NSA – No Salt Added.

Nuts – A "handful" (1/4 cup) of unsalted nuts a day, along with a Mediterranean diet rich in fish, fruit, vegetables are credited with lowering many risk factors for heart disease. Some researchers have found that adding the nuts to our life works better than the well-known olive oil associated with the Med diet. Nuts also help us "feel" full, but they do have a lot of calories, so don't overdose. Stick to the quarter cup if you want to try it and exchange that for something else you might be eating. The high antioxidant nuts that researchers are talking about for daily eating are unsalted walnuts, almonds, or chestnuts. Walnuts are top on the list with the highest level of omega-3 fatty acids at 2.27 g per ¼ cup. ¼ cup of olive oil has .428 g of omega-3 fatty acids. Almonds have none, and chestnuts have .033 g. With or without omega-3 however, these nuts have proved to help the human heart. (See: Walnuts, Almonds, Chestnuts)

Olive Oil – Olive oil reduces inflammation as well as helps reduce the risk of cardiovascular disease. For more about olive oil see: *What Can We Eat* chapter.

Omega-3 fatty acids - DHA/EPA – Considered an essential fatty acids and an effective anti-inflammatory food. They cannot be manufactured by the body but we need them to stay alive. Omega-3 fatty acids can only be obtained from foods, including nuts, salmon, tuna, and halibut. Surprisingly, it is also found in nut oils and in algae. Also known as polyunsaturated fatty acids (PUFAs), omega-3 fatty acids play a crucial role in brain function as well as normal growth and development. Provides benefits of reduced risk of cardiovascular disease and improved mental and visual function.

Organic – The Organic Foods Production Act (OFPA), enacted under Title 21 of the 1990 Farm Bill, served to establish uniform national standards for the production and handling of foods labeled as "organic." The Act authorized a new USDA National Organic Program (NOP) to set national standards for the production, handling, and processing of organically grown agricultural products. In addition, the Program oversees mandatory certification of organic production. The Act also established the National Organic Standards Board (NOSB) which advises the Secretary of Agriculture in setting the standards upon which the NOP is based. Producers who meet standards set by the NOP may label their products as "USDA Certified Organic." (Source: USDA)

Not all organic food is the same. The standards laid down by the USDA are set forth here.

1. A "100% Organic" label means that every ingredient in a product except for water and salt, was raised or farmed and harvested in an organic environment as approved and certified by the USDA. A farm field must be free of toxic pesticides and fertilizers for at least three years before a certified organic crop can be grown on it.

2. Products labeled "organic" must consist of at least 95 percent organically produced ingredients.

3. Processed products, cans, packages, frozen, that contain at least 70 percent organic ingredients can label their food with "made with organic ingredients" but must list up to three of the organic ingredients or food groups on the principal display panel.

4. Foods containing one ingredient, such as milk, eggs or fruit require an official USDA Organic label be displayed on the package or on the fruit.

Osteoporosis – Osteoporosis is a bone disease. It causes bones to break from having become too fragile. Osteoporosis generally progresses without pain – until a bone fractures or it breaks. Usually these happen to a wrist, hip, or more severely, to our spine. Hip breaks or fractures pretty much demand surgery and sometimes long hospitalization. Hip fractures generally create problems later with walking without assistance. They can also cause death. Spinal or vertebral fractures can cause shortness of height, terrible back pain, and sometimes unwelcome deformities.

Osteoporosis is four times more common with women. Men have thicker bones to begin with. Women naturally have smaller bone density and then to make matters even more challenging, they begin to lose bone mass at an earlier age than men. This process is increased by menopause. It's at that time women have to really pay attention to potential osteoporosis. Research has shown that regular exercise, and a generous calcium intake during childhood (read about milk and other dairy products), helps women and men build a supply of calcium that will be needed later in life. While bone length is established by age 20, bone strength and density continue to develop through age 30. Today there are medications and procedures to help those with signs of osteoporosis or with ways to prevent it. But it's always better to prevent it first with the exercise and youthful intake of calcium than it is to take the somewhat challenging procedures later.

Oven Temperatures – Ovens vary in actual temperatures. Even though one might say it's at 350° F, it may not be exact. All ovens rise and drop in temperature levels during baking periods. For instance they may rise to 450° F and the drop to 250° F during a baking period, a method of operation that holds to an average of 350° F.

That is one reason you don't want to keep opening your oven to check while you are baking or cooking. Opening the door causes about fifty to one hundred degrees of heat to escape rather quickly. This has been demonstrated to me by our oven manufacturer. See–through oven doors were a great addition to ovens. Thermometers in meat should be placed so that you can read them through the window.

Partially Hydrogenated (oils) – Refers to vegetable oils that have partially hardened. Less expensive than other cooking fats, partially hydrogenated oils become "shortening." The process turns otherwise safe cooking oils into highly saturated fats with a high trans fats rating. Should be avoided. Look for it in processed baked goods, shortening, margarine, whips and especially imported products.

Peanuts (unsalted) (legume) – Unsalted peanuts provide a lot of nutrients, but don't go with them. They have a lot of calories as well. One-quarter cup of unsalted peanuts contain generous portions of manganese, tryptophan, vitamin B3, folate, copper and protein. Also about 200 calories. Still, they make a good snack and all you have to do is exchange the calories with whatever your other snack was going to be. (Most commercially salted peanuts contain MSG. Unsalted don't.)

Pectin – Pectin is gleaned from ripe fruit for use in making jams and jellies. When making jam with some ripe fruits we don't need to add pectin. With others we do. High pectin levels can be found in apples, blackberries (domestic and wild) citrus fruit, and red currants. Strawberries are especially low with natural pectin and nearly always require added pectin when making jam. We don't always make jam with "ripe" fruit, so we add pectin when necessary.

Phosphorus – Phosphorus is an essential mineral required in every cell of our body to ensure normal function. It is usually found in nature combined with oxygen as phosphate. Phosphorous is found in most foods since it is an important or critical component for all living organisms. We obtain much of our phosphorus when eating fish, meat and dairy products. Phosphorus in plant seeds we eat like cereals, peas, nuts, beans, etc., are stored in the form of phosphate otherwise known as phytic acid or phytate. When we eat these seeds, we receive only about 50% of the phosphorus. The science behind that gets to be tricky. Can we get too much? Generally a slight overload will be washed out by our kidneys, but get it in excess and we can get too much, which could prove to be harmful. There is an intrinsic relationship with vitamin D in that high blood levels of phosphorus suppress Vitamin D. If you are a heavy cola drinker, you may be getting too much phosphorus in your diet.

Phyllo – A paper-thin sheet of dough or pastry. Raw unleavened flour dough used mostly by Greeks, Turks, and Middle Easterners. Popular in restaurants for pies, apfelstrudel, meats, and many other uses.

Phytochemicals – The word *"phyto"* originated from a Greek word meaning plant. Phytochemicals are non-nutritive plant chemicals that have protective or disease preventive properties. These chemicals are in plants to protect the plant. However, recent research has discovered that they may also protect us against diseases. More than a thousand phytochemicals are known to exist. Best known include lycopene (found in tomatoes especially), isoflavones, (found in soy), and flavonoids, (found in fruits.

Phytonutrients – Phytonutrients are certain organic components of plants, and these components are thought to promote human health. Fruits, vegetables, grains, legumes, nuts, and teas are rich sources of phytonutrients. Unlike the traditional nutrients (protein, fat, vitamins, minerals), phytonutrients are not "essential" for life, so some people prefer to refer to them as phytochemicals. Phytonutrient benefits include service as antioxidants, converting vitamin A (beta-carotene is metabolized to vitamin A), cause cancer cells to die (apoptosis), repair DNA damage caused by smoking or other toxic exposures, alter estrogen metabolism, and they are known to enhance our immune response.

Potassium Bicarbonate – Potassium is a mineral found naturally in nearly all foods and is necessary for body function, especially our hearts. Potassium bicarbonate is used to prevent or to treat a potassium deficiency known as hypokalemia. Many of today's "No Salt Added" products are adding potassium bicarbonate for "taste." This can prove to be dangerous if too many of these products become standard items in our diets. Especially found in no-salt soup bases. This is also the product that is dominate in Featherweight Baking Powder. (See: Ener-G baking powder). If you are prescribed diuretics (water pills) then you may also have been prescribed potassium tablets. The reason for this is that diuretics can drain your body of potassium as well as fluids.

Caution: Too much potassium, or too little can be harmful to our hearts. Elevated blood levels of potassium may cause irregular heartbeats or even a heart attack. With a proper dietary plan the body maintains blood levels of potassium within an established range. Usually, it is not possible to produce potassium toxicity from the ingestion of potassium in natural foods or even supplements. However, high intakes of potassium bicarbonate and chloride may cause serious illness. Symptoms include nausea, vomiting, diarrhea, possibly ulcers. Please avoid taking potassium tablets as supplements without first discussing it with your doctor. And also try to avoid using "salt substitutes" that are usually nothing more than potassium bicarbonate or potassium chloride. Research has shown that salt substitutes using potassium chloride can be dangerous, possibly deadly for renal patients. Potassium chloride (see below) should not be used if you have kidney failure, Addison's disease, severe burns or other tissue injuries.

Potassium Chloride – A chemical compound composed of potassium and chlorine. Also known as muriate of potash, especially used for fertilizer. (Most potassium is used for fertilizer.) However, it's used for many other things from natural gas operations to drilling for oil. For our concern, it is used medically and in food processing, especially for foods processed currently as "no salt added." Be cautious when buying processed unsalted foods like tomato ketchup, canned tomatoes, and other no salt added foods. If you have been told to cut your potassium intake down, then read the ingredient labels usually placed under or alongside the FDA panel.

Potassium Lactate – Potassium lactate is hygroscopic (absorbing moisture from the air), that is can take up and retain moisture for freshness. It is used in meat and poultry to control food-borne pathogenic bacteria and to protect and enhance meat flavor. You'll find it in cakes, ice cream, candy, jam, processed meats among other processed foods.

Potato Flour – Adds moistness to most baked goods. Necessary in gluten free breads to help texture. Exchange one flour for one potato flour if adding to a recipe not calling for it. A few teaspoons with muffins and cakes and about a tablespoon for a loaf of bread work well.

Probiotics – Probiotics are live microorganisms that are similar to the good bacteria already inside our bodies. Available through dietary supplements and foods like "living culture" yogurt, these probiotics generally restore intestinal health by increasing the number of bacteria that are helpful to us – if we need them. It's not a good idea to take any supplements without first discussing the matter with your doctor or registered dietitian.

Intestinal balance function or balance can be disturbed by more than a few things, including surgery, antibiotics, some medications and a poor diet – one that doesn't offer good nutrition. Age is another offset to a healthy intestine. Getting upset or becoming "stressed" hurts as well. And then there's traveling. It not only exposes us to harmful bacteria in restaurants, water, unfriendly restrooms, and generally stress and exhaustion, it sometimes causes great constipation and pain. Therefore, using a probiotic a day might support our digestive system and keep us "normal" at all times, however research into this supplement has not yet been extensive enough to dive in and start your own program. If however, your doctor suggests this is a good idea, then the benefits of probiotics outweigh any costs (they are usually inexpensive). They increase the number of healthy bacteria compared to the unhealthy strains. Furthermore, the probiotic strains that enter the body compete for space and nutrients with the less desirable strains you'll run into. You can pretty much get the same results from eating yogurt on a daily basis.

Prothrombin Time, ProTime (PT) – Used to measure Warfarin (Coumadin) dosage and or potential liver damage and to learn your vitamin K level. Helps to figure out clotting potential.

Protein – Adults need about 60 grams of protein a day. All of the recipes in our books and on-line list the amount of protein they contain so that you can figure out what you eat each day. Also, you can look at an FDA food data panel to find out how many protein grams are in a serving. But if you're eating a balanced diet, you don't need to keep track of it. It's pretty easy to get enough protein. Dietary proteins are involved in metabolic functions. Basically, they furnish the amino acids required to build and maintain body tissues. As an energy source, proteins are equivalent to carbohydrates while providing 4-calories per gram. Proteins play a major if not primary role in all body tissues and in the formation of enzymes, hormones and various body fluids, and secretions. Proteins aid the transport of a few lipids, vitamins, minerals, and they help maintain the body's homeostasis (The ability of an organism or cell to maintain internal equilibrium by adjusting its physiological processes.)

Refrigerator Temperatures – Most freezer/refrigerator combinations operate with the compressor working on the freezer's temperature. A gate valve opens from the freezer side and passes cold air into the refrigerator side to keep it at a preset temperature. You'll want to keep your fridge around 40° F or slightly lower. Opening either the freezer door or the refrigerator causes a great deal of the cool air to escape. That's why you'll often hear the compressor come on after you leave it open for more than a few moments. Temperatures are averaged just as they are with ovens.

Right heart catheterization – A test that allows the doctor (usually a cardiologist) to inspect the inside of your heart's right chamber. This is where your heart pumps blood returning blood into your lungs for a renewed supply of oxygen. The catheter is a long thin bendable tube. (I have watched this procedure more than a half dozen times on the monitor while they performed it on me.) The tube enters either through a vessel at the groin or neck or your arm. The procedure allows the doctor to measure oxygen, check your blood pressure in the chambers of the heart and to examine the valves between the chambers. Generally you are not "knocked out," but instead anesthetized only at the point of entry. Blood vessels do not have nerve endings so there is no pain.

Salmon – Best fish with omega-3 fatty acids, which are necessary for effective anti-inflammatory affects. Wild salmon is best. Alaska produces world's best wild salmon. Avoid imported or farmed salmon. Northern Atlantic wild salmon is acceptable but not as high in omega-3 fatty acids as Alaskan. Salt-free albacore tuna also contain omega-3s. (We prefer Merino's for canned, unsalted albacore tuna. See: www.merinoseafood.com

Salmonella – Salmonella is a strain of bacteria that occurs in many animals, especially poultry and swine. (In 2008, nationwide, only 17% of the chicken purchased in the U.S. was free of salmonella.) It can enter our system via contaminated water, soil, insects, meat, poultry and any egg that has a cracked shell. (Do not use an egg out of a carton that was cracked in the carton in the store. If you crack one in your home, use it immediately or toss it.) Salmonella can be found on kitchen surfaces, especially after raw poultry has been prepped or a spill of egg happens. Clean with a Clorox based cleaner before using countertop for any other food. After handling poultry, wash hands well before handling other food. Acute symptoms of Salmonella illness include nausea, vomiting, diarrhea, abdominal cramps, headache and fever.

Salt, Table – Table salt is 40 percent sodium by weight. Salt is "sodium chloride" with chlorine components as well as other inert materials. Six grams of table salt equal one-teaspoon. Converting 2.325 grams of salt means that one level teaspoon of salt has 2,350 mg of sodium.

You may have read recent reports that salt can kill. They are true, but it's not just the salt as much as it is the sodium in the salt. Newly born infants should not be fed any salt for at least a year. None! It's the law in the U.S. and for a good reason. Concentrated added sodium can prevent infants from breathing or excreting sodium quickly. The normal treatment for adults overdosing on sodium is to drink lots of water and "force" the sodium out. Short of that adults might find themselves vomiting it out.

Infants do not excrete sodium well through their kidneys and urine; neither do the elderly. The older we get, the less sodium we should consume.

When is it safe for a healthy lifestyle to add salt? According to Dr. Trevor Beard, never. "If you want the same blood pressure at 70 that you had as an infant, then you'll have to live like the salt-free societies do. Only they have survived without incidence of high blood pressure."[6]

Salt however, is not the only source of sodium you should be concerned about. The NIH, American Medical Association (AMA), and American Dietetic Association (ADA) strongly urged in 2006 daily consumption of dietary sodium at between 1,300 and 1,800 milligrams for healthy people. That means all forms of sodium.

Unfortunately, there are a great number of hidden sources of sodium in packaged, canned, frozen, and prepared foods as well as in dairy products, some medications and many over the counter supplements. And now we have to look out for fresh poultry and pork that is brined and watch for turkeys with additives from salt to glutamates. (NOTE: A Centrum Senior or comparable vitamin contains nearly 61 mg of sodium. In our low sodium lifestyle, that can be more than 10% of a desirable daily intake. We've seen chondroitin/glucosamine tablets listed with 2,000 mg of sodium each.) Check labels on all supplements. Some are very high in sodium levels. If sodium isn't listed on a product, ask the store manager or call the manufacturer. Many products list customer service numbers on their products. If you cannot find out, E-mail us and we'll see what we can learn.

Salt Substitutes – Most commercial salt substitutes are potassium bicarbonate (exactly the same formula as Hain's Featherweight Baking Powder) or potassium chloride. Some may add other elements, but only for flavor. According to dietitians and dietitian news, renal specialists have called for better labeling on products that use potassium chloride as a salt replacement since it could pose a hidden risk for dialysis patients. The dose of potassium is typically high when used to replace table salt. We have created a "flavor enhancer" that serves as our salt replacement and the recipe for it is in our *No Salt, Lowest Sodium International Cookbook.* We recommend against using salt substitutes for two reasons, the potassium chloride being the first, the other being the matter of using it as a crutch. If you stop eating salt altogether, within a few months your palate will heal from the damage the salt has done and you'll find yourself tasting new and fresher flavors. This is when you'll appreciate herbs and spices more and you'll find that you don't miss salt at all. Potassium chloride will do much the same to your palate as salt does. Damage it, but it is repairable by just cutting out its daily use. Too much potassium in our diets is also potentially dangerous for our hearts.

Saturated Fat – Consuming large amounts of saturated fats can result in fatty (or wax like) substances within our system. Cholesterol is one of these and it's dangerous since it adheres to the walls of our arteries. Essentially, saturated fat is a triglyceride with the maximum number of hydrogen atoms attached to the carbon atoms. Had enough science? Okay, here's the bottom line. Saturated Fats are very hard on our systems. They may lead to atherosclerosis (narrowing of the arteries) and high blood pressure. We get these fats from animal sources like beef, fowl, butter, whole-milk (instead of nonfat milk), and other dairy products. We also get it from the dark meat of poultry and the skin or fat left on the meat after removing the skin. It's no mystery any longer that we also were fed these fats by food processors in the form of partially hydrogenated palm oils and coconut oils. To reduce your risk of a heart attack, reduce your saturated fat as much as you can. Some studies suggest that replacing saturated fats in the diet with unsaturated fats will increase one's ratio of HDL to LDL serum cholesterol.

Sea Salt – Sea Salt is heavily marketed as "safer," "healthier," or "tastier." Of course, there is no difference between table salt, kosher, or sea salt when speaking about sodium content. Sodium levels are the same at 2,350 mg per teaspoon. True sea salt is produced by the evaporation of sea water. Not all of it comes from the sea, however, some comes from deep salt mines. Promoters of sea salt will list lower levels of sodium on FDA labels, but that's because they "dilute" or cut the salt with other ingredients like lycopene, etc. So, if you mix a half teaspoon of salt with a half teaspoon of lycopene, you've got half a teaspoon of sodium. No matter what flavor they add, the sodium for the salt is the same when measured teaspoon for teaspoon. And it's never "better for you."

"Salt is salt, sodium is sodium." Sodium is a base mineral and all salt (sodium chloride) structures are the same regardless of whether they came from the sea on the coast of Montpelier, France, or from a mine in Pennsylvania. When ground to finer forms (as in table salt or Kosher salt) it has a tendency to "clump," so salt producers add anti-clumping agents. They also may add sodium iodide. But that is at a very small rate. I have a can of "Baleine " sea salt in front of me right now. They add sodium iodide at the rate of 15mg/KG which can hardly be regarded as dilutional. In any case, nutritional and anti-clumping additives have already taken into account in the USDA's nutritional values, which are averages of many samples.

Any dilution effect of additives to salt among various brands will have a negligible affect on the final sodium value, thus they will not diverge in that respect from the USDA listing for "table salt" by any significant amount. (See also: Artisanal Salt)

Sepsis – A life threatening illness due to a bacterial infection. Quick diagnosis and care is important. I developed it in 2003 but thought I had the chills. I went to bed and Maureen called our son in law who heard her description and ordered me to emergency immediately. He is a doctor, so I listened and obeyed. I ended up in the hospital for 4 days with a steady antibiotic fluid through an IV. One-third of those who develop sepsis (known as "septic") die from it. Symptoms include fever (not always though), chills and shaking (my symptoms), fast beating heart or rapid breathing, confusion, agitation or a rash on the skin. Joint pain is also possible especially at wrists, elbows, knees and ankles. Your back or hips may also develop pains.

Shelf Life – Period of time any food, medicine or other perishable items have before considered unusable either for home use or in stores. Often written as "Best before," "Use by," and "Sell by."

Sodium – Often misunderstood, sodium is a mineral, and the surprise is that it's an essential nutrient. Our daily requirements for sodium are satisfied with a normal diet that does not included added salt. Sodium helps to maintain blood volume, regulate the balance of water in the cells, and keep nerves functioning. Too much sodium can cause a retention of too much fluid in the body, which in turn can bring about hypertension or at least contribute to it. The kidneys control sodium balance by increasing or decreasing sodium in the urine. One teaspoon of salt contains 2,350 milligrams of sodium, more than four times the amount the body requires per day. We suggest approximately 500 mg per day, which you can get by eating natural foods that have not been contaminated with salt. Major studies have proved that there is a direct correlation between a high sodium consumption and high blood pressure. Most dietitians agree that a high sodium intake can be harmful to us.

Sodium Alginate – Used as a thickener such as in chocolate milk, ice cream and other foods. Used in place of guar gum or other thickeners. Can be purchased for cooking at home.

Sodium Ascorbate – the sodium of ascorbic acid. It is used as a source of vitamin C, and as an antioxidant in food. You'll also find it in breakfast cereals and some processed meats.

Sodium Benzoate – *Although it occurs naturally in some foods, it is also* produced chemically and added in small amounts as a preservative to processed foods. Sodium Benzoate is effective in killing bacteria, yeast and fungi. Used especially with high acid content foods since sodium benzoate works only when pH balance is below 3.6. You'll find it in colas, vinegar, juices and salad dressings and other processed mixed ingredient products. For wine drinkers, sodium benzoate is what stops the fermentation process. You can also find it naturally in apples, cranberries, prunes or plums and other fruits. Cinnamon and cloves and a few other spices also naturally contain sodium benzoate.

Sodium Hydroxide – A caustic chemical used in everything from metal to paper. Used commercially for washing and peeling fruits and vegetables before canning. Olives are soaked in sodium hydroxide to soften them. If this doesn't make you feel uncomfortable, know that sodium hydroxide might be in your home as a drain cleaning agent for clogged drains. It is also used in the process of making illegal drugs such as methamphetamine.

Sodium Nitrate/Nitrite – See Nitrate.

Sodium Propionate – Used as a mold inhibitor in bread. It is the sodium of propionic acid.

Sodium Citrate – See Trisodium phosphate.

Sodium Labels – See FDA Panels **Spices** – Spices are typically dried seeds, fruit, roots, bark, leaves, or other vegetative substances ground or grated into a powder. Where herbs are basically from the leaf, spices are from other parts of a plant. They are used for flavoring or coloring foods or recipes.

Splenda, Splenda Granulated, Splenda Brown Sugar Blend, Splenda Confectioner's – Splenda has become the most popular of the artificial sweeteners available today. The caloric and carbohydrate content for SPLENDA Brand Sweetener is as follows:

SPLENDA Granulated

1 tsp = 0.5 gm carbohydrate = 2 calories

one half cup = 12 gm carbohydrate = 48 calories

1 cup = 24 gm carbohydrate = 96 calories

*1 tsp. = 1 serving
SPLENDA Packet or Café Stick
1 packet/stick = .9 gm of carbohydrate = 4 calories
*1 packet/stick has the sweetness of 2 tsp of sugar
Note: Per U.S. labeling laws, anything with less than 5 calories per serving, is properly labeled as "zero" or no-calorie.
Note: The calories and carbohydrates in SPLENDA No Calorie Sweetener come from dextrose and/or maltodextrin, which are added for bulk. Sucralose, the sweetening ingredient in SPLENDA Brand Sweetener, has no calories and is not a carbohydrate.
Granulated - sucralose, maltodextrin (0.5 gram per serving)
Packets/Sticks - sucralose, maltodextrin and dextrose (less than 1 gram per packet) Since you need to use only half the volume of sugar called for in your recipe, SPLENDA Sugar Blend for Baking and SPLENDA Brown Sugar Blend provides half the calories and carbohydrate that sugar would ordinarily provide.
SPLENDA Sugar Blend for Baking (use ½ as much as sugar)
one half cup = 96 gm carbohydrate = 384 calories
one half teaspoon = 2 gm carbohydrate = 16 calories
SPLENDA Brown Sugar Blend (use ½ as much as Brown Sugar)
One half cup packed = approximately 95-105 gms carbohydrate = approximately 380-420 calories
One Cup packed = approximately 190-210 gms carbohydrate = approximately 760-840 calories
Starch – A naturally abundant nutrient carbohydrate that is found primarily in potatoes, wheat, oats, pasta, yams, and rice and this may surprise you, bananas when still green at their tips. When bananas ripen (brown) the starch converts to sugar. Starch varies in appearance according to its source (seeds, fruits, tubers, roots, and stem pith of plants), but it's normally prepared as a white amorphous tasteless powder. Starch takes much longer to digest than simple sugars, such as sucrose (table sugar). Consequently, starch provides a steady stream of glucose into the bloodstream and is less likely than sucrose to cause blood glucose swings which can provoke the secretion of excess insulin.

Stereotaxis – Stereotaxis technologies are changing how clinicians treat cardiac arrhythmia and perform other cardiovascular interventions. Physicians with Stereotaxis achieve exceptional clinical outcomes without compromising safety, enabling them to confidently treat areas of the heart unreachable or potentially unsafe with manual techniques or alternative technologies. Visit: *www.stereotaxis.com*

Stevia – Stevia Rebaudiana is an herb in the Chrysanthemum family that grows wild as a small shrub in parts of Paraguay and Brazil. The glycosides in its leaves, including up to 10% Stevioside, account for its incredible sweetness, making it unique among the nearly 300 species of Stevia plants. (Excerpted from: *stevia.com*)

Stomach Cancer – Research in many countries warn of the clear association between stomach cancer and the consumption of salt-preserved foods such as anchovies, olives, salt pork – essentially foods with high concentrations of salt, which has proved to be powerful irritant to the sensitive lining of the stomach.

Sucralose – Sucralose is the only low-calorie sweetener that is made from sugar. Sucralose is highly stable under a wide variety of processing conditions. Thus, it can be used virtually anywhere sugar can including cooking and baking. Currently, sucralose has been approved in over 25 countries around the world for use in food and beverages. In the US, sucralose is USDA and FDA approved for use as a tabletop sweetener and in 15 different food and beverage categories, including carbonated soft drinks, low-calorie fruit drinks, apple sauce and other products.

Sucralose is not Splenda. For more see Splenda on the previous page.

Sucrose – Often referred to as "empty calories," sucrose is formed from fructose and glucose and is thereby known as a double sugar. Known as a viable energy source (each 100 grams of sucrose yields about 400 Kcal of energy) it has no other nutritional value. Refined sucrose is generally the "sugar" sweetener added to processed foods, or added as a flavor booster and sometimes as a preservative. Sucrose is naturally found in some vegetables and fruits.

Sugar – A simple carbohydrate. Water soluble. Sugar is sweet and pretty much all sugars are the same. A variety exists for the consumer ranging from sucrose, raw sugar, turbinado sugar, brown sugar, molasses, honey, to corn syrup. No significant nutritional difference exists except for the sodium levels. Sucrose (sugar) is rated at zero sodium by the USDA, while brown sugar ranges up to 86 mg per packed cup. Each provides the same level of energy as well. Importantly, there is no available evidence that our body can distinguish between natural or added sugars in our food.

Sulfites – Sulfiting agents are sometimes used to preserve the color of foods such as dried fruits and vegetables, and to inhibit the growth of microorganisms in fermented foods such as wine. Sulfites are safe for most people. A small segment of the population, however, has been found to develop shortness of breath or fatal shock shortly after exposure to these preservatives. Sulfites can provoke severe asthma attacks in sulfite-sensitive asthmatics. For that reason, in 1986 the FDA banned the use of sulfites on fresh fruits and vegetables (except potatoes) intended to be sold or served raw to consumers. Sulfites added to all packaged and processed foods must be listed on the product label. (All wine has sulfites in it. Even if the label does not state this.) . Generally those who complain of headaches from sulfites have concurrently consumed red wine, which does cause headaches for some people, although as of this writing, research has not determined exactly what in red wine could be the cause. Sulfites are also known to destroy vitamin B1 (thiamin, also spelled thiamine), a vitamin essential for metabolism of carbohydrates and alcohol.

Supplements – Usually means over the counter vitamins or enzymes, or antihistamines, etc. If you are taking prescription drugs, please check with your doctor first before taking any supplements. Some do interact with prescribed medications and some actually render prescription medications ineffective. You might want to seek the advice of a qualified nutritionist or doctor regarding the safety and appropriate doses of nutrients via supplements you want to take. Also seek out any potential drug interactions. Although research into supplements hasn't been in depth, some have shown that the benefits of taking vitamins and minerals probably outweigh the risks for many of us.

– See Salt, Table

Trans fats (trans fatty acids) – *Trans* fats are unsaturated fatty acids formed when vegetable oils are processed and made more solid or into a more stable liquid. This processing is called hydrogenation. Trans fats also occur naturally in low amounts in some foods. However, the trans fats we hear about these days are created in the food processing industry when they add hydrogen to liquid vegetable oils to make then solid, ala margarine, Crisco, etc. This practice is waning and be ended in the U.S. shortly. However, many imported baked goods will contain hydrogenated oils, especially coconut or palm kernel.

Partially hydrogenated vegetable oils were developed in part to help displace highly saturated animal and vegetable fats used in frying, baking and spreads. However, *trans* fats, like saturated fats, raise blood LDL cholesterol levels (bad cholesterol). High consumption of *trans* fats may also reduce the HDL or "good" cholesterol levels. Many restaurants used trans fats extensively, but that practice is also fading away. In January 2006, FDA revised food labeling regulations to require that the amount of *trans* fat in a product be declared on the Nutrition Facts panel.

Triglycerides (Metabolic Syndrome) – When you get a "cholesterol" level blood test, make sure you also get your triglyceride number. Our body's energy calories come from food. If we eat too much food or too much fat, and don't use it immediately, then the calories convert into triglycerides and these are then stored in fat cells to be used later. It doesn't matter what kind of food we eat, either. If we don't use it up burning the calories via outputs of energy, then it all converts to triglycerides (fat). If we produce a normal amount of triglycerides, then we're on track. It's when we produce more than our body needs that we develop problems. High levels of triglycerides become part of a condition known as metabolic syndrome. When we have a blood test, they'll measure our HDL, LDL, and high triglycerides. It is the reading of this combination that we want to know since an off-kilter or abnormal combined reading could mean we're on our way to heart disease, diabetes or even a stroke. Normal triglyceride readings are below 150 with high levels registering above 200. There are new tests going on as I write this that have already proved to some that finding potential heart disease will become much easier.

Trisodium Phosphate (Sodium citrate) – Sodium of citric acid. Used as a food additive for preservative or flavor. Used in some colas and energy drinks as well as antacids.

Tryptophan (amino acid) – Often blamed for people "crashing" on the sofa after a big Thanksgiving turkey dinner. But alas, turkey doesn't have much tryptophan. Those of us who don't overeat don't usually find it necessary to crash. Maybe the sleepiness has more to do with a few too many calories. Tryptophan is an amino acid that serves as a niacin precursor in the body, and niacin helps to reduce activation of free fatty acids.

Unsaturated Fat – Unsaturated fat is fat that is not fully saturated with hydrogen. There are two kinds of unsaturated fats. Monounsaturated (double bond) and polyunsaturated (two or more double bonds). We find monounsaturated fats in peanuts, peanut butter, olives, and avocados, to name a few. Polyunsaturated fats, are usually liquid at room temperature. We usually find these in vegetable oils such as olive, corn, sunflower, and soybean. Unsaturated fats are inclined to be healthier in the diet than saturated fats because they could help lower the level of cholesterol in our blood. Substituting unsaturated fats for saturated fats helps to lower levels of total cholesterol and LDL cholesterol in the blood. One way to do this? Use extra virgin olive oil instead of butter or hardened oils like margarine, etc.

U.S. Department of Agriculture (USDA) – The United States Department of Agriculture is comprised of many agencies charged with different tasks related to agriculture and our food supply. Among these is ensuring a safe, affordable, nutritious and accessible food supply. It is responsible for the safety of meat, poultry and egg products. The

USDA also enhances the quality of life for the American population by supporting production of agricultural products; caring for agricultural, forest and range lands; supporting sound development of our rural communities; providing economic opportunities for farm and rural residents; expanding global markets for agricultural and forest products and services; and working to reduce hunger in America and throughout the world.

Vegetarian – According to the Vegetarian Resource Group, less than one-percent of Americans are true vegans. A vegan eats only plant-based food, with a diet that is balanced enough to make sure they get all the nutrients needed including protein. Vegans do not eat honey, so when you see a recipe without meat or fish or animal products like milk but it does have honey, you'll find it marked as Flexitarian. Vegans can often exchange sugar or Splenda for the honey in these instances and convert the recipe for their use. Vegetarians fall into three other groups, however. Lacto-Vegetarians do consume milk (generally nonfat or 1% fat) but don't eat eggs The rest of their diet comes from plant-based foods. The next would be the lacto-ovo vegetarians who eat plant-based foods and eggs, milk or milk products like cheese and yogurt. Semi-Vegetarians, known as Flexitarians follow the plant-based diet but sometimes eat small portions of meat including fish and poultry and honey. Many of our recipes fall into one of the first three categories. Our meat recipes would have to be cut back substantially to fit into the fourth category. (See: Meat Alternatives for Vegans)

Vital Wheat Gluten – A wheat grain that has all of its starch removed and is then dried. It is a wheat protein. Used to supplement many other flours to increase protein. Gluten content is usually forty-five percent with a higher protein level of about seventy-five percent. We recommend using it in our bread recipes. Since we also recommend a high gluten flour. Our use of vital wheat gluten is below the usual recommendation of up to two teaspoons per cup of flour. Vital wheat gluten increases the protein in our recipes, but at a very low level.

Vitamins (Supplements) – Naturally obtained vitamins are nutritionally essential, usually in small amounts needed to manage metabolic processes. Vitamins are usually classified by their solubility. The fat-soluble vitamins A, D, E, and K have a special, usually individual physiologic role. Several vitamins (as with spices and herbs), have antioxidant properties to depress the effects of metabolic by-products called free radicals. Free radicals may cause degenerative changes related to aging. Nearly all of the water-soluble vitamins are components of essential enzyme systems and are not normally stored in our bodies for more than a day or so. Instead, they are usually excreted in our urine. Since they are involved in the reactions supporting energy metabolism a daily dietary supply is desirable to avoid depletion and interruption of normal physiologic functions.

Vitamin A (Retinol) – *Water soluble.* Important for maintaining good vision. An initial sign that you may be vitamin A deficient can be loss of your night vision. Vitamin A is important for the maintenance of healthy skin and for the mucous membranes that line our nose, sinuses, and mouth. Although our bodies can make vitamin A from beta-carotene, it is obtained primarily from animal-based foods. Dietary sources include dark green leafy vegetables, and colorful (bright and deep colored) fruits and vegetables. Best are yams or sweet potatoes, pumpkin, winter squashes, apricots, peaches, mangoes, and cantaloupe, and carrots. It is also available in milk that has been fortified with Vitamin A (and sometimes vitamin D). The USDA states that milk with vitamin A is rated at 102.9 mg of sodium, while milk without it is higher. Vitamin A can work against us if we consume more than is needed, so make sure you consult with your doctor or an R.D. before taking supplements.

Vitamin B1 (Thiamin) – *Water-soluble.* Vitamin B1 is a vitamin that the body requires to break down carbohydrates, fat, and protein. All B vitamins help our body to convert carbohydrates into glucose (sugar), which in turns become the energy we burn. There are eight (8) water soluble B vitamins known also as complex vitamins. They are necessary in the breakdown of fats and protein. Vitamin B1 is also essential for the proper functioning of nerve cells. Thiamin is thought of as an anti-stress vitamin since, it is believed, it enhances the function of our immune system and offers our bodies the ability to deal well with stress. Found in plants and animals, it plays an important role in some metabolic reactions, especially the conversion of carbohydrates into energy. Dietary sources include nuts and green vegetables, beets, carrots, turnip, lettuce, cauliflower, beans, whole-grain, enriched cereals and rice, bran, blackstrap molasses, and wheat germ. Yeast and egg yolks contain about 100 IU of vitamin B1 (thiamin). Meat is a poor source but thiamin can be found in pork and lamb (mutton).

Vitamin B Complex – Foods that contain vitamin B1, B2, B3, B5, B6 and B12 are in effect good source of what are known as "vitamin B complex," a combination of important vitamin B elements. Dietary sources include whole grain cereals, wheat, nuts, green leafy vegetables, molasses, beef liver, and yeast. Before taking any vitamin B supplements, check with your doctor.

Vitamin B2 (Riboflavin) – *Water soluble.* Vitamin B2 is a water-soluble vitamin that helps the body process amino acids and fats. It is essential for growth. B2 activates vitamin B6 and folic acid, and converts carbohydrates to sugar that is then burned up as energy. Under some conditions, vitamin B2 can act as an antioxidant. Riboflavin is not easy to find in food, and because of that B2 deficiency is more prominent if our diets exclude those foods where it is found. It has been added to some processed foods. Elderly especially have to take care that they get enough. Symptoms of riboflavin deficiency include fatigue, digestion problems, sores around our mouth, eye fatigue, lip soreness and a sensitivity to light. A lack of riboflavin is also blamed for some headaches. B2 is therefore important for people who get migraines, have anemia or eating disorders, or cataracts. Dietary sources include yeast, almonds, milk, egg, liver, (organ meats), whole-grains, wild rice, mushrooms, soybeans, green leafy vegetables, and broccoli. Raw spinach is good too, as well as cereals fortified with riboflavin.

Vitamin B3 (Niacin) – *Water soluble.* Vitamin B3 is also water soluble and helps to convert carbohydrates into glucose (sugar/energy). Niacin helps rid our bodies of toxic (harmful) chemicals. It is used in the synthesis of sex hormones, as well as treating schizophrenia and other mental illnesses. Some use it as a memory-enhancer, but there's little proof it works. Basically, it helps improve blood circulation and the reduction of cholesterol in our blood; it also reduces the mobility of free fatty acids. Our bodies are able to convert tryptophan, an amino acid found in the protein in many foods, into niacin. You might spot a shortage of vitamin B3 if any of the following symptoms appear: Canker sores, diarrhea, fatigue, halitosis, headaches, indigestion, insomnia, loss of appetite, low blood-sugar, muscular weakness, skin eruptions, and inflammation. There are other symptoms as well. Dietary sources include beets, brewer's yeast, fish, beef liver, beef kidney, pork, turkey, chicken, veal, salmon, tomatoes, peas, beans, cereals, green vegetables, swordfish, tuna, sunflower seeds, and peanuts. Also available in supplement, but be careful. Usually we don't need to take this vitamin. Check with your doctor or registered dietitian first.

Vitamin B5 (Pantothenic Acid) – *Water soluble.* Vitamin B5 is a water-soluble vitamin that ignites the adrenal glands. It is absolutely necessary in transporting and releasing energy from fats. It enables the synthesis of cholesterol, vitamin D, and steroid hormones. It works best when consumed along with foods containing vitamins A, C, E and other B group vitamins. Vitamin B5 is very important for the production of red blood cells as well as sex and stress-related hormones that are produced in the adrenal glands). Pantethine, a by-product of B5, has been shown to lower cholesterol and triglycerides in the blood. It has not shown to be toxic in high dosages although one can exhibit digestive upsets and diarrhea with too much. Top level for daily ingestion should not exceed ten grams a day. Dietary sources abound in unprocessed foods. They include fresh meats, unprocessed (raw) grains, yeast, corn, cauliflower, kale, broccoli, tomatoes, avocados, lentils, molasses, wheat bran, yams/ sweet potatoes, liver, egg yolk, kidney, and milk. Lobster and salmon also contain Vitamin B5.

Vitamin B6 (Pyridoxine) – *Water soluble.* Part of the vitamin B complex. Vitamin B6 plays a role in the synthesis of antibodies by the immune system, which are needed to fight many diseases. Vitamins B6, B12, and B9 work together to control blood levels of the amino acid homocysteine. It helps maintain normal nerve function and also acts in the formation of red blood cells. Vitamin B6 is also needed for normal brain development and function. B6 plays an important role in making brain chemicals called neurotransmitters. Additionally, it aids in the production of DNA and RNA, our body's genetic makeup. In order for vitamin B12 to be absorbed, we must also have B6. B6 is another anti-stress vitamin. Low vitamin B6 consumption has been linked to heart disease. *Dietary sources* include, fowl, salmon, beef liver, lentils, nuts, avocados, bananas, carrots, bran, sunflower seeds, wheat germ, whole-grain flour and brown rice.

Vitamin B9 (Folate / Folic Acid) – *Water soluble*. Known also as folate or folic acid, B9 is required for cell replication and growth. Folic acid helps build up our RNA, which is needed for protein synthesis. It also serves to build our DNA, which holds the body's genetic information. Folic acid is necessary for growing tissues quickly, especially with a fetus—folic acid is critical during pregnancy. B9 regenerates our body's red blood cells and immune cells. If we develop anemia, we can start the reversal process quickly with folic acid supplements. *Taking folic acid for heart disease is not recommended.* Consult with your doctor before deciding to take this supplement. We need only 400 mcg a day and a good diet rich in fruits and vegetables, along with whole grains, and fat-free dairy products like milk and yogurt will give us all we need. Additionally, citrus fruits, and tomatoes are good sources of B9. Today's wheat (bread) flour is fortified with folic acid. There's enough in the flour to add an estimated 100 micrograms per day to our average diet.

Vitamin B12 (Cobalamine) – *Water soluble*. Vitamin B12 interacts with B9 (folic acid) and B6 to control homocysteine levels. Vitamin B12 deficiency is known to cause fatigue. B12 injections are available for deficiency but a relationship between B12 injections and the energy level of people who are not vitamin B12-deficient is inconclusive due mostly to a rarity of research into the subject. Oral B12 supplements most likely do not produce the same results as being injected with

B12, since our bodies have a relatively poor absorption rate for B12. Food sources for B12 include venison, salmon, beef, lamb loin, low fat yogurt, scallops, halibut, snapper and lean beef tenderloin. Animals contain more B12 than plants since plants cannot store B12. Some plants that do contain B12 are kelp, and fermented plant foods as well as brewer's yeast. However, plants are inconsistent with their content of B12 and can't be counted on as a good source. *Important.* Vitamin B12 along with B9 will help enhance our memory. The older we get the more important it is for these two interactive vitamins. How to get them together? *Eat fish and beans at the same setting.*

Vitamin C (Ascorbic Acid) – *Water Soluble.* Vitamin C is an essential vitamin that has an extensive range of functions for us. If you like to eat, then C is one of the more enjoyable vitamins to seek out. It's in more foods than you might imagine including kale, cauliflower, Brussels sprouts, bell peppers, oranges, cantaloupe, kiwifruit, papaya, strawberries, and many more. Vitamin C works strongly as a serious antioxidant sentry guarding us against a high cholesterol levels. In other words, vitamin C protects our cells from free radical damage. It also regenerates our Vitamin E, improves iron absorption, and for some, reduces cancer risk. Ergo, make sure you get your ascorbic acid every day. Vitamin C may also protect against heart disease by fighting platelets that coagulate in our veins, which causes a stiffness of arteries. It is credited with powerful antioxidant properties, as a producer of collagen, aids in the formation of liver bile, and as we age, if we take vitamin C supplements to replace the C we aren't otherwise making or getting, it could help in the prevention of cataracts. There are many benefits of this vitamin, too many to list them all here. If you want more information, plenty is available at your local library or on-line. Other Food Sources include parsley, fresh lemon juice, Romaine lettuce, cabbage, tomatoes, asparagus, raspberries, celery, spinach, green beans, watermelon, cranberries and more.

Vitamin D – *Fat soluble.* Vitamin D helps increase calcium absorption from food, which helps maintain blood levels of calcium. This helps keep calcium stored in bones instead of the body having to draw it away from bones, which paradoxically, vitamin D can also do. Calcium drawn from bones can weaken them. The complex workings of many naturally produced and dietary vitamins is a good reason for supplements if you're not getting the correct amounts. Your doctor may ask you to get a blood test for these conditions. Vitamin D is absolutely needed for healthy bones and teeth. Fortunately, we produce vitamin D when exposed to UV rays from the sun. But those rays are sometimes difficult to get if you work or live indoors most of the time. Also they are difficult to absorb during seasonal changes like winter, cloud cover, dirty or smoggy air, and if you put on sunscreen. Sunscreen helps protect against skin cancer, but it also blocks out vitamin D absorption from the sun. All of the above make vitamin D scarcer for people in northern latitudes than in southern. For those of us who live in the northern hemisphere, we might want to consider taking a vitamin D supplement. Vitamin D plays many other roles. For instance Vitamin D is necessary for the maintenance of sufficient blood levels of insulin. Some researchers have found that vitamin D supplements may increase insulin secretion for some patients with adult-onset diabetes. We wish we could list all of vitamin D's benefits here, but we can't, so we suggest you do a search for more information on the Internet, or at your local library. Food Sources include Sockeye or Chinook salmon (broiled or gilled), unsalted/non brined shrimp, cow's milk (nonfat, low fat), cod (bake or broil it), or a whole egg, hard-boiled or poached. One serving of salmon by the way, provides over one-hundred percent of our daily requirements.

Vitamin E (Tocopherol) – *Fat Soluble.* Vitamin E is an antioxidant with the power to protect us from radical damage. A Johns Hopkins analysis of many studies concluded that taking 400 IU of vitamin E supplements did not prevent cardiovascular disease or cancer. In fact, 400 IU a day may cause harm that could lead to death. The Johns Hopkins report also stated that taking 200 IU or less a day may offer benefit in heart health, but they did not confirm that it would. Vitamin E is known to "thin the blood" or work as an anticoagulant. If you are taking Coumadin or Warfarin, and you want to take vitamin E supplements, you may want to check with your doctor first. Vitamin E helps our body process glucose. Vitamin E has also been linked as an anti-inflammatory, and to blood cell regulation, tissue growth (connective), and genetic control of cell division. Cooking oil nearly always contains added Tocopherol (vitamin E) to help keep the oil from becoming rancid. It is wise to read all FDA labels and the ingredients labels before purchasing food when on a restricted diet. Food sources include vegetable oils, parsley, kale, papaya, bell pepper, kiwifruit, tomato, blueberries, broccoli, Brussels sprouts, collard greens,

Vitamin K (Phylloquinone) – *Fat Soluble.* Coagulant. Vitamin K is necessary for proper bone growth and it serves as a natural blood coagulation. (If you're taking Warfarin or Coumadin, you will want to keep your vitamin K intake balanced. Vitamin K helps our bodies transport calcium, which is what helps with the coagulation. Vitamin K is used to treat overdoses of Warfarin (Coumadin). Emergency room personnel might give you a shot of vitamin K if you need immediate surgery due to an accident or other event. Let them know you are taking a blood thinner. It is best of you're taking Warfarin or Coumadin, that you maintain a balanced diet of K foods. Try not to "bounce" the K. If you do bounce, your next blooddraw might show it and you could end up readjusting your medications. Food sources include green leafy vegetables, kale, collards, spinach, cabbage, turnip greens, and to a lesser degree, milk, eggs, beef liver, cereals and some fruits and other vegetables. Don't fear Vitamin K however. Just keep your diet balanced and you'll be okay. (See also: Blood Thinners)

Walnuts (nuts) – Studies have shown that a few unsalted walnuts a day might benefit each of us. An excellent source of omega-3 fatty acids. A quarter cup of unsalted walnuts a day would provide you about 91 percent of your daily value for omega-3 essential fatty acids. Exchange something else for this daily treat. The calories are about 160 Kcal. Walnuts include manganese, copper, tryptophan and other nutrients. These help protect our cardiovascular system and promote cognitive function as well as serving as an anti-inflammatory for asthma, rheumatoid arthritis, eczema, and psoriasis. Walnuts also have anticancer properties and they support our immune system.

Wayzata Bay Chili Powder – Good unsalted chili powder available at http://healthyheartmarket.com/wbchilipowder-hot.aspx for a hot version and http://healthyheartmarket.com/wbchilipowder-hot.aspxhttp://healthyheartmarket.com/wbchilipowder-med.aspx for a medium heat version.

Whole grains – The whole kernel of grain that includes the outer shell, which is known as bran. *Following is the official definition of whole grains, approved and endorsed by the Whole Grains Council in May 2004.* "Whole grains or foods made from them contain all the essential parts and naturally-occurring nutrients of the entire grain seed. If the grain has been processed (e.g., cracked, crushed, rolled, extruded, and/or cooked), the food product should deliver approximately the same rich balance of nutrients that are found in the original grain seed."

The health benefit provided by whole grains includes a reduced risk of cardiovascular disease. This benefit is derived from the combination of fiber, vitamins, minerals and phytochemicals found in whole grains. Whole grains include amaranth, barley, buckwheat, corn (cornmeal and popcorn included), millet, oats (including oatmeal), quinoa, rice (wild, brown and colored), rye, sorghum or milo, teff, triticale, and varieties of wheat including spelt, emmer, faro, einkorn, durum, bulgur, cracked what and wheat berries. (This list is not complete.) For more about whole grains, visit the Whole Grains Council Web site at: http://www.wholegrainscouncil.org/

Zinc – Zinc is an essential micro mineral with a wide variety of functions within the human body. Zinc is necessary on a daily basis, but only in small amounts (about 50 mg or fewer). Zinc is needed to repair wounds, and to maintain fertility in adults and growth in children. It's important for vision, reproduction of cells, boosting our immunity and it works as an antioxidant to protect against free radicals. Here's a fact about zinc you can use during your next trivia game. Zinc regulates many of our genetic activities. Each cell of our bodies have a unique compartment known as the nucleus. Inside that nucleus are about one-hundred thousand genes. Zinc is needed for the cells to ready genetic instructions. If you fail to get zinc daily, then your genes are not getting their instructions. Zinc therefore becomes important for many other activities. As an aside, in a few trials, zinc lozenges proved to reduce the length or duration of colds contracted by adults. They have not yet proved this affective in children. You can get too much zinc, so don't overload by taking supplements unless your doctor has recommended them. If you do overdose on zinc you might develop a metallic taste in your mouth or develop stomach pain, nausea, vomiting cramps, or diarrhea that contains blood. To learn more about zinc, visit your library or search Google online. Food sources: Calf's liver, crimini mushrooms, boiled spinach, beef tenderloin, lamb loin, summer squash, asparagus, venison, dark leafy vegetables, pumpkin seeds, low-fat yogurt, broccoli, maple syrup and other foods.

[1] Beard, Dr. Trevor, *Salt Matters*, pge. 165, Hachette Publishers, Australia/ New Zealand.

[2] University Of Rochester Medical Center (2005, January 26). Grapefruit Juice And Medication Can Be A Dangerous Mix. *ScienceDaily*.

[3] We understand that Losartan in Cozaar may interact with grapefruit. Grapefruit can boost some medications substantially while having no affect on other medications. Check with your doctor or R.D.

[4] Asthmatics and some diabetes patients in particular are subject to reactions to MSG and other glutamic acids.

[5] FDA, *http://www.fda.gov/FDAC/features/2003/103_msg.html* For a counter presentation see *www.truthinlabeling.org*

[6] Beard, Dr. Trevor, Salt Matters, pge. 168, Hachette Publishers, Australia/ New Zealand.

[7] In some rare cases, patients need more sodium in their diet than less. For this, sodium tablets are sold.

8 Beard, Dr. Trevor, Salt Matters, pge. 169, Hachette Publishers, Australia/ New Zealand.

Index

Living Well Without Salt

C

E

F

G

H

I

J

L

R

S

T

V

W

Y

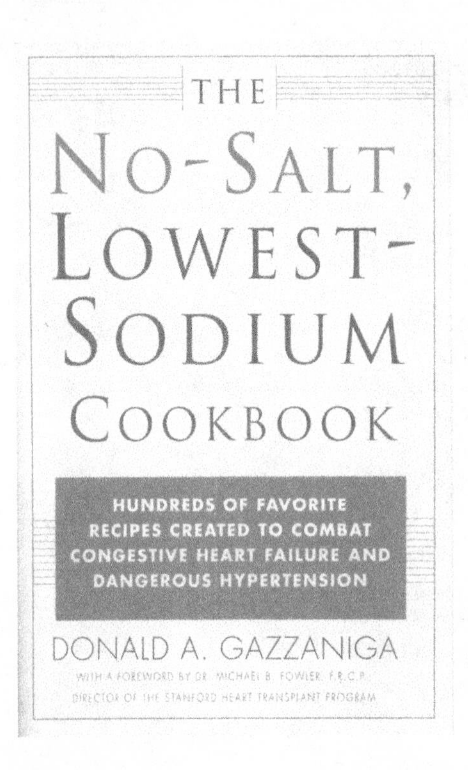

ISBN-10: 0312291647
ISBN-13: 978-0312291648

The first no-salt cookbook to help patients who have to cut salt out of their lives. The original dietary approach to a no salt life with a 28-day meal planning guide in the back of the book for you to use as a guide to build your own program with your own tastes. Recommended by doctors for heart failure, Meniere's Syndrome, hypternsion, Nephrotic Syndrome and other maladies requiring a no-salt lifestyle.

ISBN-10: 0312335024
ISBN-13: 978-0312335021

Third in the no-salt, lowest-sodium cookbook series. This book contains 25 incredible soups and stews, 25 salads and dressings, 25 sandwiches and lots of spice mixes to make and store as well as bread recipes for the sandwiches.

Visit Megaheart.com and click "Testimonials" to read what users think of this and the other books.

Available in Kindle and other electronic formats. Author available 24/7 via the Web site, Megaheart.com

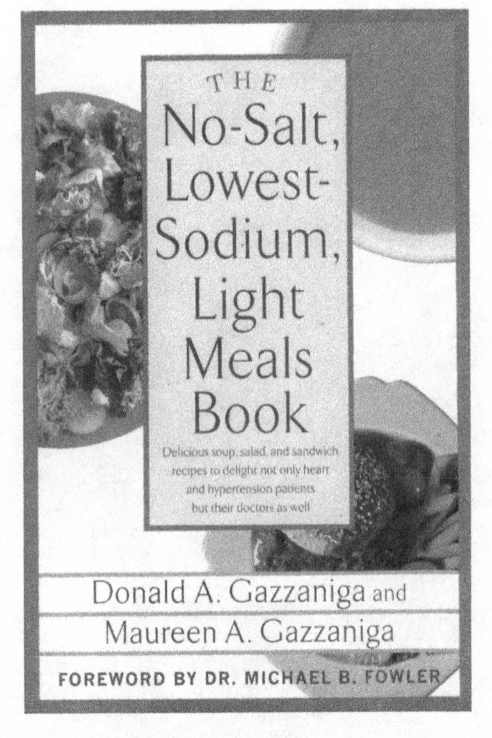

ISBN-10: 0312335245
ISBN-13: 978-0312335

When Don first began developing no-salt recipes he found himself battling an old myth that "bread cannot be made without salt." Even bread machine manufacturers were printing that warning in their manuals.

It didn't take Don long to figure out the formula for making salt-free bread while keeping the flavors as well.

Today Don's recipes are seen throughout the Internet. "Basically, stick to the chemistry of good bread making and salt is never needed," he wrote.

Want a special bread, check out this book and each of the others and find reicpes at Megaheart.com

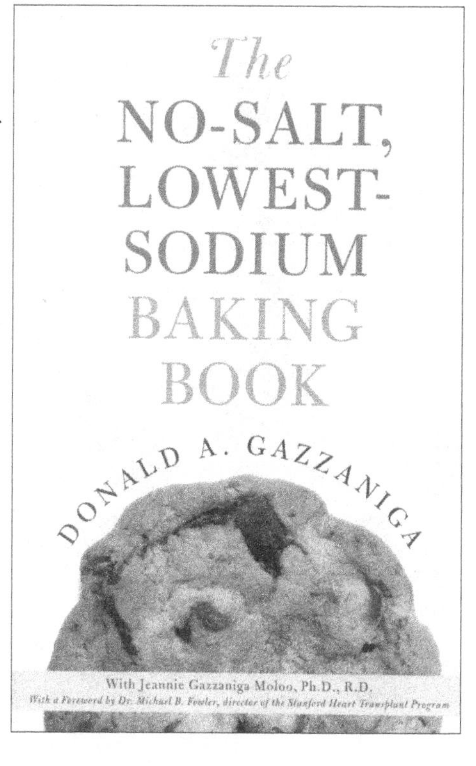

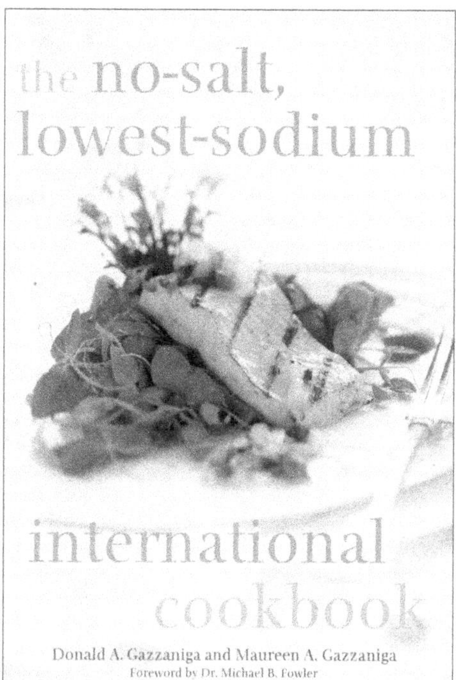

ISBN-10: 0312355718
ISBN-13: 978-0312355715

200 great recipes from around and no salt nor any high sodium products like baking powder or baking soda. A wonderful soy sauce replacement, entrees from Asia, Afirca, Europe and America's deep south.

Don's favorite Ethiopian Spice Bread and Chinese Sesame Chicken as well as the only bread native to China—a steamed bun

From Hoison sauce to British Bangers and international spice mixes, this book is the only of its kind in the world. Found at Amazon on Kindle and in print form, it's worth it just to enjoy meals you thought you'd never eat again.

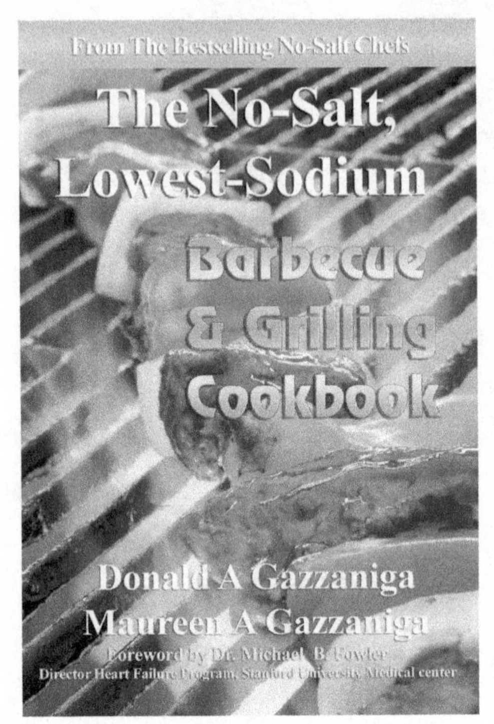

ISBN-10: 1512325392
ISBN-13: 978-1512325393

With a complete index to each recipe, this book has two-hundred plus low-sodium and salt free recipes for outdoor living including grilled meat, vegetables, side dishes, desserts, Dutch Oven recipes and more. Don's No-Salt, Lowest-Sodium Cookbooks have been featured in national magazines, on TV and in newspapers around the world. See more about this book and others at Megaheart.com.

CPSIA information can be obtained
at www.ICGtesting.com
Printed in the USA
LVHW050956090523
746507LV00004B/23